The
HEALTHY
BONES

Nutrition Plan
and Cookbook

The
HEALTHY
BONES

Nutrition Plan
and Cookbook

How to Prepare and Combine
Whole Foods to Prevent and Treat
Osteoporosis Naturally

Dr. Laura Kelly
and Helen Bryman Kelly

Foreword by Sidney MacDonald Baker, MD

Chelsea Green Publishing
White River Junction, Vermont

Disclaimer

This book is intended as information, not medical advice. You must not rely on the information in this book as an alternative to medical advice from your doctor or other professional healthcare provider. If you have any specific questions about any medical matter, you should consult your doctor or other professional healthcare provider. If you think you may be suffering from any medical condition, you should seek immediate medical attention. You should never delay seeking medical advice, disregard medical advice, or discontinue medical treatment because of information in this book.

Acquisitions Editor: Makenna Goodman
Developmental Editor: Fern Marshall Bradley
Copy Editor: Laura Jorstad
Proofreader: Helen Walden
Indexer: Margaret Holloway
Designer: Melissa Jacobson

Printed in the United States of America.
First printing June, 2016.
10 9 8 7 6 5 4 3 2 1   16 17 18 19

Our Commitment to Green Publishing

Chelsea Green sees publishing as a tool for cultural change and ecological stewardship. We strive to align our book manufacturing practices with our editorial mission and to reduce the impact of our business enterprise in the environment. We print our books and catalogs on chlorine-free recycled paper, using vegetable-based inks whenever possible. This book may cost slightly more because it was printed on paper that contains recycled fiber, and we hope you'll agree that it's worth it. Chelsea Green is a member of the Green Press Initiative (www.greenpressinitiative.org), a nonprofit coalition of publishers, manufacturers, and authors working to protect the world's endangered forests and conserve natural resources. *The Healthy Bones Nutrition Plan and Cookbook* was printed on paper supplied by Thomson-Shore that contains at least 30% postconsumer recycled fiber.

Library of Congress Cataloging-in-Publication Data

Names: Kelly, Laura, 1967– author. | Kelly, Helen, 1942–
Title: The healthy bones nutrition plan and cookbook : how to prepare and combine whole foods to prevent and treat
    osteoporosis naturally / Laura Kelly, Helen Kelly.
Description: White River Junction, Vermont : Chelsea Green Publishing, [2016]
Identifiers: LCCN 2016008928| ISBN 9781603586245 (paperback) | ISBN 9781603586252 (ebook)
Subjects: LCSH: Bones—Diseases—Prevention. | Osteoporosis—Prevention. | Nutrition. | BISAC: COOKING / Health
    & Healing / General. | HEALTH & FITNESS / Diets. | HEALTH & FITNESS / Diseases / Musculoskeletal. |
    HEALTH & FITNESS / Nutrition. | LCGFT: Cookbooks.
Classification: LCC RC931.O73 K45 2016 | DDC 641.5/63—dc23 LC record available at http://lccn.loc.gov/2016008928

Chelsea Green Publishing
85 North Main Street, Suite 120
White River Junction, VT 05001
(802) 295-6300
www.chelseagreen.com

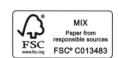

Dedication

To my mother, who worked tirelessly
to help me focus and guide my passion; to my
grandmother, on her 100th birthday; to you, who
read this book, for your curiosity and your strength;
and to Nick, who has supported me in all ways,
above and beyond, with love and patience.

—Laura

For my daughter Laura, indefatigable in her search
for root causes and truth and unshakable in her integrity,
who has given of her time steadfastly and lovingly to restore
my skeletal health; and to my husband, Chris Titterington,
for driving two hours every two weeks to buy raw milk and
supporting me staunchly in my quest for bone health.
My heart belongs to Chris.

—Helen

■　■　■　■　■

To the people who bring wholesome food to market:
the farmers who do not use pesticides, the pickers who are
careful not to bruise, the transporters and the sellers,
each taking care of the food so we can take care
of ourselves and our families. Thank you.
We offer our deepest respect and appreciation.

—Laura and Helen

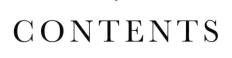

CONTENTS

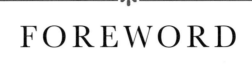

FOREWORD

It sure would be nice if "the experts" didn't keep changing the truth about what's good for us and what isn't. The truth about bone health has recently changed from *calcium pills are good for you to calcium pills are bad for you*. When the truth changes, professionals like me are in an awkward spot. I am invited to break an implicit rule of my art—I should always inspire my patients with confidence in my knowledge. This rule demands that silence replace certain words, such as "Oops" and "I don't know," which could lower exam scores and, presumably, the confidence of patients.

The loud "Oops!" merited by calcium supplements tumbling from the shelf where we keep our medical truths might go unnoticed in the racket over other recent medical flip-flops, including the reversal of the long-held consensus that fat is bad and the emergence of the new truth that fat is good and sugar and carbs are bad.

We may feel more comfortable—or even joyful—about saying "Oops" when the truth moves in the direction of common sense. For example, consider that neither of the authors of the book you are holding are "bone specialists" in the framework of the medical establishment. One of their key messages is *it's not that complicated*. It's a powerful message that can help you join a positive trend in information technology, medical practice, and health outcomes.

The Healthy Bones Nutrition Plan and Cookbook is part of a sweeping change in how scientists, practitioners, and writers are thinking about health care and how people can shift their state of being from chronic illness to good health. These paths rise above the flat landscape of name-it, blame-it, tame-it prescription-pad medicine to a lofty view of a multidimensional web that constitutes living systems. Once we have the vantage point of this interconnected system, we can see proximity in elements that previously seemed distant—so that goings-on in your gut or brain become relevant to problems in your bones. The new way of thinking says: Let your personal health data talk to you about your personal lifestyle and treatment options. Those data will remind all of us of the ancient message to let food be our medicine.

The most significant lesson you may take from this book is that, in the realm of chronic illness, the target of treatment is not the disease but the individual. If you are chronically ill, the common-sense question is this: Is there something you need to add or something you need to avoid in order to favor Nature's buoyant impulse toward healing? Laura Kelly and Helen Bryman Kelly apply this idea to osteoporosis, making the point that in most cases osteoporosis is not disease; rather, it is deficiency.

Common sense says that steel and lumber are the framework for the structures we inhabit. Upon reflection, though, we realize that bolts and nails are key components upon which the size and structure of buildings ultimately depend. This book will help you understand that critical elements in the foods you eat—just like the bolts and nails in a building—are essential players in keeping your skeleton both strong and flexible.

This elegant book is a timely pioneer in a migration of expertise from an exclusively top-down direction to one in which we listen to the data. The voice of medical authority will be heard from insightful thinkers such as Laura Kelly, who can gather the facts and fashion them to fit the body of truth.

When a health practitioner says that osteoporosis is the cause of a patient's problem and chooses a treatment aimed at curing it—as if it were a disease—the practitioner is bypassing a lot of information about the patient. To grasp the diagnostic *name* as if it were a *thing* capable of *causing* illness is to stumble into confusion about the nature and causes of chronic illness. In matters concerning *acute* illness such as a strep throat or a broken arm, the confusion of names, ideas, and things doesn't make much difference. But with chronic conditions such as bone health, it is especially important to be reminded that osteoporosis is only the name used to describe the condition, and neither the cause nor the target of treatment.

If you grasp the distinction between treatment aimed at a disease versus treatment tailored to you as an individual, you will share my admiration for how the authors of this book prepare you for maintaining healthy bones by owning the data, as opposed to using it to name your condition and then treat the name. If you and your practitioner follow the path of owning your data, the treatment options change to become a collaborative process of tailoring in which the facts (symptoms, signs, lab test results) of the matter are tried on, adjusted, and made to fit. This change, called personalized medicine, is currently catching on, and for good reason. It has to do with precisely the kinds of information this book provides. Readers who follow the guidance provided by Dr. Laura Kelly and Helen Kelly to create a personal nutrition plan will be empowered to interact with medical professionals in a new, more rational, safer, and less costly way. And they will enjoy much better health outcomes, relying on truths that are highly likely to endure.

Sidney MacDonald Baker, MD
Sag Harbor, New York
May, 2016

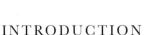

INTRODUCTION

Why Supplements Alone Won't Save Us

Despite the millions consumers spend on calcium pills and the number of prescriptions for bone loss drugs they fill, worldwide there is an osteoporotic fracture every three seconds. These cracked bones are not the sole the province of the hunched-over elderly. Fifty percent of Americans over the age of 50 have osteopenia,[1] a term that describes significant bone loss—and by percentage more fractures occur among people with osteopenia than among people with osteoporosis. Globally one in three women over age 50—and notably, one in five men in the same age range—endure osteoporotic fractures. Of those women and men who crack a hip, one in three becomes dependent on full-time care for a year and one in five dies during that time, many within the first month. The outcomes for osteoporotic spinal fractures are grimmer still.

To put the risks starkly in context, each 10 percent loss of bone mass in the hip can result in a 2.5 times greater risk of hip fracture. Each 10 percent loss of bone mass in the vertebrae can double the risk of vertebral fractures.

Clearly calcium pills and pharmaceuticals aren't enough to keep bones healthy; however, there is plenty of evidence that diet is. In nations that are shifting from traditional diets and natural food toward fast food, processed foods, farmed seafood, factory-farmed eggs, sugary drinks, and chemically treated plants and meat, bone health shows sharp declines.

For instance, at the time of this writing, health industry economists project that China's osteoporosis numbers will double by 2035;[2] by 2050, osteoporotic injuries will cost the Chinese the dollar equivalent of over $25 billion. The projections are drawn from statistics: From the 1960s to the 1990s there was a 300 percent increase in hip fractures; by 2010, 2.3 million Chinese people—70 percent women and 30

1

percent men in this increasingly Westernized country—had sustained osteoporosis-related hip, vertebral, and wrist fractures that required treatment, at a dollar-equivalent cost of $10 billion.[3] There are similar though less dramatic figures for other nations.

The science is unequivocal: Eating the wrong foods increases your risk of osteopenia and osteoporosis; eating the right foods for bone health reduces your risk of osteopenia and osteoporosis and can help you build bone reserves before menopause, control bone loss after it, and arrest bone loss if not restore it at any time of life. We know this firsthand because some of the recipes in this book were Helen's starting point for arresting severe osteoporotic bone loss at age 70.

Healthy Bones: Your New Paradigm

The pain, suffering, hospitalization, disability, and death due to bone density loss are ringing alarm bells worldwide, and scientists agree that more must be done to treat bone loss in the early stages. Yet even medical professionals disagree about the best treatment, and few report a focus on prevention.

To help you evaluate recommendations for preventing and treating bone density loss and prepare to speak with your doctor about them, in this book we set out information about how bones grow, what happens when they lose density over time, how nutrients take center stage in both processes, and how you can harness the power of nutrients to build and sustain flexible, dense bones. There are genetic factors that appear to relate to bone density, however it is key to note that genes can be turned on and off by lifestyle choices and nutrition. This book does not address the genetic side

of bone loss because for the vast majority, targeted nutrition and exercise are enough.

The modern Western medical paradigm offers testing technology and powerful medicines that eradicate diseases and improve the lives of many people. Our appreciation is boundless; our respect immeasurable. Yet every paradigm has limits, and we see the Western paradigm straining against its present limits when we consider the approach to the epidemics of chronic illness facing American society. Instead of considering root causes or fully exploring prevention, the discussion tends to focus on treatment and pharmaceuticals. But pills should be the last option rather than the first, especially where established nutritional therapies can address the condition harmlessly and for the long term.

Let's look at some examples of the pharmaceutical paradigm in distress:

- In a large study, 50 percent of postmenopausal women who took statin developed diabetes.[4] Statin therapy appears to increase diabetes risk by 46 percent in the general population.[5]
- Adverse drug reactions cause hospitalization of approximately 1.5 million Americans every year.[6]
- Bisphosphonates can arrest bone density loss in the short term, but these pharmaceuticals can also cause the jawbone to deteriorate and the femur to snap.[7]

These are serious enough, but when we also consider that as of 2014 over eight million children were prescribed psychiatric medication in the United States[8] when for many, dietary changes would do the trick, we are rightly distressed.

Make no mistake: Pharmaceuticals are justified in those cases where there are no options;

Of Doctors and Diet

From the original Hippocratic oath (late 5th century BC):

With regard to healing the sick, I will devise and order for them the best diet, according to my judgment and means; and I will take care that they suffer no hurt or damage. Nor shall any man's entreaty prevail upon me to administer poison to anyone; neither will I counsel any man to do so.

In the amendment for modern American doctors in 1964, the commitment to diet was removed and these words were substituted:

I will apply, for the benefit of the sick, all measures which are required, avoiding those twin traps of overtreatment and therapeutic nihilism.

where illness unqualifiedly demands a pharmaceutical. Nevertheless, there are newly suggested limits on bisphosphonates[9], and reliance on pharmaceuticals as the go-to solution for issues that might be addressed in a timely way by diet or other nonpharmaceutical interventions has gotten out of hand.

Reclaiming *Natural*

We propose a new paradigm for addressing bone health: evidence-based prevention and treatment that includes specific groups of natural food.

In the food industry and other realms, the word *natural* has been overused, used frivolously, and sometimes used to create false impressions.

To help highlight the new paradigm, we have reclaimed the word *natural* as it applies to food. By *natural* we mean food from plants and animals that grew unaltered in habitats and on farms without use of chemical pesticides and fertilizers. We've reclaimed this word because it deserves standing and because we want it to represent the power of its true meaning. *Natural* is one of the few words in English that describes life in harmony and balance in nature. Natural food is, we believe, the medicine best placed to promote bone health for a lifetime.

Helen's Story

After 22 years of consecutive bone loss leading to severe osteoporosis and many years eating what the doctors said was the right food, a new approach to combining nutrients and foods arrested my bone loss. Here's my story. In the run-up to menopause my first bone scan showed advanced osteopenia, so I started in meticulously taking care of my bones. I did not trust pharmaceuticals, so I declined them, but I did wholeheartedly trust the experts on food and supplements. I drank soy milk and ate greens and cheese, organic whole-grain bread, olive oil instead of butter, sweet potatoes instead of white potatoes, and berries and raw kale galore.

Pretzels were out; raw organic nuts were in. Red meat was out, turkey was in. I took my calcium supplements every day, 1,200 milligrams as directed with vitamin D, and followed all this faithfully for several years—until my charge toward bone health came to an abrupt and devastating end: My bone density scan showed full-blown osteoporosis. How could that be? I had done everything the experts recommended.

It turned out I wasn't alone in finding out that the touted route to bone health was a set of deleterious steps on a long dead end. Women around the world were earnestly adhering to the same heavily hyped eating regime, and millions of enlightened, diligent women succumbed nonetheless to dangerously thin bones.

Why did things go wrong? For more reasons than I could have imagined.

First, it turns out that to build bone tissue, bodies need not only calcium but also other minerals in the right ratio along with vitamins and enzymes. So calcium pills alone, even those enriched with vitamin D, could never have helped me preserve my bone density.

Second, I was eating my raw nuts, seeds, and leafy greens, which are all rich in calcium, but the calcium was not available for digestion. It turns out there are natural substances in raw plant-based foods that bind calcium and other minerals into large calcium-rich but nondigestible molecules. (These substances protect the plant: They safeguard a delicate developmental pattern, prevent seeds from sprouting when conditions are unfavorable for growth, and ward off enemies.) Although I was eating plenty of calcium-rich food, once in my gut, the protective chemicals in those grains and seeds and berries and greens, sticky as spiderwebs, were binding up the calcium along with other essential minerals. All that calcium, but none of it reached my bones.

The biggest surprise, though, was yet to come. It had to do with milk and other dairy products. A wonderful source of calcium, right? Not necessarily. When milk is pasteurized, bacteria in the milk are killed. The intent is to destroy bacteria that could cause illness. But in fact, pasteurization also kills the plentiful bacteria in milk that are beneficial for digestion, and it kills the enzymes that make the abundant calcium in milk fully available to bones. Without those enzymes,

all the calcium in pasteurized milk, organic or not, and all the calcium in pasteurized cheese, won't bring but a farthing's worth of goodness to your bones, and actually can make things worse.

So there I was, years into absolute compliance with a rigorous routine and feeling disheartened and like a real fool. I had relied on a diet of foods rich in calcium that had either been boiled out or locked up, and I had in addition taken the supplements faithfully, never knowing that my regimen had in the end denied my bones the much-needed calcium I had worked so hard to provide.

That is where my daughter Laura, this book's lead author, stepped in.

I was still set against pharmaceuticals. Doctors in two countries had prescribed bisphosphonates, the baby boomers' wonder drugs, but the scant research on long-term outcomes did not satisfy me, so over my doctors' objections I ruled them out.

Laura brought me back to food—this time with a new approach. Patiently she taught me the science of bone building and bone loss. She believes that solid information helps people step back from fear-mongering marketing hype to make objective, informed decisions. She was right. I found it satisfying to know what was going on inside my body, and even more satisfying to know I could take some control over what happens there.

Laura and I set out to combine foods that supplied all the minerals plus the vitamins and enzymes required to ensure calcium reached my bones, and to learn how to prepare edible plants so that the minerals would be available during digestion. As a side note, I was humbled to learn that virtually all pre-Western civilizations, back even to the ancients and primitives, knew about the substances in plants that bind minerals and how to weaken these substances when preparing the plants for consumption in order to unleash the minerals. I was respectful, too, when I learned that forest animals also know instinctively that they must weaken substances that bind minerals, and they know how to do it. So in this book we include methods for preparing plant-based foods for optimal digestion of nutrients, with due respect to those who knew before us.

Why I Wrote This Book

Until Laura devised my diet, I felt caught between the devil and the deep blue sea. Pharmaceuticals designed to prevent or treat bone disease could produce acute side effects and ultimately injure my bones. Calcium supplements, fortified processed food, and pasteurized dairy hadn't worked—the calcium hadn't reached my bones. Still, doing nothing carried a fracture risk—and in the case of osteoporosis, hip fracture carried a risk of death.

The turning point was learning that getting calcium to my bones and keeping it there is a synchronized set of chemical steps that require a large cast of nutrients. It's like producing a stage show: There are star players, but the show can't go on without many others combining forces to set the stage and then manage it.

If I'd none nothing, would my bones have thinned naturally? Yes, they would have, typically almost invisibly after age 30 and then more as hormone levels wane. Does that mean being stuck with taking drugs as a short-term fix or risking a shrinking skeleton, especially after menopause? No, not at all. Women of any age—and the 20 percent of osteoporosis patients who are men—can strengthen bone, prevent bone loss, and build new bone by choosing, preparing, and combining foods correctly. Which is why Laura and I wrote this book.

Laura's Story

This book came to life when my mother wanted to treat osteoporosis without the use of bisphosphonates. I could find no structured guidelines for arresting bone loss without pharmaceuticals, yet I was confident we could arrest my mother's bone loss naturally.

I was confident because in my work as a Traditional Chinese Medicine practitioner, food is medicine; and my experience in healing fractures and traumatic injury to bones and muscles is supported with current research on the success of Chinese medicine at speeding up fracture healing.[10] So I reasoned that helping my mother would simply be a matter of applying what I already knew about how the Chinese use food and herbs as medicine for bone restoration in order to find a new solution.

I set about planning the intervention with attention to metabolic science and a rigorous examination of current research. I developed a nutrition plan and recipes. Each recipe includes essential elements required for bone health. The nutrition plans we developed, along with specific supplements, allowed my mom to achieve a balanced intake of all the bone health elements every day.

After 14 months following the plan, we found that we were successful. My mom's bone loss stopped. We wish to share our experience with you—what we learned and what we did—so you, too, can take charge of your bone health and hopefully avoid potentially harmful medications.

Although we began by tackling the problem of declining bone health, we recognized and learned that diet can provide prevention, too. So even if you did not build an ideal peak bone mass when you were in your teens or twenties, with the help of this book you can begin to improve your bone health whatever age you are now.

We hope you will share the ideas and information in this book with men and women of all ages. Nutrigenomics, the study of how food affects gene expression, shows that what your ancestors ate affects your health, and what you eat will affect the health of subsequent generations. So let's start everyone on the road to healthy bones safely, naturally, and effectively—and with any luck, without pharmaceuticals. Our planet has provided us with everything we need to live long and healthy lives. Knowledge of how and what to use is the key. In this book, I hope we provide helpful information about one part of what will sustain you on your journey to a long life in good health and in happiness. Remember—your bones are part of a larger system, that of your entire organism. This body as a whole does not operate in independent factions—what is good for your bones is good for the rest of your body.

Why I Wrote This Book

Bone loss drugs can have severely deleterious consequences. Their use is increasingly limited by regulators, and Western medicine has no non-pharmaceutical alternatives. However, virtually everyone can address the matter of bone density decline naturally by eating the right food in the right form. It is inexpensive, and there is a huge payoff for the long term.

I wrote this book in part to share that knowledge as widely as possible. And since prevention *is* the better part of cure, I wrote it in the hope that women and men will tell their mothers and sons and daughters that natural food can save years of heartache, lifestyle limitations, disability, and death.

I wrote this book because it is just and fair for people to know that there are safe, natural,

effective alternatives to pharmaceuticals. And because I feel it is essential that people become equipped to make informed choices and become prepared to take a rightful place as an equal participant in substantive discussions with healthcare providers.

The book reflects the satisfaction and happiness I experience personally and professionally helping people live the longest life possible in the best possible health.

This Above All

It is the saddest of ironies that so many people put years of heartfelt effort into learning about food and health (and buy what advertisers insist doctors say will lead to long life in good health) only to end up ill, or very ill, or dead, because the information they trusted was slickly packaged for quick sale—and was dead wrong. The unrelenting low-fat diet crusade may be partly responsible for the epidemic of heart disease[11] in the United States. The calcium pill campaign is a triumph of mass marketing that has resulted in soaring rates of osteoporosis and osteoporotic fracture among women and men; confused, worried consumers who take more and more when a modicum doesn't work; and a death rate among people who have a normal calcium intake from food and simultaneously take high-dose calcium supplements that is 2.5 times the normal rate among people who obtain calcium from whole food.[12] And amazingly enough the US Preventive Service Task Force recommends *against* daily supplementation of vitamin D_3 and calcium for primary prevention of fractures[13]—because independently it appears that they don't work.

The glut of half-truths, manufactured food, and ineffective nutrients is pervasive, yet we may attain better health—and in this case better bone health—by stepping back from the promotional fearmongering and learning which natural foods in what forms meet the well-defined needs of bones. The good-nutrient road to bone health is very much less expensive, very much more pleasurable and satisfying to the senses, and a very much simpler and more reliable way to protect bone health for life. In this book you'll find detailed information about why natural foods strengthen bones and why pharmaceuticals can weaken them. There's information about which foods make bone-friendly combinations, why they strengthen bones, and how to prepare and cook them. You'll learn about some challenges that natural food presents and how to meet them, and you'll find recipes for delicious dishes that help to prevent and redress bone loss.

Above all, what we've written in this book sheds light on a few big ideas that underpin the rationale for deciding on diet as the road to bone health.

Calcium Pills Aren't Enough

Calcium pills alone do not and cannot prevent or treat bone loss. That's because calcium cannot make the journey from the digestive system through the bloodstream and into bone without a large supporting cast that stars vitamin D, vitamin K_2, magnesium, phosphorus, silicon, and trace minerals. Each member of the company plays a part in calcium absorption and calcium transport to bone. Without them, calcium can settle where you don't want it—in joints and blood vessels.

The Wonders of Sunshine and Mushrooms

Since vitamin D plays a key role in bone health, we humans are exceptionally lucky that nature offers a ready source of it that we can take every day at little cost or for free: sunshine. And mushrooms make vitamin D just the way your skin does—by sitting in the sun. If you set mushrooms in the sun for two days running, they make vitamin D that remains full strength for a year. You can sun a few mushrooms at a time, cook and eat them right away, or sun 10 pounds of mushrooms at a time, dry and store them, and you'll have supplemental vitamin D on hand for months to come. Note that mushrooms generate vitamins D_2 and D_3. Your body can metabolize only the D_3 form, and so must convert the D_2 into D_3 (more on this in chapter 6). Maitake mushrooms have the special ability to make vitamin D while they grow whatever the sun quotient, so if you can find maitake mushrooms, they're guaranteed to be vitamin D–ready.

You can gain a day's vitamin D_3 dose by exposing most of your skin (not just hands and feet) to the sun for 20 minutes per day—outdoors if you have the luxury of privacy or in a sun-filled room such as a conservatory. Be cautious, though; while exposure to sunshine can decrease your likelihood of death from all diseases significantly, overexposure can damage your skin. So please do not exceed 20 minutes' direct sun exposure—not because you can make too much vitamin D (you can't), but because if you don't have sufficient vitamin C (more on that later) longer exposure can damage the skin. If you don't wish to sit in the sun or don't have an opportunity to do so on a regular basis, dine in the sun when you can on natural calcium-rich food. And wherever you are, sun your mushrooms and add a few to your meal. You gain calcium and D plus dozens of nourishing nutrients—and there goes that calcium-with-D supplement pill right out the window.

Magnesium and K₂: Essential, Yet Elusive

Magnesium is another wheel in the calcium transport machinery. Without it, there's a standstill. And vitamin K_2 also keeps calcium on track for deposit in the bones. Your body makes neither one, and neither is abundant in the modern Western diet. Beyond that, even in a healthy gut magnesium digestion is less than ideal. Magnesium is best applied as a spray and absorbed through the skin. You can buy a magnesium spray, or make one following the directions we provide in chapter 6. You can't spray on vitamin K_2, but a few foods offer it, and you will learn about them, too, later in the book.

Herbs Contain Concentrated Nutrients

A great many herbs contain every ingredient you need to build bone and in the right ratios. If you combine apple cider vinegar and certain herbs and let them sit for a few weeks, then put a tablespoon of this delicious herbal vinegar in some hibiscus water or anything else you like to drink or eat, you've supplied nearly half your daily calcium along with vitamins, trace minerals, phytonutrients, and myriad benefits. Herbs are a concentrated food with highly concentrated nutrients. Another occasion to toss the calcium pill.

Supplements Can't Match Food

Nutrients from natural foods function differently in your body than the same nutrients isolated and packaged as supplements. Imagine planting a calcium pill. It would not grow into a bone! Nutrients in isolated form are not functional. Natural food comprises enzymes, vitamins, minerals, proteins, phytoestrogens, and many other elements that interact to produce the nutrition show.

A Healthy Gut for Healthy Bones

The health of your gut bugs is no small matter. Without an intact and healthy gut lining and gut barrier, nutrition absorption is radically compromised. A large portion of your immune system is actually located in your gut, so keeping this healthy is of paramount importance to overall good health, as well as bone health. We explain this fully in chapter 5.

Professional Advice About Supplements Is Wise

Supplementation is a sober matter—a medical decision best made based on your own metabolic profile. Ingesting too much calcium—which typically occurs in people who eat a balanced diet *and* take calcium supplements—has been shown again and again to be not only dangerous but deadly. Too much vitamin A without enough vitamin D can cause bone loss. Too little K_2 and calcium won't bind properly to bone.

Your physician or licensed healthcare provider can order a simple test that shows your baseline levels in the nutrients required for the optimal bone health. This test, a nutrition evaluation, is the starting point of discussion about the road you will take toward bone health and a key tool in understanding what supplementation you may need. Then you will supplement in the context of your own body's health—and begin to exchange supplementation for natural foods as your nutritional profile improves.

New Ways, Bit by Bit

You can begin to cook for bone health immediately by choosing recipes that appeal to you. However, tailoring your personal nutrition plan is something to learn gradually, savoring the new knowledge. Your plan will include a list of essential nutrients and good sources of them, combinations ideal for your own nutritional requirements, and ultimately your own recipe collections.

There's a lot of information about bone health to take in, and trying to keep it all in your head would reduce the pleasure of developing the knowledge, confidence, and skill to take charge of your bone health. But by spending time gradually learning about foods and combinations of nutrients that support bone health—and if you're so inclined, learning the scientific whys and wherefores—it will eventually become instinctive to choose foods that help you curb if not eliminate the need for pharmaceuticals. This knowledge, along with a personalized plan for supplementation that you develop with your doctor or healthcare provider, will lead you toward enduring good health, including good bone health.

As choosing food for bone health becomes second nature, you'll ignore the hawking and fearmongering designed to sell supplement pills. You'll shed the stress that accompanies the awful feeling that there are no alternatives to prescription drugs that may build up bone for a short time yet can render bones so fragile they break. That does not mean you won't take any supplements at all; it doesn't even mean you'll never take a bone health prescription drug. It does mean that whatever you choose, you will have criteria for evaluating options, and be well informed about the likely consequences of each one.

So here's what we hope you'll take away from exploring this book: that over time choosing, preparing, cooking, and eating food with bone health in mind will become second nature. We hope you'll enjoy the confidence that comes with being equipped to discuss options with your doctor as an equal partner in decision making. We hope that you'll feel gratified to take charge of

---

Staying Current

Our recipes and text reflect scientific information that is current at the time of this writing and is aligned with fundamental principles of nutrition and health that have stood a rigorous test of time. However, science and research will continue to provide new information that may improve the application of these basic known principles. The interest in bone health these days is robust, and scientists are working globally to find agents that safely prevent and treat porous bones without harmful side effects or risk down the road. As new research and information becomes available, we will post it faithfully to the book's website.

---

your bone health, confident that you have the understanding to make informed choices about protecting your bones or addressing bone loss if it occurs. We hope you'll experiment with creating your own recipes and meal plans using the foundation principles we've set down. We hope you will choose natural foods whenever possible: organically grown plant-based foods, pastured meat, raw dairy, and eggs from pastured hens.

And maybe this above all: We hope that eating for health, along with exercise, will one day soon be each person's principal route to bone health and overall health for a lifetime.

How to Use This Book

This is more than a cookbook. Part 1 provides information about the science of bone metabolism and the individual and systemic factors that influence bone health. We also explain how to create a Personal Nutrition Plan (which you can also find online at www.medicinethroughfood.com). Should you decide to create a Personal Nutrition Plan, you'll find suggestions for measuring your baseline nutrient profile, analyzing the gap between where you are and what nutrients you need, and what you can do in the kitchen to close the gap. Using the Personal Nutrition Plan worksheets, you can track your intake and strengthen your bone health nutrient profile, progressing at your own pace and mapping your progress over time.

However, if you prefer to just get cooking, try diving right into part 2. Reading through the recipes, you'll gradually gain a clear idea of what cooking for bone health is all about. We've assembled a collection of recipes for appetizing, sometimes adventurous, and always delicious dishes that supply bone growth nutrients in a form your body can absorb, digest, and use. As such, part 2 is neither a diet in the traditional sense nor a diet plan. Rather, it is a set of bone health recipes along with guidelines for using them.

With this information at your fingertips, shopping, cooking, and eating in support of bone health—whether at home or in restaurants—slips unobtrusively into your routines. And that sets the stage for naturally preventing and treating bone density loss starting at any age and continuing for your lifetime.

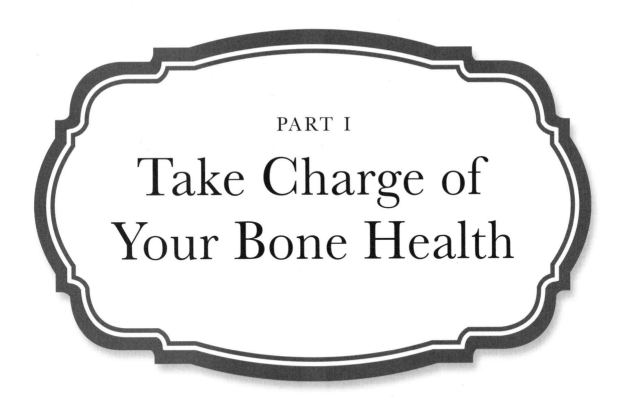

PART I

Take Charge of Your Bone Health

Untreated, bone loss due to aging averages about 10 percent per decade of a person's life.[1] This gradual loss is essentially equivalent in men and women, except for the approximately 10-year period of increased bone loss in women after menopause. This hormone loss does cause bone density decline, ordinarily between 5 and 10 percent—but this does not have to become osteopenia or osteoporosis. Rather the culprit in the worldwide epidemic of severe bone density loss resulting in osteopenia and osteoporosis—and associated fracture—is nutrient deficiency aided and abetted by lack of exercise, stress, consumption of processed food, smoking, alcohol excess, a gut in poor health, and inflammation—all of which can trigger bone density loss. Certain compounds in plant-based foods also play a role because they trap minerals and can inhibit mineral absorption.

Thus we think of osteopenia and osteoporosis as deficiency rather than as disease in the traditional sense, and we'd like to explain why. While bone is growing, collagen, calcium, phosphorus, magnesium, and trace amounts of other minerals like silicon assemble to make new bone. But new bone is not built, or not properly built, without the full nutrient complement present. For example calcium, one of the principal ingredients in bone, cannot make the journey from digestive system to bone without assistance from vitamin D_3, vitamin K_2, magnesium, phosphorus, silicon, zinc, boron, protein, and trace minerals plus enzymes and others. If absorption is weak, calcium can be excreted. If nutrients are missing and calcium is absorbed but not transported to bone, excess in circulation can settle where you don't want it—in joints and blood vessels. A deficiency in calcium at the site of bone could be due to a deficiency in elements necessary for absorption, lack of enzymes to transport or metabolize calcium, presence of chemicals that kidnap the calcium, or lack of the other elements that allow calcium to play its part in forming bone.

It is a complicated story about genes, lifestyle, environment, and gut function—all set against a backdrop of hormones, enzymes, and food—yet one thing shines through: Nothing in your body operates in isolation. By learning which foods contain what you need and how to prepare them—and then making those foods a key part of your diet—you can gradually reduce the nutrient deficiencies that are almost always the root cause of osteoporosis.

In this part of the book, we set out information about bone metabolism—how bones grow and what happens when they lose density. We explain how and why each of the bone health nutrients, separately and collectively, can help you maintain bone density, prevent bone density loss, and treat it starting at any age. To understand why bones lose density—and why food can counteract bone density loss—it is useful to know these metabolic mechanics. But bone metabolism, the many chemical processes that keep bone alive, is multifaceted and quite complex. So we also re-explain key points at several places later in the book as well. Over time you'll find that your understanding of the interplay of vitamins, minerals, and other nutrients required for bone health settles into a coherent big picture of nutrition and healthy bones.

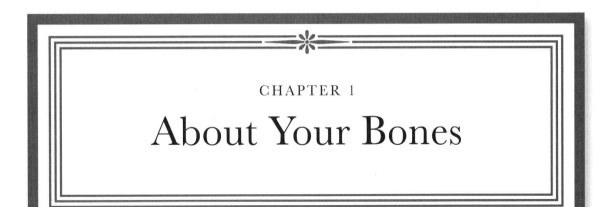

CHAPTER 1

About Your Bones

Bones keep us upright and defend against knocks; they store calcium and make platelets and red and white blood cells, and stem cells reside in the marrow. And like all living tissue, bone turns over. That is, old cells break down and new cells arise in a natural process called bone remodeling.

That's where the problems of density decline begin. When you're young, your bone cells break down and the bone replaces them with new ones. Overall bone density remains fairly constant. With age, the balance shifts and breakdown outpaces replacement.

To understand why this happens, and how you can counteract it through food, take a look at how bone metabolism works.

Bone Matrix: The Collagen–Calcium Connection

A high-level look at bone shows an outer shell called periosteum, which surrounds cortical bone. This surrounds and protects trabecular bone matrix and also, at the center, marrow, which creates blood and other cells, as shown in figure 1 on page 1 of the color insert. Cortical and trabecular bone are made of the same materials in different combinations—essentially collagen, calcium phosphate, and calcium carbonate plus sodium, magnesium, and trace minerals.

The matrix of the trabecular bone is a scaffolding built of collagen that in healthy bone holds a dense population of calcium phosphate crystals. The trabecular scaffold is exquisitely fit for purpose: It is lightweight and very strong. It has great tensile strength, which means that under pressure the scaffold will flex rather than snap. Mineral salts are deposited on top of this flexible scaffold, adding density to the bone. As generally measured, bone loss refers to a drop in the density of calcium phosphate crystals occupying the scaffold, causing a thinning of trabecular bone. In the case of osteoporosis, cortical bone also thins. Cortical bone, the harder outer bone,

Osteoporosis, the Hidden Killer of Men

Bone health is typically presented as an issue involving women who are fading in middle age, not something with which any man worth his self-esteem would identify. But we are sorry to say, gentlemen, that losing bone density is a part of aging for you, too. Men can lose hormones just as women do, and in both cases hormone loss correlates to lower bone density. Other triggers for bone loss are also blind to gender: steroids, illness, lack of exercise, obesity, drinking a lot, being stressed and worried, job loss, divorce, social alienation, loneliness. You may be even more startled to learn that the figures show that consequences from osteoporosis are more dire for men than for women. When it comes to hip fractures, only 25 percent of total hip fractures occur in men, but 31 percent of those men die within a year, against only 17 percent of women who succumb after the same kind of fracture.

Less-than-wonderful lifestyle habits and a stressful life aren't the only factors that account for a man's osteoporosis. There are genetic factors and predispositions that are gender-blind, and there are genetic inheritance factors as well. If a man's grandfather suffered a hip fracture, he is much more likely to develop osteoporosis than the grandson of someone who didn't break a hip.

Men tend to develop osteoporosis later than women do, but 20 percent of people in the United States who suffer osteoporotic fractures are men, and worldwide that number is 30 percent. The statistics for people who smoke a lot are even more sobering. One 2015 study in *Annals of the American Thoracic Society* reported that 58 percent of pack-a-day people who smoke for 10 years have low bone density, and 55 percent of these smokers with low density are men. The same study reported that 37 percent of the same population had vertebral fractures—and 60 percent of the fractures were in men. Add in chronic respiratory illness and the figure goes up to 84 percent—every one of them with osteoporosis.

Cook for your bones, gentlemen. You and everyone who loves you will be very glad you did.

will lose about 3 percent density per decade in both men and women. Trabecular bone loses 7 to 11 percent per decade, which is why it is primarily responsible for osteoporotic states. See figure 2 on page 1 of the color insert.

The crystals that settle into the matrix scaffold are 85 percent calcium phosphate, 7 percent calcium carbonate, and small amounts of sodium, magnesium, and other trace minerals. The salt these minerals form is called hydroxyapatite. Hydroxyapatite makes up most of the calcium stored in your bones. It breaks down to release calcium when your body needs calcium—or when, in the normal process of bone tissue turnover, there's more bone cell breakdown than bone cell growth.

Over time humans also lose some density of cortical bone, though the density readings typically report more on the status of the trabecular matrix. However, in the hip, density of cortical bone appears to play a more significant role in osteoporotic fracture than in other bones.[1]

Density of hydroxyapatite in the matrix is the focus of mainstream medicine's attempts to strengthen bone. But it is important to remember that density does not necessarily equal strength. Japanese women tend to have lower bone density than Caucasian women, yet they have far fewer fractures. Collagen health, which maintains flexibility, is almost always overlooked yet, we feel, it is of equal importance. (To learn more about collagen, see "Collagen" on page 25.)

Losing the Balance

Your bones can't manufacture the calcium or phosphorus that form hydroxyapatite or all the amino acids needed to make collagen. You have to ingest these nutrients, and the most beneficial source overall is natural food—by which we mean whole, unprocessed, chemical-free food. It supplies the vitamins, minerals, proteins, enzymes, and fats that regulate the metabolic process of calcium deposition into the bones and keep the breakdown-to-growth ratio under control.

If any of the essential nutrients for bone turnover is insufficient or missing, collagen scaffolds can be weak, and calcium can go elsewhere in your body and not into your bones—even if your bones are in desperate need of it. Instead, calcium can contribute to plaque in your arteries or deposits in your joints; it can mineralize outside the bones as stones that form in your gallbladder or kidneys.

Some factors play a pivotal role in bone mineralization and growth. A healthy gut—that is, having the right bacteria in your gut for proper digestion and absorption—is the first line of defense for effective mineral absorption. Amino acid absorption is easier for your body than absorbing minerals. To stay healthy, gut bacteria need the nutrients from natural foods you bring to them via your diet. We delve into gut health more in chapter 5.

Sometimes what you eat can cause calcium to leach from your bones. Excess salt, sugary drinks, bicarbonate, caffeine, and alcohol can draw calcium from bone. Some plants considered healthful, such as spinach, contain chemical compounds called anti-nutrients that lock onto calcium and other minerals, making the minerals unavailable for digestion. You can weaken the anti-nutrient hold on a plant's minerals by preparing the plants properly for cooking, as explained in chapter 6.

Less often bone density declines due to inadequate exposure of the skin to sunshine, low hormone levels in adolescence, body-wide inflammation, or medication.

Bone Turnover: Key Players

When bone tissue breaks down to release calcium, the process is called bone resorption. Androgens—the hormones estrogen and, to a lesser extent testosterone—play a primary part in bone turnover in both women and men. These hormones signal bone to maintain new growth in a healthy balance with bone breakdown. Exercise and manual labor—any activity that pulls muscles against bone—signals bone to strengthen. And micro-damage such as bones experience in day-to-day life triggers self-repair, too.

Specific cells are dedicated to making and breaking down bone tissue (bone remodeling, as shown in figures 3 and 4 on page 2 of the color insert). Those responsible for making bone are the osteoblasts; those responsible for breaking down bone are the osteoclasts. Both take orders from a variety of sources including hormones, vitamins, and minerals (see figure 4)—along with other nutrients—that control the timing and amount of building and breaking down. When breaking down outpaces building, the result is bone density loss.

Osteo is from the Greek word for bone; *blast* is from a Greek word for germinate. The osteoblasts function in groups of connected cells called osteons and have two functions: They produce the collagen fibers that form the matrix scaffold, and they secrete the enzyme alkaline phosphatase, which binds with collagen as preparation for formation and which creates the sites on the collagen scaffold where crystals of hydroxyapatite can be deposited.

The osteoclast is the osteoblast's opposite. *Clast* is from the Greek word for broken. Osteoclasts travel along the surface of the bone and secrete acid phosphatase, an enzyme that unglues the calcium in order to break down the bone. Since bone is the body's calcium storehouse, when there isn't sufficient calcium in circulation for all the metabolic processes that involve calcium, the body sends a request via the central nervous system for osteoclasts to break down some bone.

A third type of bone cell, the osteocyte, does not play a direct role in bone turnover. Osteocytes are old osteoblasts that retire to the interior of the bone and help the bone tissue maintain oxygen and mineral levels and call for strengthening of bone in response to stress or damage such as the pull of muscle against bone when you exercise.

Stealing from the Storehouse

Beyond its function in bone health, calcium is required for other vital life processes such as secreting insulin, managing blood pressure, and transmitting nerve impulses that in turn allow muscles to contract. When there is sufficient calcium in circulation, all is well. But when your body needs calcium and there isn't enough in circulation, or what's in circulation isn't available, hormone messengers tell your bones—the body's calcium storehouse—to release calcium.

And take note: When calcium for metabolic processes is in short supply, and your bones need to restock it, metabolism wins. Some bone mineral is broken down to free up calcium (and phosphorus) for the body.

This forced choice is not generally a problem during the first half of a human's lifetime. In the early years, bones grow extra-dense with calcium, a bit like stockpiling nuts for winter. There's enough calcium to fund the body and refill the bones. Past midlife, bone density declines gradually. But we are not stuck with shrinking bones. While it is ideal to start shoring up bone mass before you reach age 30, you can take action to strengthen bone at any age. In Japan, where people traditionally followed a diet that naturally protects bone density, even after midlife bone loss rates were just 40 percent of ours in the West.[2]

Building Blocks

The collagen scaffold requires a good supply of amino acids (protein), the presence of vitamin C, and trace minerals copper and zinc to help in the building process and silicon for stabilization. The mineralization process—hydroxyapatite deposition—requires primarily calcium, phosphorus, magnesium, vitamin D, vitamin K_2, and trace minerals manganese, boron, and fluoride.

Calcium and the Road to Bone

Once you have eaten foods containing calcium, your body takes many steps to get the calcium deposited into your bones. In a healthy gut, enzymes and bacteria allow the foods you eat to be broken down properly and taken into the bloodstream. Once that happens, the freed calcium can be absorbed in the intestines in two ways. The first path needs the presence of vitamin D. The second main site of calcium absorption does not require vitamin D, but absorption is greatly increased in the presence of a simple sugar such as lactose (milk sugar). Once in the bloodstream, calcium must be joined with phosphorus and trace minerals in order to form hydroxyapatite to be deposited on the scaffold. Thus, phosphorus must be present, but also vitamin D, magnesium, and vitamin K_2 present to activate the protein, called *osteocalcin*, that carries out this joining. Osteocalcin is released from healthy osteoblasts. Trace minerals help strengthen the hydroxyapatite crystals. The hormones parathyroid hormone (PTH), calcitonin, and estrogen also play a background role. For an overview of the road to bone, see figure 5 on page 3 of the color insert.

Since calcium is central to so many metabolic processes, the body keeps a very tight rein on calcium levels. It is also the main component of bone, which is why calcium supplementation became the focus of the fight against osteoporosis—though as you now know, calcium cannot act alone.

The Interplay of Calcium and Hormones

A finely tuned arrangement—one that relies on hormonal signaling—detects calcium and regulates the levels of calcium in circulation.

The parathyroid gland has a delicate calcium-sensing membrane that monitors calcium levels in circulating body fluids. When the membrane senses falling blood calcium levels, it signals the gland to release parathyroid hormone (PTH).

This hormone is a quick-response system that pulls three organs—kidney, gut, and bone—into a beautifully orchestrated choreography. PTH triggers a growth spurt among osteoclasts, the cells that break down bone, which releases calcium from bones.

The kidney increases synthesis of vitamin D_3, which in turn leads to improved calcium absorption in the gut.

Conversely, if there's too much calcium, the thyroid gland secretes the hormone calcitonin. Calcitonin plays opposite PTH. It slows down both growth and activity of osteoclasts, which has the effect of pulling back on bone breakdown. This is a short-term solution, though, because osteoclasts get wise to calcitonin pretty quickly and stop responding after a few days. This helps to explain why calcitonin as a treatment for osteoporosis seemed promising but hasn't proven successful. (See chapter 7 for more on calcitonin as a treatment for osteoporosis.)

Calcium balance is a key to health. Calcium binds and operates with a vast array of molecules in the body—for example, it binds with a protein, calmodulin, that activates enzymes that provide energy for muscle contraction. It is a stabilizer of proteins and enzymes, optimizing their performance. In the same way that vitamin D is required for most of the calcium absorption in the small intestine, the enzyme Ca ATPase is necessary for the release of the calcium into the body for nerve conduction.

Calcium is central to bone metabolism, but it alone can't be effective for bone health. Phosphorus, magnesium, and trace minerals—zinc, copper, silicon, boron, fluoride, and manganese—play major roles, too, along with enzymes, vitamins, and collagen.

Phosphorus

Phosphorus is the second most abundant mineral in your body. It filters waste in the kidneys, balances the activity of vitamins and other minerals, and relays cellular signals. It is an integral part of cell membrane structure and plays a role in tissue growth, maintenance, and repair. It assists in the formation of the genetic building blocks: DNA, the chemical structures that contain genetic information, and RNA, the structures that translate genetic information.

Phosphorus combines with calcium to make hydroxyapatite (calcium phosphate), the principal player in bone density. So it is essential to bone health—85 percent of a body's phosphorus is stored in bones. Phosphorus also funds plant growth once a seed germinates. Yet while phosphorus is highly bioavailable—the body can easily absorb and use it—most mineral-rich highly nutritious plant-based foods contain phytic acid, a chemical compound that keeps

phosphorus locked up until the seed germinates. (See chapter 4 for more on phytic acid.)

When phosphorus levels are in balance—that means in the ideal ratios for life—calcium and phosphorus naturally form calcium phosphate when it is needed, and balanced levels of both minerals in the body leave calcium in the bone where it is needed. A phosphorus overload in circulation, however, triggers the release of PTH, which in turn triggers bone breakdown to release calcium. High phosphorus levels are implicated in cardiovascular disease, especially when calcium phosphate is deposited outside of bone. Meat, poultry, processed foods, and carbonated sodas contain very high levels of phosphorus. Soda has 10 to 20 times more phosphorus than calcium, so drinking one serving of soda can trigger the body to break down bone.

Magnesium

Magnesium is central to all phases of skeletal metabolism, including both formation of the collagen matrix and mineralization, and transport of minerals across cell membranes. Magnesium converts vitamin D to its active form, which promotes transport of calcium to the bones. Magnesium also stimulates calcitonin production, which increases deposition of calcium in bones. Magnesium is part of the cycle that ensures calcium does not get deposited in soft tissue. Magnesium also has a direct effect on bone through its influences on hormones; low magnesium levels cause both osteoblasts and osteoclasts to slow down, with a net loss in bone density. Stress causes magnesium loss, and very low magnesium levels trigger PTH secretion, which starts bone breakdown.

Hundreds of enzymes require magnesium in order to function. Energy production, protein synthesis, and cell signaling also depend on magnesium. It improves the sensitivity of insulin and appears to support stroke recovery. Magnesium deficiency can interfere with vitamin D and calcium balances.

The adult human body contains about 25 grams of magnesium. Inadequate blood magnesium levels are known to result in low blood calcium levels, resistance to PTH action, and resistance to some of the effects of vitamin D—deficiencies that deplete bone matrix.

Low magnesium levels appear to contribute more to causing heart disease than cholesterol or saturated fat do.[3] Magnesium also helps balance the enzyme that creates cholesterol in your body.

Trace Minerals

For a long time, science did not recognize that trace minerals are necessary to human health and that deficiency is a factor in bone loss. In fact they are vital, and all are vital to bone health. There are chemical and electrical processes ongoing in your body every second, and these processes rely on the well-known bone health minerals but also trace minerals such as boron, chromium, copper, fluoride, iodine, iron, sulfur, manganese, molybdenum, selenium, and zinc. All are present in the earth's crust, and everything in the world, including humans, contains them.

They are so important nothing in your body would be built or processed properly without them. They are mediators of inflammation and participate in transporting oxygen, normalizing the nervous system, and simulating growth, maintenance, and repair of tissue. They are also vital to the maintenance and repair of bones.

Silicon is one of the most important trace minerals for bone health, and it is essential to healthy bone formation. It appears that silicon regulates the deposition of calcium and phosphorus in the bone tissue. There are some indications that the full benefit of silicon is found only in the presence of estrogen. If this is shown to be the case, phytoestrogens can stand in for estrogen to reap the full benefits of silicon (see "A Deeper Look" on page 76).

Boron is linked to healthy bone metabolism. Boron levels are often low in people with arthritis, as well as osteoporosis. Boron appears to raise estrogen and testosterone levels, which then allows more productive mineral deposition. It also influences the effectiveness of vitamin D and helps to prevent calcium loss through the urine.[4]

Copper is necessary for the formation of the links that bind the collagen scaffold. People who have osteoporosis have a copper deficiency.

Manganese is required to stimulate osteoblast activity, but also osteoclast activity. When there is a manganese deficiency, bone deposition quality is reduced, and weak bone does not break down. This can leave brittle bone in place.

Fluoride stimulates osteoblast growth and the formation of new bone. It increases hydroxyapatite crystal density, helping to stabilize the bone mineral. Too much fluoride greatly reduces proper bone mineralization, leaving bones more brittle and subject to fracture.

Zinc enhances bone formation by stimulating osteoblasts, assisting with collagen synthesis, and enhancing the effects of vitamins necessary in bone health.

People obtain trace minerals by eating food plants that were grown in good soil. Some widespread farming practices, including use of pesticides and leaving soil uncovered (which leads to soil erosion), contribute to the depletion of these vital minerals in the human diet.

Trace Mineral Absorption and Proton Pump Inhibitors

Trace minerals require the presence of adequate stomach acid for absorption. Heartburn drugs sold over the counter—such as Prilosec, Nexium, Prevacid, and others—interfere with mineral absorption and negatively affect bone health. These drugs, called proton pump inhibitors, have seen skyrocketing sales. They inhibit production of stomach acid in part by affecting the movement of protons within stomach membranes. They are very strong drugs and very effective at inhibiting production of stomach acid.

Twenty-one million prescriptions for these drugs were written in 2009; in 2013, Nexium alone took in over $6 billion for AstraZeneca.[5] Collectively, the result of inhibited stomach acid production is severely decreased mineral absorption and decreased nutrient absorption overall. As the intake of these drugs increases, bone health worldwide will continue to decline.

And it isn't just bone health that suffers among people who use this type of proton pump inhibitor. In June 2015, Stanford University researchers data-mined 16 million health records. They found that taking this type of proton pump inhibitor *increases* the chances of heart attack by 16 to 21 percent.[6]

This is such a strong link that, eventually, there will have to be changes in how these drugs are sold. For the moment, however, please be careful. If you take these drugs for longer than two weeks consecutively, you run much higher risk of a heart episode, and an FDA drug safety communication recently recommended "for the shortest duration possible," not to exceed three 2-week treatments per year.

Enzymes

Typically enzyme names end in *-ase*. Enzymes catalyze every chemical reaction in the body. They prepare nutrients to play their part in metabolism by breaking down protein, carbohydrates, and fats into forms that your body can digest and by activating vitamins.

Many foods in their natural forms contain the enzymes needed for their own breakdown. Milk is an example. The enzyme lactase is found in milk; it breaks down lactose, or milk sugar, the carbohydrate in milk. Lactose is a relatively large molecule—too large for the human intestine, which can only absorb small molecules. So lactase, which breaks the lactose into smaller units, is essential for digestion. Some but not all people produce lactase in the gut.

This information about lactase and lactose helps to answer questions about lactose intolerance—something that affects far fewer people than advertisers would like you to believe. Here's the lowdown.

The heat of pasteurization destroys enzymes including lactase and alkaline phosphatase. Phosphatase activity assists calcium absorption, destroying it lessens calcium absorption in the intestines. It is my experience that patients who describe themselves as lactose intolerant have no trouble digesting raw milk.

So the large numbers who are self-labeled lactose-intolerant almost certainly aren't; they are, I believe, lactase-deficient, and that's thanks to pasteurization much more often than to true lactose intolerance. Of course the end is the same: Many people can't drink pasteurized milk without suffering gastric distress. We think it is much better to drink natural raw milk from a licensed farm than to drink pasteurized lactose-free milk that has been even more denatured to make it suitable for people who can't digest pasteurized milk.

Actually molecules of any protein—a protein is a chain of amino acids—are too big for the small intestine to absorb. Proteases are enzymes that break down amino acid chains to create free amino acids that are small enough for your body to absorb. Fats—chains of lipids—are prepared for digestion in the same way by the enzyme lipase.

In addition to preparing food for absorption, enzymes convert inactive vitamins to active ones and, in the case of bone, facilitate the transport of minerals to and within bone.

Enzymes play a role in resorption (bone breakdown), too. Collagenase secreted by the osteoclast membrane breaks down the bone matrix, releasing the components calcium, phosphorus, magnesium, trace minerals, and collagen into the bloodstream.

Heat kills enzymes so highly processed foods will generally be devoid of enzymes.

Vitamins

Vitamins are molecules with wide-ranging functions in the body. They serve primarily as coenzymes—that is, they help enzymes to function.

Vitamins are soluble in either fat or water: Vitamins A, D, E, and K are soluble in fat; B vitamins and vitamin C are soluble in water. Fat-soluble vitamins are stored in the body's fat cells and can accumulate. Water-soluble vitamins circulate and are either used or excreted.

Vitamins are listed here in their relative importance to bone health, although the whole body needs all vitamins to function properly.

Vitamin D

Vitamin D increases the absorption of calcium (and phosphate) in the intestine by increasing the permeability of the intestinal membrane, leading to higher levels of calcium in the blood, which signals the body to slow bone breakdown. Without vitamin D, sufficient calcium cannot be properly absorbed or transported to bones.

Vitamin D induces the creation of proteins in the gut that bind to calcium, also assisting with proper absorption.

The primary site of calcium absorption is in the duodenum, the upper small intestine, and this site requires the presence of vitamin D. If you do not have enough vitamin D, there will be some through insufficient absorption throughout the intestine. There is increased absorption at a secondary site, the ileum, which does not require vitamin D. Absorption here increases in the presence of a simple sugar, such as lactose. If the proper combination of simple sugars and calcium makes it to the ileum, you will absorb up to double the amount of calcium.[7]

Among vitamin D's many jobs in the body, and of great importance to us, is generating osteoblasts, the cells that grow new bone. Also, as the body processes vitamin D, the final end product is a repair-and-maintenance steroid hormone that stimulates production of cathelicidin, one of the body's naturally occurring antibiotics.

Without the presence of vitamin D, only about 10 percent of the calcium you eat will be absorbed.

Vitamin K_2: The Dark Horse Star

Vitamin K_2, also called menaquinone, is a bone health celebrity. Its star turn is nothing less than enabling calcium to be deposited where it should be, in the matrix of bones, and not in the joints or arteries. It participates in making proteins that bind calcium in bone. Japanese and Dutch research reports that adequate K_2 cuts osteoporotic fracture rates in half.[8] The most potent K_2 forms for bone health are MK7 and MK4. It is thought that MK7 helps clear plaque from arteries.

Some gut bacteria can produce a minimal amount of vitamin K_2. However, these bacteria do not produce enough K_2 naturally for our bone health requirements, and thus we need to get it from food or supplements.

Like other nutrients, K_2 wears many hats. It seems to stimulate bone formation and suppress bone resorption, and slow down osteoclast growth.

Perhaps most important, vitamin K_2 is a necessary component of the protein osteocalcin. Osteocalcin is secreted by osteoblasts, and among other important jobs appears to regulate the deposition of calcium into the bone. Higher osteocalcin levels correlate with higher bone density. This protein is vitamin K–dependent, meaning if you do not have vitamin K_2 present, this all-important protein will not function properly.

Comparative studies indicate that people who have osteoporosis often have excess vascular plaque, putting them at risk for a cardiovascular event—plaque that K_2 appears to disperse, possibly due to the activation of the osteocalcin. Cells in vascular plaques often turn on the same genes for bone formation.[9] See chapter 6 for more details about vitamin K_2.

The Other K Vitamins

Vitamin K_1, phylloquinone, is typically referred to as vitamin K. It functions differently than vitamin K_2; it plays different parts in maintaining health. Vitamin K, found in leafy greens, helps blood to clot. Most doctors recommend that anyone taking blood thinners avoid or exclude vitamin K entirely. However, the new recommendation is that regulating the amount of vitamin K (1 and 2) in the diet is a better strategy—having the same amount each day. If you take blood-thinning medication, speak with your doctor about vitamin K in your diet. Long-term anticoagulant treatment (heparin, warfarin) appears to induce bone density loss,[10] due to the inhibition of vitamin K and the resulting reduction of active osteocalcin. Soft tissue calcification is also associated with long-term anticoagulant treatment;[11] it appeared in warfarin-treated experimental animals within two weeks.

Ordinarily K_2 alone does not interfere effectively with blood clotting. In a study using very high doses of K_2 there was a slight reduction in blood thinner effect; however, it did not promote blood clots.[12]

Vitamin K_3 is a synthetic product, not useful for promoting bone health. The natural K vitamins are fat-soluble.

Vitamin C

Vitamin C is housed in the skin and transported from there to the bloodstream. It plays a part in wound healing and immunity. It is a strong antioxidant (there's more about antioxidants in "Natural Defense: Antioxidants" on page 29) and a natural sunscreen that protects skin from UV damage. Most importantly in our context, vitamin C is involved in every step of collagen formation. In the building of the bone scaffold, collagen fibrils are linked together in a process called cross-linking. Vitamin C as well as trace minerals are necessary for proper cross-linking.

Keeping up vitamin C levels will help you promote ideal collagen growth[13] and make it possible for you to take advantage of the sun to produce vitamin D. The benefits of vitamin C are enhanced by the presence of vitamin E and zinc. At the end of the collagen formation cycle, vitamin C is destroyed, so it is important to consume this vitamin regularly in order to build bone.

The B Vitamins

The B complex is a group of vitamins: B_1, B_2, B_3, B_5, B_6, B_7, B_9, and B_{12}. Each has a distinct role in metabolic activity. One of the B vitamins' many jobs is to regulate homocysteine, whose high levels are directly correlated with bone loss (see "Homocysteine, Sodium, Thyroid Hormones, and Acid/Base Balance" on page 31 for more on homocysteine). Magnesium and the B vitamins appear to work in concert to alleviate anxiety, PMS symptoms, and migraines. Most B vitamins are known popularly by other names. Table 1.1 summarizes the most important functions of each B vitamin.

There is a genetic mutation among humans in a gene named MTHFR. This mutation affects the body's ability to use vitamin B_9, folate. As this mutation is relatively common, it is a good idea to ask your healthcare provider for a test to see if you carry it. If you do, you will need to take a specific form of folate in order for it to work in your body. This is critical for handling homocysteine breakdown.

Vitamin A

Vitamin A is essential for the growth of osteoblasts, the bone builders, in the early stages of their growth. In fact it helps regulate the growth and life of virtually all cells in the human body. Vitamin A is necessary for hormone production that in turn influences bone health. Vitamin A interacts with vitamin K_2 to create the conditions for proper calcium deposition. The three active forms of vitamin A in the body are retinol, retinal, and retinoic acid. These compounds are referred to collectively as retinoids.

Vitamin A is found in food in the form of retinyl esters in animal products and beta-carotene (β-carotene) in plants. Beta-carotene and other compounds that can be converted by the body into retinol are referred to as carotenoids. Plants synthesize hundreds of different carotenoids, but only about 10 percent of them can be converted to retinol. Different forms of carotenoids have different values in this regard. For example, 12 mcg of beta-carotene are needed to produce 1 mcg of retinol, but 24 mcg of alpha-carotene and beta-crytoxanthin are needed to produce that same amount. The precursor to retinol is found in animal-based foods, whereas plants contain only carotenes.

Protein

Protein, chains of amino acids, keeps the body's 100 trillion cells doing all the jobs assigned to them, ranging from translating genetic

Table 1.1. The B Vitamins

Common Name	Chemical Name	Key Metabolic Functions
Vitamin B$_1$	Thiamine	· assists with the flow of electrolytes in and out of nerve and muscle cells · nervous system and muscle function · digestion · carbohydrate and energy metabolism
Vitamin B$_2$	Riboflavin	· converts pyridoxine, niacin, and folate into useful forms · an antioxidant (attacks free radicals) · assists energy metabolism · assists building tissue · assists eyesight
Vitamin B$_3$	Niacin	· facilitates electron transfer for molecular synthesis of fatty acids and lowers cholesterol · fosters DNA repair and genome stability
Vitamin B$_5$	Pantothenic acid	· serves as main component of coenzyme A, which facilitates enzyme activity · generates energy from food · participates in synthesizing molecules, neurotransmitters, and hormones · accelerates wound healing
Vitamin B$_6$	Pyridoxine	· synthesizes heme, a component of hemoglobin · participates in formation of enzymes vital to protein metabolism · reduces homocysteine levels
Vitamin B$_7$	Biotin	· fosters DNA packaging/histone modification (histones are proteins found in chromosomes)
Vitamin B$_9$	Folate	· plays a central role in formation of nucleic acid and in gene methylation · promotes healthy nervous system function and homocysteine balance
Vitamin B$_{12}$	Cyanocobalamin	· plays a central role in folate metabolism · fosters DNA integrity · preserves the myelin sheath around neurons · helps to reduce homocysteine levels

instructions to transmitting pain signals to the brain. A complete protein consists of 20 amino acids. Nine of these are the essential amino acids, which means your body cannot synthesize them so you must take them in through the food you eat. A tenth amino acid, arginine, is considered essential during times of growth; although you can make some, you can't make enough. The rest of the amino acids are termed non-essential. This doesn't mean your body doesn't need them; it does mean your body is able to synthesize them from byproducts of metabolism. All 20 amino acids must be present to build protein, so complete amino acid intake is an absolute requirement whether you obtain the essential amino acids from animal products, plants, or a combination.

Lately, there's been a fair bit of speculation about a correlation between protein intake and bone density. Some studies seemed to show that increased protein intake led to unwanted calcium loss through the urine. Taken as a whole, however, the research shows that increased protein intake is positive for bone health, as long as there is enough calcium in circulation and enough stored in the bone.[14]

Collagen

Collagen is the principal structural protein in connective tissue and the bone matrix scaffold. Healthy bone scaffold is rarely discussed, but it is a key component to bone health. Collagen makes up about 25 percent of a human body's protein and is part of organs, arteries, veins, skin, ligaments, tendons, bones, and marrow. Collagen works together with the structural protein elastin to maintain connective tissue elasticity. Inflammation can destroy collagen (more about this in chapter 2). Vitamin C is essential to collagen formation. It works with anthocyanins (which are antioxidant compounds found in dark red/purple fruits) and with copper to ensure strong collagen formation.

The cooked form of collagen, gelatin, is a perfect way to supplement and thereby increase the body's collagen. Gelatin is easy to digest even for people with gastrointestinal conditions and food sensitivities.

Regular consumption of gelatin helps replenish the mucosal barrier of the gut and stop inflammation. This is increasingly important because it appears that intestinal permeability issues are paramount in allergies, food intolerances, autoimmune conditions, and many other inflammatory chronic health conditions.

By now, you're probably getting the picture that the food choices you make for bone density are also good for many other aspects of your health—and vice versa.

CARTILAGE

Cartilage is primarily collagen and elastin proteins. The cartilage in bone broth is found mostly in the joint tissue, helping us to reduce joint deterioration in our bodies and support strong connective tissue.

GLYCINE

It has been recently found that high-glycine/low-methionine diets directly increase longevity. Bone broth is rich in this amino acid, which plays a wide variety of important roles in the body including glucose production and regulation. It is one of the three amino acids that make up glutathione, a tripeptide that acts as our body's most prominent antioxidant. It is also crucial for protecting muscle, in muscle recovery, and in wound healing. It is thought to be an inhibitory neurotransmitter, helping with sleep and recovery from seizures.

Glycine increases gastric juices, assisting in the prevention of ulcers and digestive-related conditions, and it is essential for liver detoxification.

PROLINE

This is the primary amino acid required for collagen formation, and so is essential for healthy cartilage, tendons, bones, ligaments, and skin. Proline also helps keep the arteries flexible and producing collagen, reducing arteriosclerosis and blood pressure and repairing damaged tissue.

For collagen formation proline is best taken with vitamin C.

CHAPTER 2

Systemic Factors
That Promote Bone Loss

In chapter 1 we discussed the nutritional building blocks of bone. If your diet doesn't include all the building blocks, you won't make bone efficiently or effectively. That is, you will suffer bone loss due to nutrient deficiency. However, other factors can also affect bone turnover. These factors, such as inflammation and stress, are considered systemic, in that they tend to affect the entire metabolic system rather than just the bone-building process.

Treatments for these systemic issues is beyond the scope of this book, but we wish to share some specifics on how important the larger environment of your body is in combating bone loss. Changing how you eat is one big part, and positive dietary changes can improve mood, reduce inflammation, mitigate free radical damage, and help to regulate hormone production. But if these systemic factors remain at play, bone building can be stunted or interrupted. These systemic

factors can affect the degree to which your nutrients can help to build bone. These detrimental extra-nutritional factors often start with stress, which can lead to inflammation.[1] Emotional stress such as anxiety, anger, grudges, and untreated emotional or physical pain can compromise or counteract your best efforts to eat right for your bones. So can other stresses, such as pesticides and environmental toxins, which challenge your health at a cellular level.

Inflammation

Sometimes inflammation is visible. Something is red, swollen, and/or painful. Inflammation is the body's response to damage or threat, and it is protective. The inflammation trigger might be a toxin such as a pesticide residue, a splinter, a bacterium or virus, or chronic emotional stress. The unwelcome visitor interferes with the body's everyday metabolic activity and causes an aggravated response—the capillaries dilate and become porous to allow immune factors to get to the damage, the area swells, and inflammatory molecules may activate a pain response. All of this occurs, the invader or damage is fixed, and things return to normal.

However, if the infiltrator remains in the body and the response continues, the inflammation becomes chronic, and it can turn nasty. The inflammatory response causes tissue damage that must be repaired. And this isn't straightforward. Each type of tissue has an individual repair mechanism. For example, skin has excellent regenerative capacity. But when inflammation occurs in a neuron, which has very little regenerative capacity, there can be long-term damage.

The body has a range of responses to inflammation, including sending cholesterol as a repair substance if there has been tissue damage; while defense is under way, however, the body suspends ordinary immune system response and some metabolic processes in order to concentrate cellular energy on eliminating the threat. This emergency response, which is different for each type of attack, is part of our living system survival kit and, of course, highly desirable. However, with the immune system focused on a particular inflamed area, a sustained attack can leave the body vulnerable to many and varied dysfunctions that ultimately may cause serious health problems including excess breakdown of bone tissue.

Chronic, low-level inflammation appears to be a factor in most chronic disease—and eliminating this low-level inflammation must be part of the recovery process for all maladies, including osteoporosis.

Glucocorticoids, Stress, and Bone Loss

Steroids are chemicals that affect cell activity and response. Glucocorticoids are naturally occurring steroid hormones sometimes used as medication. Glucocorticoids arise as part of a coordinated response system to imbalances caused by stress. In a stress situation, the immune system triggers the hypothalamus, a brain region, to signal the adrenal glands to secrete glucocorticoids, which reduce inflammation. Synthetic glucocorticoids such as prednisone are often used to treat inflammatory conditions, an overactive immune system, and sometimes cancer.

Though glucocorticoids do decrease inflammation, they too often lead to further health problems. When used for more than a week, glucocorticoids begin to impair the adrenal glands, suppress the immune system, and induce bone loss. If taken extensively they trigger a condition that doctors call glucocorticoid-induced osteoporosis.

Here's how that works. Inflammation promotes the growth of osteoclasts, the cells that break down bone matrix and simultaneously suppresses osteoblasts, the bone matrix makers. Because of this, even low-level chronic inflammation increases fracture risk.

Inflammation also affects hormone function, potentially increasing the release of parathyroid hormone (PTH), which increases bone breakdown.

Free Radicals

Sometimes chronic inflammation can give rise to an excess of free radicals, which are atoms that have an incomplete number of electrons in their outer shells. Scientists describe them as highly reactive because they will take any opportunity to regain their missing electron and become stable. And indeed free radicals are scavengers. They invade cells and tissue randomly; they are not particular about where they pinch an electron and are relentless in the drive to find one. When healthy tissue loses electrons to free radicals, the tissue becomes unstable and vulnerable. And since free radicals will latch onto any type of cell, the bones, joints, organs, and even DNA are all equally subject to attack.

Free radicals arise as byproducts of normal metabolism—for instance, powerful free radicals called superoxides are a byproduct of the body's conversion of oxygen to energy—and ordinarily the body's response system is sufficient to demobilize most of them. But free radicals also arise when the body is called upon to metabolize unnatural or exceptional compounds such as processed food, air pollution, preservatives and synthetic coloring in food, gasoline, toxic and carcinogenic chemicals in groundwater, and synthetic chemicals in personal care products. Formation of free radicals can even be stimulated by the anxiety created by health-and-wellness hype, among other unnatural or exceptional events the body was not designed for and is not equipped to handle.

Free radical overload and indiscriminate attack on systemic cells is called oxidative stress, which causes inflammation, interferes with genetic expression, can render otherwise healthy tissue damaged, and opens the road to disease.

To deal with free radicals, the body produces antioxidants, principally enzymes, that scoop up the free radicals and neutralize them. But if free radical production exceeds the body's ability to neutralize them, the excess radicals can cause very serious damage. A free radical overload can overwhelm the body's natural defense force.

Natural Defense: Antioxidants

The body's natural defense against free radicals are antioxidant enzymes. Superoxide dismutases (SOD) are enzymes that partition the very toxic superoxide radical (the byproduct of oxygen metabolism) into less harmful subunits that can be broken down further by other enzymes.

The *-ases* are mighty, but though our natural provision of them is enough to balance our natural production of free radicals, it is not sufficient to fight off the army of free radicals most of us now encounter in our daily lives. Fortunately, though, many enzymes in whole, unrefined foods have the capacity to disable free radicals. Nutrients such as vitamin E, vitamin C, and beta-carotene act as antioxidants. Polyphenols are naturally occurring chemicals that in plants protects cells against environmental damage and directly affect metabolism, cell signaling, and oxidants. In food, plant polyphenols are the main source of antioxidants.

The best antioxidant sources are spices such as star anise and cloves, herbs such as rosemary and oregano, black elderberries, hazelnuts and pecans, celery seeds, chocolate in the form of cocoa powder and dark chocolate, and fruits including plums and apples.

In some instances free radicals and the presence of superoxides actually appear to positively impact life. This is a complex idea beyond the scope of this book, but in general continually forcing the body to deal with an overload of free radicals is detrimental to health.

Smoking and Free Radicals

Smoking a single cigarette generates a considerable free radical load. As you can imagine, smoking many cigarettes each day generates a voluminous free radical load that can overwhelm and damage cells and entire organs—and, perhaps most damaging, prompting the liver to produce enzymes that can destroy precious hormones.

Smoking also is a trigger for these deleterious reactions:

- Destruction of osteoblasts (cells that build bone) by free radicals.
- Destruction of osteoblasts by nicotine.
- A rise in cortisol levels, which prompts bone breakdown.
- Interference with the hormone calcitonin.
- Damage to blood vessels, which impedes circulation and interferes with oxygen supply.

When a smoker suffers a fracture, healing is slow and poor, partly due to damaged blood vessels and reduced oxygen supply.

Stress

In the quest to control bone loss, managing chronic stress is key. That's because any kind of stress, emotional or environmental, produces not only free radicals but also chronic cortisol release, which, like excess free radicals, raises inflammation in the long term.

Cortisol is a hormone secreted by your adrenal glands. It is an efficient anti-allergy, anti-inflammation agent. Cortisol levels peak in the morning, ready for the stresses of a day, and decline steadily to a low during deep sleep. Any sudden stressor at any point in the cycle elicits an acute cortisol surge that triggers an increase in blood sugar, sends energy to muscles, sparks the need to escape, and raises blood pressure. The signal to raise blood sugar will prompt the body to break down amino acids, especially if the system is low on carbohydrates. This system is called gluconeogenesis, and is a backup mechanism that allows the body to form fuel even in the absence of food. What's also important here is that the body's responses to cortisol take priority over the immune system, so normal immune response is temporarily diverted and your body is open to attack.

Acute cortisol release does not cause damage, but chronic cortisol release does. Chronic cortisol release is a state of sustained high alert brought on by a habitually stressful life. It alters the body's

A Note About Antidepressants

Chronic stress can lead to depression. The most widely prescribed antidepressants are SSRIs, selective serotonin reuptake inhibitors. These drugs work on the neurotransmitter serotonin, leaving it in the system longer. There is evidence that SSRIs affect bone metabolism[2] due to the fact that serotonin produced in the gut affects bone mass. High levels of serotonin outside of the brain (approximately 95 percent of our serotonin is produced in the gut and circulates in our platelets) lead to lower bone density.[3] If you are taking SSRIs and suffer bone density loss, discuss this with your healthcare provider.

inflammation response, desensitizing immune cells to cortisol's anti-inflammatory effects.

Chronic cortisol release weakens the immune system, delays wound healing, damages the learning response and memory retrieval, and—you guessed it—directly and immediately reduces calcium absorption in the intestines, which slows bone formation. Collagen can be a direct target of chronically elevated cortisol, transforming it so it cannot be used to strengthen bone.

Directly, cortisol attacks the outer layer of the bone (periosteum). The result of this is an inhibition of osteoblast formation, and thus decreased bone building.

Other Systemic Factors

Four other factors play a role in bone loss: homocysteine levels, sodium levels, levels of thyroid hormone, and acid/base balance.

Homocysteine

Homocysteine is an amino acid that is produced naturally in the body when the amino acid methionine breaks down. Homocysteine can build up in the body, causing damage—not only to bones but also to arteries, raising the risk of heart attack,[4] stroke, and blood clots. Folate and the other B vitamins help the body maintain safe levels of homocysteine. However, some people (perhaps 30 percent of the population) have a genetic mutation—MTHFR—that affects their absorption and use of folate. This mutation leaves the body vulnerable to high homocysteine levels. Lack of B vitamins and a high intake of the amino acid methionine can also lead to this potentially dangerous imbalance.

High homocysteine correlates to higher incidence of hip fracture. And listen up, men: Men with the highest homocysteine levels suffer hip fracture nearly four times more than men with the lowest levels. Women with high homocysteine had nearly a doubled risk of hip fracture.[5] Homocysteine levels can be tested, and in cases of bone loss without obvious factors, testing is highly recommended.

Sodium

Everyone has heard doctors decry high sodium intake. It's worth taking note. Once the body has all the sodium it needs, the excess is excreted. But every gram excreted pulls a whopping 26 mg of calcium along for the ride.[6] In other words, all it takes is slightly more than 1 teaspoon of sodium to pull circulating calcium into the urine. And if there isn't enough calcium in the bloodstream, the body raids its calcium store in the bones. Even a little excess sodium every day can cause up to a 1 percent loss of bone annually.

Processed foods are generally considered the culprit, because eliminating processed foods from the diet appears to eliminate this problem. In adult women, studies published in the journal *Nutrients* looking at this relationship found that bone mineral density could be maintained simply by reducing sodium to 2,300 mg per day and keeping calcium around 1,000 mg per day.

Thyroid Hormones

A properly functioning thyroid gland producing balanced thyroid hormones is a key to healthy bone turnover. Hyperthyroidism—a condition which is characterized by overproduction of thyroid hormone—can lead to severe bone loss. Thyroid hormones increase the activation of new bone remodeling cycles, appearing to increase bone breakdown in relation to bone building by causing an increase in osteoclast production. Laboratory tests[7] show that high thyroid

A Long-Standing Link

The first documented case of hyperthyroid bone disease dates back to 1891. A doctor named von Redklinghausen described "worm eaten" bones of a young woman who died from hyperthyroidism. "The ribs showed multiple fractures, and could easily be crushed between two fingers . . . [bone] was almost translucent when held up to the light."[8]

hormone levels increased the release of calcium from bone by up to 60 percent.

In the case of hypothyroidism, a condition characterized by lower-than-normal levels of thyroid hormone in the body, adults show an *increase* in bone density. However, the bone quality is poor, and hypothyroidism also results in an increase in fracture rates. Intake of seaweed has been shown to positively affect thyroid function, increasing thyroid-stimulating hormone production.[9] Please discuss this with your healthcare provider if you suffer from thyroid conditions.

Your body will exercise any measure at any cost to keep your blood within a specific pH range. Consider the case of soda: Too much phosphoric acid leaves an acid residue. That residue signals your body to pull calcium from your bones to restore pH balance. Likewise if your diet is high in acid foods, such as meat and grains, which disrupts the acid base balance in favor of acid, your body signals the need to restore the pH balance and again pulls calcium into play.

Because dietary acids found in meat and grains are excessive in the Western diet, the blood momentarily tends towards acidic, so the body releases minerals that balance the pH of the blood. This means the body will signal the bones to release calcium. Diets higher in alkaline foods, such as fruits and vegetables, help to keep minerals in the bones where they belong.

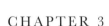

CHAPTER 3

Choose Natural Food
for Healthy Bones

The foods we recommend in this book help restore the balance of breakdown and renewal that characterizes turnover in bone. But all food is not equal. The more we learn about human health, the more it is clear that natural food is the safest—both for health and as medicine: food that is untreated, unheated, and delivered in safe containers; food grown from seed that has not been genetically modified; food that has never been exposed to synthetic chemicals during growing, transport, storage, or display for sale. Natural food has not been processed; it is as it grows, naturally.

Foods, Forms, Combinations

Our planet's living systems all arose from the same earthly elements. By eating the foods that are naturally available—those that evolved over time rather than those scientists create—we can maintain and sustain strong and healthy bodies and a viable planet. However, if plants have absorbed pesticides during growth or been sprayed with chemicals to artificially preserve color and shelf life, or have been stored in packaging that contains harmful chemicals such as bisphenols (BPA and BPS) that can disrupt hormone balances, these harmful substances remain in the plants even through heating and can disrupt biochemistry, affect cells, and even change DNA. If animals have been plied with antibiotics and growth hormones, fed grain that their bodies are not built to digest, and crowded into such confined spaces that they can barely move, the animals become extremely stressed, flooded with cortisol, and the animals as food are severely compromised. Their biochemistry is altered, their nutrient and hormone balances shift, and consumers eat the lot. If that meat has been further sullied with carbon monoxide to

Methylation

In some cases, the human body can't use nutrients that are essential for life and good health in their raw forms. For example, vitamins must be converted into usable forms once inside the body. A metabolic process called methylation transforms nutrients into usable forms. Substances called methyl donors do the transformation work; thus the process name, *methylation*. A healthy body produces methyl donors, though production declines with age.

Fortunately natural food provides methyl donors. For example, lightly cooked vegetables are highest in dietary methyl donors. However, people whose diet is heavy in processed foods are usually short of methyl donors, and thus they run a heightened risk of disease.

If you are moving away from a diet high in processed foods, consider supplementing with trimethylglycine. This substance is naturally formed in the body and provides a safe way to increase methyl donors. (See "Supplemental Trimethylglycine" on page 73).

artificially preserve red meat color, risk goes up and nutritional benefit fades.

As with all things, natural is the starting point for bone health food, but it is not the only requirement. Calcium, phosphorus, and magnesium are the foundation nutrients for bone health because they make up bone matrix (as explained in chapter 1), and you need a steady supply of all three along with other nutrients that play a part in bone health metabolic processes outside and inside the bone. So no matter how much of any single food, nutrient, vitamin, or mineral you take in, even if local and natural, it won't be effective on its own. That's why learning about the nutrient content of foods is the basis for learning how to combine foods in ways that provide sufficient amounts of all the essential bone health nutrients.

Why Natural Foods Are Best for Bones

Left to itself, a chicken clucks around fending off pecks, eating grass and weed seeds, scratching for insects, and sunning itself in a dust bath. That's what chickens do when they're not cooped up. And that's the pedigree we want for chicken we eat.

Why? All living systems draw from a common source of available nutrients. When a chicken does what comes naturally, its body retains a full complement of nutrients required for good health. So if we eat the chicken, there is a rich source of nutrients we can easily absorb.

That's why as a society, we are conscientious about feeding children wholesome food—and for good reason. Wholesome food, natural and nutritious, does contribute nutrients in a form we can digest and absorb and does not interfere with natural patterns of growth and development. Introduce artificial ingredients—those that aren't naturally digested and absorbed—and the body reacts with random biochemical responses that affect physiology, behavior, development, stress levels, and genes. For example, animals fed synthetic growth hormones don't metabolize or excrete the chemicals; they conserve the hormones in muscle cells even after death, and we in turn ingest those hormones when we eat the meat of those animals.

Human health, including bone health, depends on the proper absorption of specific groups of nutrients that coexist in natural foods. When food plants and animals are not grown naturally, the plants and animals experience high levels of stress that cause epigenetic and biochemical changes that deplete many nutrients. So we choose natural foods rather than processed foods—and suggest that you do, too—because natural foods are not only much more likely to be properly absorbed but also much less likely to disrupt our own metabolic processes.

To see the effect on an animal living naturally compared with the effect on one living an unnatural life, consider the nutritional content and action in the body of eggs, meat, milk, and vegetables grown naturally.

Eggs

An egg from a pastured chicken offers four times as much vitamin D, twice the omega-3, three times more vitamin E, and seven times more beta-carotene than an egg from a chicken raised in a cage on a factory farm.[1] Eggs from pastured chickens also contain more trace minerals (depending on environment, feed, and so on) and 35 to 80 mg vitamin K_2, the vitamin that helps guide calcium to bones.

Meat

For optimal nutrition, seek beef from pasture-raised cows—animals that grazed on natural green grass and on plants that grew organically from their own untreated, unheated natural seed. Grass-fed meat has many other benefits. It contains less total fat, saturated fat, cholesterol, and calories than meat from confined animals. It also provides more vitamin E, beta-carotene, vitamin C, and health-promoting

---

CLA

Conjugated linoleic acid (CLA) is an omega-6 fatty acid that has been shown to lower body fat, increase insulin sensitivity, and is anti-tumor, anti-asthmatic, anti-inflammatory, and anti-osteoporotic.[3] Grass-fed beef and raw dairy products are excellent sources of CLA. Swiss and Colby cheeses are especially rich in CLA, as are pomegranate seed oil and grass-fed lamb.

---

fats that include omega-3 fatty acids and conjugated linoleic acid (CLA).[2]

And importantly for bones, pasture-raised animals naturally produce vitamin K_2. It is most abundant in organs such as liver, which you may believe you wouldn't wish to eat (though we hope our recipes will change your mind). But organ meats aside for now, enjoy drumsticks, thighs, and eggs from pasture-raised chickens and you'll be giving your body a small supply of that precious K_2, which will help the calcium you consume reach your bones.

Animals kept in confined animal feeding operations (CAFOs) have to endure cramped conditions and are fed what costs the least to fatten them. They are often treated with antibiotics, and we imagine they are miserable. And just as physical and mental stress can harm your health and disrupt your metabolism, it can do the same to livestock.

This is why we encourage you to eat meat, organ meats, and eggs from pastured animals. In life, the animals will be content doing what comes naturally. Their hormones will flow as planned, their bodies have the best chance of being healthy, and the nutrients we need from the foods they produce will be present in a form we can use.

Yes, grass-fed meat and eggs from pastured chickens cost more than the conventional meat and eggs sold in supermarkets. We hope that where possible you will make the effort to save some extra for your meat and eggs so you can buy pasture-raised meat and eggs from pastured chickens. And please avoid bargain meat; it's no bargain for your health.

Milk: Processed Versus Natural

Milk that comes straight from an animal's udder is often called raw milk, but we call it natural milk. That's because natural milk is not processed: not pasteurized (heated to high temperatures), not homogenized (a process of mechanically breaking down fat particles to keep cream from rising to the top), or in any other way altered from its natural state. And when it comes to promoting calcium transport from your blood to your bones, there is a world of difference between the two.

In fact, they are essentially different foods. The enzymes in natural milk help your body break down the milk into its separate elements— proteins, calcium, phosphate, enzymes, and sugars. The enzymes also help the body absorb these components via the gut into the bloodstream and send them to their allocated destinations. With vitamin D present, natural milk is a formidable force for bone health. But when milk, even organic milk, is pasteurized it's a different story. The naturally occurring enzymes perish in the heat, and the milk protein becomes what scientists call denatured—protein that is much less useful to your body. [4]

So natural milk has the minerals, including the calcium, for which it is highly prized, and protein required for life processes in all cells, but processing destroys the enzymes that facilitate mineral absorption and alters the protein on which so many people depend.

This helps to explain the rain of reports that milk does not actually contribute much to strong bones and teeth. The journalists aren't making a distinction between pasteurized and natural milk. Straight-from-the-udder milk has the enzymes and protein that render milk a rich contributor to strong bones and teeth, but high temperatures and artificial processing render those precious resources largely powerless.

We think of unpasteurized milk as natural milk, and we think of pasteurized milk as denatured milk product—and in both cases wish the USDA would do the same.

Although many US states and some other countries prohibit the sale of unpasteurized milk, we would like you to know that Laura advises all her patients to drink unpasteurized milk they obtain from licensed farms, because natural milk appears to make a profound positive difference to bone density. And we would like you to understand the nature of the benefit to bone density in the event you are in a position to obtain natural milk or choose to work for approval of its sale in your home state.

HOW MILK IS DIGESTED

Alkaline phosphatase is a naturally occurring enzyme that helps the body break down many types of molecules. It is present and necessary in all tissues throughout the body, and in bone. It is found to be high during bone formation, and low in postmenopausal osteoporosis. The test used to determine whether milk has been pasteurized is a test for alkaline phosphatase. The enzyme is supposed to be *absent* in pasteurized milk. Thus, it's clear that bone health potential is destroyed in the pasteurization process.

Another important difference between natural milk and the pasteurized product—even if organic—is the shape of the proteins. Your body recognizes proteins, and their function, by shape and the presence of specific protein-degrading enzymes. Pasteurization can alter the shape of the milk protein and inactivate the enzyme that breaks down the milk protein for proper absorption. Heating above 135°F (57°C) destroys lactase, the enzyme in milk that is responsible for the proper breakdown of lactose. Pasteurization of milk is generally carried out between 161 and 300°F (72–149°C). Since lactase is always destroyed by pasteurization, lactose may not be digested properly. People experience this as a lactose intolerance. Please note, some people are intolerant of whey and casein (milk proteins) and are generally advised to avoid dairy.

HOW TO FIND UNPASTEURIZED MILK

In many areas of France, raw milk is dispensed for sale from raw-milk vending machines and much of the cheese sold throughout the country—and in many other European countries—is made from raw milk. The situation is quite different in the United States. In some states you can buy raw milk at the local supermarket; in others, only at a licensed farm. In still others, you must own a share in a cow (see the resources section on page 267) in order to get raw milk, and in some states raw milk is sold only for consumption by pet animals. In addition, especially but not limited to states that forbid the sale of raw milk in retail establishments, cheeses made with raw milk must be aged at least 60 days, and the sale of raw cream and butter is strictly forbidden. So viewed from some perspectives, raw milk is one

way and another widely available—but the subject is inculcated with as much scare-mongering as opponents can muster, availability is uneven, often fraught with restrictions such as those concerning pets, and reports of benefits are subordinate to overblown, exaggerated often unconfirmed reports of illness among people who buy unpasteurized milk from unlicensed, unregulated farms. US cheese masters decry the 60-day age rule that forbids them to make the fabulous Brie, Camembert, and other soft cheeses that are available overseas.

Of course you must purchase natural (raw) milk only from dairies that adhere to mandated, strict-testing protocols. In US states that allow the sale of natural milk for human consumption, the safety testing of the milk is uncompromised, systematic, and rigorous. This helps to explain why the number of illnesses attributable to natural milk is negligible compared with the hundreds of illnesses that result from consumption of everyday foods such as deli meat, chicken, and even spinach.[5] Furthermore people in the tiny-number samples who claim they became ill from unpasteurized milk end up reporting that it was not the milk after all; that they had eaten a contaminated food.

How Plants Influence Health

Plants are among our best friends and most steadfast allies. Flowers and their fragrances inspire us at even the darkest times. Essences and oils calm and relax. Plants produce oxygen that keeps us alive; they make our life easier and more pleasing by serving as dyes for paint, rubber for tires, fibers for clothing, and wood for homes. Herbs and spices contain concentrated amounts of beneficial plant substances that heal even as they enliven meals we prepare. As food, plants can provide complete protein, and variously produce every vitamin and mineral humans need.

Plants are sustenance when we are well and medicine when we are not. Plants and humans are inextricably, synergistically connected and all our lives are possible because of it; better for it.

The particulars of our synergistic ties emerged over time as traditional approaches to diagnosis and treatment illuminated the peaceable as well as the antagonistic properties inherent in plant life. Over millennia rigorous observation and systematic testing documented nutrients, metabolic roles, and toxic and healing properties we could put to use in the enduring search for immortality, or at least good health into old age.

Understanding the connection provides a deep sense of peace, harmony, and well-being. But we get downright excited about the plant–person connection when looking at it through the lens of genetics. A study published in *Genomics* in 2014 reported that snippets of RNA from plants, fungi, and bacteria are present in human blood. RNA molecules play many roles, among them coding and conveying genetic information that influences gene expression. Why does that matter? It provides evidence that plants can have a direct influence on our genes.

Recent research has confirmed this by establishing that what you eat influences gene expression. The scientific term is *epigenetic influence*: influence on top of the inherited genes. What you eat can act as a mechanism affecting whether your genes are turned on or off. We postulate that the regulatory activity of these plant-coded sequences helps damp down the expression of harmful mutation and turns on genes geared toward health. Everyone always told you to eat your veggies. This is why.

Fungi and animals appear to share an evolutionary history that diverged from plants a billion years ago. The genetic similarities may explain why mushrooms and other fungi provide humans such wide-ranging nutritional benefit. For example cordyceps, one of the most widely used mushrooms in medicine, appears to act naturally at the genetic level to slow down cellular response to inflammation.

Plant medicine is one of the oldest and widely used on the planet. Western pharmaceutical medicine began by isolating effective elements from plants, and still does today. We are again looking to plants to help with the growing burden of sickness in the United States, and studies of traditional plant remedies fill journal pages. Our recipes include many plant-based foods and a diversity of fresh herbs and spices.

Plant medicines are often herbs and spices, as these contain higher concentrations of beneficial plant substances. We urge you to find the herbs and spices you like best and cook with them liberally. Most fresh herbs are naturally high in calcium, and offer anti-inflammatory and antioxidant benefits, among others.

As you look through this book, you will see a preponderance of plant recipes and ingredients along with vegetarian/vegan options. This is part of the philosophy of eating not just for bones but for life. There are many meat recipes, too, as we both thoroughly enjoy meat, but the balance we tried to create is the balance we like to use in our own overall approach to eating.

The Danger of Pesticide Residues

The Environmental Working Group has released a list of the foods most likely to be contaminated by pesticide residues (based on tests by the USDA). The foods on this list tested positive for

---

Salt

Salt was once the most highly prized commodity. Roads were built to transport and trade it. At ancient sites, archaeologists have found salt extraction vessels that are more than 8,000 years old. Salt was used to seal agreements and to make covenants with gods. Now people are not quite so sure that salt is a prized commodity. Some studies show—and the US Centers for Disease Control holds—that sodium increases blood pressure; some studies negate that proposition. As usual, it's all about balance.

In the United States hypertension levels are high, and the current advice is to achieve an optimal weight for your frame. We think that's good advice, especially if you eliminate processed foods as part of this regimen. Why? Studies show that when a person increases consumption of natural plant-based foods and cuts back on processed foods, blood pressure levels drop.

It is possible that the problem with sodium is the balance with potassium, rather than the sodium itself. The proper balance of sodium and potassium is fundamental to cell function. That balance allows cells to function like a battery, with different charges inside and out making it possible to transmit signals. Nerve cells communicate this way.

Looking at evolutionary diets, our ancient ancestors probably ingested about 16 times more potassium than sodium. The Standard American Diet clocks in at about 2,500 mg of potassium and 3,600 mg of sodium. The imbalance is clear.

Too much sodium and too little potassium drastically increases your risk for a cardiovascular event. One of the largest American studies to evaluate the relationship of salt, potassium, and heart disease deaths showed that those who ate a lot of salt and very little potassium were more than twice as likely to die from a heart attack.

The bottom line? Cut out the processed foods and enjoy the full taste of fresh foods—with good, natural salt, such as sea salt. The fresh whole foods will provide you with enough potassium as well as other whole-food nutritional benefits.

---

more than 60 chemicals. We believe that all should be organically grown, and then the organic produce should be universally available.

Apples	Lettuce
Celery	Nectarines
Cherries	Peaches
Domestic blueberries	Potatoes
Imported grapes	
Spinach, kale, and	Strawberries
collard greens	Sweet bell peppers

On its website the Environmental Working Group has posted a list of foods that absorb very little pesticide (see the resources section on page 267). This organization has also warned that even washing produce before consuming it reduces but does not eliminate pesticide exposure.

The Downside of Processed Foods

In nature, a food chain is a set of interlinked alliances that rely on complementary nutrients: Flowers need to be pollinated, and so they offer nectar to attract hummingbirds, which pollinate the plants while consuming the nutritious nectar. Alliances like these have been precisely honed over millennia, and even a tiny departure from the natural order can be disruptive. Modern food production relies increasingly on synthesizing. Artificial sweetener comes to mind; so do genetically modified seed and hydrogenated fat. However, the underlying assumption—that what we replicate in the laboratory will function the way it does in nature—is groundless. It turns out that in order to digest food and make best use of it, the body requires the complex chemical mix in food as it grew in nature, consumed intact.

Consider the widely documented effects of consuming refined sugar, high-fructose corn syrup, and hydrogenated fats. Natural sugar in fruits and naturally occurring fats can benefit metabolism and longevity, but process the same raw substances into a form not found in nature and they may cause the likes of insulin intolerance and atherosclerosis.

In that light, contemplate the effects on our bodies of ingesting synthetic pharmaceuticals, pesticides, artificial sweeteners, unnaturally fortified food, and genetically altered food. In these synthesized products, atoms and molecules are combined in new ways that do not exist in nature or are an isolated re-creation of a natural substance. So it is not surprising that even small amounts of synthetic material ingested can cause toxic side effects, disruptive behavior, developmental anomalies, infertility, and birth defects; and it is not surprising that they can interrupt

---

Is Natural Food Affordable?

Do you think that organically grown food plants, natural milk and meat and eggs from pasture-raised animals are probably too expensive as a replacement for conventionally grown and processed food? Before you give up on whole foods, try this experiment. Look at the per-ounce costs of every processed food in the pantry and buy an equal weight of fresh organic vegetables and fruit. You'll probably end up with more than you can consume, plus you'll be substituting available nutrients for depleted ones and perhaps doing away with calcium-leaching chemicals at the same time.

---

and distort the activity of genes and important body functions such as absorption and gut health.

Chemical Changes in Processed Food

There is another very serious concern about processed foods: the change in chemistry when the foods are subjected to high heat. Two potentially detrimental types of chemicals—advanced glycation end products (AGEs) and heterocyclic amines (HCAs)—form naturally when food is cooked dry and at very high heat. Other detrimental end products of some cooking processes include polycyclic aromatic hydrocarbons (PAHs).

AGE

Acrylamide, a chemical used in the manufacture of plastics, is also present in many foods cooked at high temperatures, and it is an AGE, also known as glycotoxin. This is a group of molecules that form when sugar attaches to protein, as when starchy foods such as potatoes and grains, as well as red meats, are cooked in the absence of water at very high temperatures.

According to Professor Helen Vlassara, an AGE researcher from the Mount Sinai School of Medicine, "AGEs are ubiquitous and addictive, since they provide flavour to foods. But they can be controlled through simple methods of cooking, such as keeping the heat down and the water content up in food and by avoiding pre-packaged and fast foods when possible."

AGEs create oxidative stress and inflammation[6] and are implicated in the present epidemic of diabetes and cardiovascular disease.[7] Diabetics then also form AGEs because high blood sugar levels cause sugar to stick to the protein in cell membranes, and it appears that these AGEs cause the side effects of diabetes such as nerve damage, blindness, and kidney damage. AGEs can damage any and every tissue in the body, and modern processed food diets contain very high levels of them. AGEs disturb bone remodeling during aging;[8] this process is accelerated in the presence of diabetes. Lower systemic levels of AGE appear to lower the risk of diseases such as Alzheimer's, kidney, cardiovascular, and diabetes.[9]

The higher the cooking temperature, the more AGEs are formed. They do not form when food is cooked in or with water. Cooking with water prevents sugars from binding to proteins. So steamed and boiled vegetables, whole grains, beans, and fruits cooked with water will not contain significant amounts of advanced glycation end products. This is another reason that a large portion of your fruits, vegetables, whole grains, and beans should be eaten raw or cooked with water. Using an acid such as lemon juice or vinegar (marinating steak, for example) reduces the formation of AGEs.[10]

Acrylamide and AGE levels in starch-based foods cooked at high heat—potato chips, french fries—are considered dangerous. Potato chips contain 500 times the maximum allowable amounts of acrylamide, and french fries contain more than 100 times the maximal allowable amounts. Tortilla chips, breakfast cereals, breads, cookies, crackers, and other bakery products contain smaller but significant amounts of acrylamide/AGEs.

AGEs can be produced during pasteurization, drying, smoking, frying, microwaving, and grilling. Any food that contains sugars, fats, and proteins will produce AGEs under high dry heat.

High-AGE foods. The foods highest in AGES are butter (pasteurized—unknown if unpasteurized), margarine, mayonnaise, meats, processed cream cheese, refined oils (canola, safflower, corn, soybean), and roasted nuts.

Low-AGE foods. The foods lowest in AGE content are fruits, legumes, milk/yogurt products, unprocessed grains, and vegetables (especially with no added fats).

To immediately start consuming 50 percent fewer AGEs, poach, stew, or steam meals. This 50 percent reduction can decrease plasma levels of AGEs by 30 percent within a month. Diets with more raw foods typically contain minimal AGEs, as they are not present in the foods themselves. In addition, raw foods help the body detoxify AGEs that we ingest.

HCAS

HCAs are formed when creatines (a compound that helps supply energy to muscle cells) and amino acids react together with heat. HCAs are genotoxic, causing mutations in DNA that can lead to cancer.

The most concentrated sources include grilled/charred meats and fish. Ready-to-eat commercial breakfast cereals, processed carbs, refined fats/oils, and tobacco smoke also contain high levels. The minimum recommended intake to support the body's fight against cancer development is a ratio of 2:1 plants: meat. The more plants, the less cancer.

PAHS

PAHs include compounds formed by the incomplete burning of organic matter (including foods) at temperatures in excess of 392°F (200°C).

HCAs and PAHs are one of the reasons that in studies by the International Agency for Research on Cancer (IARC),[11] processed and red meats are associated with cancer. Pickled, smoked, barbecued, and processed meats (such as bacon, ham, sausage, hot dogs, salami) seem to be the worst offenders.

With all three of these chemicals, temperature is the most important factor. Problems begin at 212°F (100°C), with highly toxic HCAs forming at about 572°F (300°C).[12] As with AGEs, the advice is to slow-cook, use indirect heat, and use cooking methods with water such as poaching, stewing, braising, or steaming.

USE YOUR JUDGEMENT

Now, a little charred meat or a few roasted nuts seem very unlikely culprits in aging and disease. However, if you examine your diet you may find that with the steak, the breakfast cereal, the Danish, and that deli meat sandwich, you are suddenly overrun with these sly chemicals. Add a little bit of alcohol, some air pollution, and some stress, and suddenly the rising levels of illness seem far less mysterious. I believe these chemicals to be a silent factor in the disease and aging processes.

So as you cook your way to bone health, use your judgment. If your diet is low in processed foods and relatively little of your food is cooked

> ## Plastics, Chemicals, and Hormone Disruption
>
> We note that medical science has acknowledged the detrimental effects of chemicals used in food production. Exposure during the prenatal period can trigger obesity in later years, and some disruptors lead directly to type 2 diabetes. The recommendations are to eliminate as much plastic from your food as possible—don't microwave the food in the plastic wrapper, don't buy water in plastic bottles. Nearly everyone has been exposed to one or more of these chemicals, which include bisphenols (BPA and BPS) found in food-can linings and cash-register receipts, phthalates found in plastics and cosmetics, flame retardants, and pesticides.
>
> A literature review presented recently at the European Association for the Study of Diabetes (EASD) 2015 meeting in Stockholm linked exposure to pesticides to a 60 percent increased risk of type 2 diabetes.

by high heat, go ahead and grill that steak or bake that chicken. If your diet is low in plant-based foods that help detoxify your body, as you begin to move away from processed foods you might want to enjoy stew more often and a more desirable ration of properly prepared plant-based foods to meat.

Things to consider:
- Green tea inhibits the formation of AGEs.[13]
- Microwaving increases AGE content more rapidly than conventional ovens.

- Commercial soft drinks that contain high fructose corn syrup also contain high levels of glycotoxin.

Genetically Modified Ingredients

The evidence we've read about the likely impact of genetically modified food on human health could raise hairs on the back of your neck. While there is almost no research concerning the before-and-after state of humans who have eaten genetically modified food, here's a sampling of research results from animal tests and the impact of genetically modified organisms (GMOs) on the environment—of which the latter is less harrowing at first yet equally destructive and deserving of equal attention and call to action.

A 2009 White Paper by the American Academy of Environmental Medicine reports that "GM foods pose a serious health risk in the areas of toxicology, allergy and immune function, reproductive health and metabolic, physiologic and genetic health and are without benefit" to humans.

Looking across multiple studies, research suggests that the unexpected health risks are those listed by the Center for Food Safety: toxicity, allergic reaction, antibiotic resistance, immunosuppression, cancer, and loss of nutrition.

The American Academy of Environmental Medicine reported in 2009 that health risks associated with genetically modified food consumption included infertility, immune dysregulation, accelerated aging, dysregulation of genes associated with cholesterol synthesis, insulin regulation, cell signaling, and protein formation, along with changes in the liver, kidney, spleen, and gastrointestinal system. They announced their conviction that there is a causal relationship between consumption of genetically modified food and disease. And there are multiple studies showing that the inserted genes can produce allergic response.

Shall we be graphic? Reported in *GMO Myths and Truths* 2012, an evidence-based examination of the claims made for the safety and efficacy of genetically modified crops, "Rats fed Flavr Savr tomatoes developed stomach lesions, mice fed GM soy showed disturbed liver, pancreas and testes function and had abnormally formed cell nuclei and nucleoli in liver cells which indicates potentially altered patterns of gene expression"— which means which genes, including those that protect us from disease, are turned on or off.

The Center for Food Safety says that GM crops "may be the greatest threat to sustainable agriculture on the planet." This center also reports that "a significant percentage of processed foods purchased today contain some genetically engineered (GE) food products. As a result, each day tens of millions of infants, children and adults eat genetically engineered foods without their knowledge." At the time of this writing, the FDA rarely requires safety testing before genetically modified foods go on the market. This despite a 10-year study following three generations of rats fed genetically modified corn, as called Bt corn. The study reported many changes to normal tissue, organ weights, and chemical abnormalities, including infertility.

And what about the presumed benefits of genetically modified crops such as corn and soy as a way to feed hungry and starving populations? These don't pan out. The website Failure to Yield reports that after more than 20 years of research and 13 years of commercial investment, genetic modification of agricultural products has "done little to increase overall crop yields."

In Europe and in some US states genetically modified food and food containing genetically

You Can't Fool Mother Nature

Animals and plants that grow naturally contain a full complement of nutrients required for their own good health. But do we know for a fact that to digest food and make best use of it, the body requires the complex chemical mix in food as in the plant and animal sources of it, consumed intact. Why wouldn't foods re-created exactly in the lab be just as good for us?

Here's one study that demonstrated conclusively—although unintentionally—that the laboratory version of a food doesn't match up to the natural version.[14]

This study dealt with epigenetics, a field within genetics that studies how environment interacts with genes to influence the extent of a gene's activity. In this study, researcher Robert Waterland of Baylor College of Medicine and the USDA/ARS Children's Nutrition Research Center was looking at how a mouse mother's diet affected the weight of her pups.

As part of an experiment concerned with obesity and inheritance, Dr. Waterland tested the epigenetic impact of three diets: a natural diet with naturally occurring methyl donors (chemicals that influence the activity of genes), a synthetic diet with comparable levels of methyl donors, and a synthetic diet without methyl donors. He expected that the methyl-donor-rich synthetic diet would properly activate the genes, as well as the natural diet. But to his surprise it did not. Only the natural diet resulted in normal epigenetic outcomes.

Clearly, mimicking Mother Nature can be tricky.

---

modified ingredients must be labeled. The law is strictly enforced. Whether we can influence the remaining states of the US government to follow suit is another matter entirely.

As we are editing this book the US Food and Drug Administration has approved the introduction of genetically modified salmon for wholesale and retail sale. Many people including Helen have worked locally to promote reflection and extreme caution until systematic research has definitively determined the short-, medium- and long-term effects of genetic manipulation on a natural genome. The best way to keep genetically modified food off your table is: buy products labeled non-GMO, encourage companies selling products that are now routinely genetically modified to label those that contain food from non-GMO seed, and encourage the FDA to require labeling. The non-GMO project (nongmoproject.org) is a nonprofit third-party verification organization that has verified nearly 35,000 products.

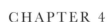

CHAPTER 4

Disarm Anti-Nutrients in Plant-Based Foods

In most plants that people eat—seeds, beans, grains, and greens—one or both of two natural chemicals are present: phytic acid and oxalic acid. Both act against mineral absorption unless you prepare the food in a manner that weakens the chemicals. Looking back in time, even in the 3rd century BCE Egyptians were preparing their plant-based foods for consumption in these ways. At the time bread was a mainstay, and bread was prepared by fermenting the grains; then in the 1st century BCE, yeast came into use. In this chapter we will explain why the Egyptians, as well as most other traditional cultures around the world, prepared their plant-based foods, and how.

Phytic acid locks up phosphorus and other minerals a young seedling will need for germination, but that same action renders the minerals unavailable for human digestion or absorption.

When phytic acid binds with a mineral, the two become a compound called a phytate.

Oxalic acid is a component of leafy plants that binds with calcium and can irritate human tissue. When oxalic acid binds to calcium it forms an insoluble salt called oxalate. When insoluble salts like oxalates become too concentrated, they can form stones, especially in the approximately 20 percent of humans who are genetically disposed to form stones.

Phytic and oxalic acids are called anti-nutrients, so named because each in its own way inhibits mineral absorption from the many and varied plants people eat. Fortunately this anti-nutrient downside to plants as a source of minerals is readily addressed by weakening the acid before consuming the plant.

Lectins are another anti-nutrient found primarily in beans and grains that can trigger the immune system.

Weakening Phytates

Wet, warm conditions signal a seed to germinate and also to release an enzyme, phytase. Phytase uncouples minerals from phytic acid so the seedling can use the minerals as food. If you soak, sprout, or ferment seeds, you create conditions that mimic germination. Then the seed releases phytase, which disengages the minerals and frees them for digestion. The same holds true if you soak whole grains. Phytic acid is stored in the bran and outer skin of grains. If you enjoy whole grains, it is best to soak them before cooking or eating to simulate early germination conditions.

The need to weaken anti-nutrients can't be overstated. Flax, chia, sunflower, and pumpkin are among the seeds people enjoy in part because of their highly touted abundant nutrients. Pulses, some nuts, and beans are also seeds—and all of them contain some level of phytic acid. People who rely on high-cereal diets of unsprouted grains, or who eat diets high in legumes, beans, nuts, and seeds because they are good sources of calcium and other bone health minerals, are actually at risk of deficiency and problems associated

The Anti-Nutrient Wars

The controversy about anti-nutrients, legumes, and grains is not just about chemicals that inhibit mineral absorption. Legumes, which are principally pulses (think lentils) and beans (think black and pinto), are prized for protein. People who decry meat choose legumes in combination with rice and grains to consume the nine essential amino acids (see chapter 3 for more about essential amino acids). People who decry legumes and grains point to the many chemicals in plants that have adverse effects on our bodies: They bind up minerals, create leaky gut, interfere with key hormone receptors, and introduce sometimes high levels of phytoestrogens (chemicals in many plants that in the human body behave in much the same way human estrogen does—a concern we consider in more detail in chapter 7).

Grains provide vitamins, minerals, protein, and protective compounds. People who embrace grains say just sprout them first and enjoy. People who decry grains say humans were never meant to eat them. Nuts are also a subject of scrutiny because they are very high in chemicals that prevent absorption, though mysteriously nuts are allowed, or at least are not prohibited, in the popular primal diets, perhaps because we don't eat so many of them.

Looking back at traditional and ancient diets around the globe, we see in every culture the same food preparation methods. Dozens of legumes are abundant and form a staple diet, especially in regions where money and/or meat aren't plentiful. Peoples from Persia to Nigeria to Peru soak, sprout, and prepare beans and grains before cooking and consuming. These practices arose intuitively, long before scientific testing confirmed their value.

with bone density loss—unless they prepare the foods properly to weaken phytic acid's hold on the minerals. The amount of phytate in a dish or meal is called phytate load.

Oxalic acid kidnaps the calcium in most greens. The amount of this anti-nutrient varies with the vegetable. Oxalic acid ties up about 95 percent of calcium in spinach but much less in kale. Swiss chard, chocolate, beet greens, and tea, widely known as superfoods, are all very high in oxalates, and there is so much oxalic acid in rhubarb leaves it is corrosive, so we treat them as poisonous. Human bodies do manufacture some oxalic acid. It stimulates peristalsis, the action of constriction and release that makes the gut move its contents forward.

Enzymes That Help Weaken Anti-Nutrients

Phytase is principally a plant enzyme. Some bacteria in a healthy human gut produce a tiny quantity of phytase, though not nearly enough to meet the need for weakening anti-nutrients. Interestingly, although high levels of phytates prevent mineral absorption, *small* amounts of phytates in the intestine show a protective effect against tumors. And in case you are wondering about pasture-raised animals, you're right: Ruminant animals, which naturally graze in pastures and fields and enjoy a diet rich in seeds, are favored with resident gut bacteria that do produce phytase copiously. Thus ruminants can eat unsprouted seeds and have immediate access to the minerals they contain.

Soak, Sprout, and Ferment

Whether you plan to prepare and then cook a plant-based food or eat it raw, you can start to disarm the anti-nutrients by soaking and sprouting to release the minerals, or you can disempower the anti-nutrients by fermenting, which means introducing bacteria to help.

When it comes to preparing beans for optimal nutrient release, each type of food requires a slightly different plan. You can soak or soak and sprout seeds and legumes—or soak and ferment beans and grains—to fully optimize nutrition. Processing grains to make them better for digestion and safer for bones is anything but new, though the practices eluded the West for generations as people opted for convenience.

Weakening anti-nutrients by introducing bacteria is a very effective method yet changes the plant's taste. Your preference for method—soak, sprout, or ferment—will develop over time as you experiment with preparing these foods and learn tastes and combinations you most enjoy.

Soaking is simple: Let the food sit in water in a dark place. Sprouting pulses, beans, seeds, and nuts also increases protein and nutrient content and availability, and beneficial plant hormones.

Soaking Beans

A rule of thumb is that 1 cup of dried beans becomes 3 cups of cooked beans. Do not add salt to the soak; it will make the beans tough. You can add lemon juice or whey to the help ferment the beans. Whey is the liquid remaining when you prepare milk for making soymilk (see "How to Make Soymilk" on page 246) or cheese.

For sprouting, use only dried beans. (Canned beans won't sprout.) You will need a stockpot or other large pot and a food thermometer such as a candy thermometer that can measure temperatures in the range of boiling water.

1. Add water to a large pot (at least 3 cups for each cup of dried beans you plan to use).

Bring the water to a boil. Remove the pot from the heat, and add cool water until water cools to 140°F (60°C).

2. Put the beans in a second large pot. Pour the warm water over the beans to cover completely. Add whey or lemon juice—1 tablespoon per 3 cups of water. Set the pot in a warm place and allow the beans to soak at least 18 hours and up to 24 hours. A longer soak releases more minerals from their chemical bonds.

3. As the beans absorb the water, add more warm water as needed to keep the beans covered. You don't have to maintain the 140°F water temperature continuously, but do keep the beans warm.

4. After soaking, pour off the soaking water, rinse the beans with fresh water, and cook them according to your recipe.

Sprouting Beans

Sprouting beans means leaving them in water until a primary shoot appears. (See figures 6 and 7 on page 4 of the color insert.) With the exception of organically grown mung and adzuki beans which you may eat immediately once they sprout, cook sprouted beans before eating them because they will still contain phytic acid and lectins (toxins that can damage the gut lining). It is imperative to cook red kidney beans, as their very high levels of lectins can cause poisoning.

1. Fill a widemouthed glass jar one-third full with dry beans (except mung and adzuki beans: For them, fill only a quarter full).

2. Cover the beans with warm filtered water (you can use cool water, but warming it a bit hastens the sprouting). If you wish, you can add 1 tablespoon whey or lemon juice per quart of water. Fill to top of the jar.

Vitamin C

Vitamin C appears strong enough to overcome phytic acid. In one study,[1] adding 50 mg of vitamin C counteracted the phytic acid load of a meal. In another study, 80 mg of ascorbic acid (vitamin C) counteracted 25 mg of phytic acid.

Consume vitamin C–rich foods with meals that contain phytic acid. Dense sources of vitamin C include guava, bell pepper, kiwi, oranges, grapefruit, strawberries, brussels sprouts, cantaloupe, papaya, broccoli, sweet potato, pineapple, cauliflower, lemon juice, and parsley.

---

3. Place cheesecloth or a small piece of metal mesh screening over the mouth of the jar and secure it in place with a screw-on ring or a rubber band.

4. Allow the seeds to soak overnight, then pour off the water. Rinse well in the jar: Without removing the top, fill with water, swirl gently, then pour out the water through the mesh lid. Repeat twice more.

5. Invert the jar and let it sit at roughly a 45-degree angle so it can drain and also allow air to circulate. For example, you can lean the jar against a cake pan or set it in a dish-draining basket.

6. Rinse the seeds every 6 to 12 hours, per instructions in step 4. The seeds will be ready in 1 to 4 days.

MUNG AND ADZUKI BEANS

Rinse these beans four times each day. Typically the beans sprout in four days. Mung beans are

Mung Beans

The mung bean seems to be a bit of magic—a food-as-medicine exemplar. These tiny beans contain high levels of biologically active proteins, amino acids, oligosaccharides, and polyphenols—a whole food for human host and beneficial gut bacteria. The beans have antioxidant, antimicrobial, anti-inflammatory, and anti-tumor activities as well as anti-diabetic and lipid-lowering properties. Mung beans are one of the strongest cancer-fighting foods on the planet, and are high in vitamins K, C, and B, phosphorus, and iron. Mung beans have been a staple in India for millennia. From there they became known to Southeast Asia, Africa, and China soon after. In Asia people eat sprouted mung beans to protect against cancer. In ancient books, writers celebrated mung beans for their power to detoxify.

ready to cook or eat freshly sprouted when the sprout is 2 inches long. Adzuki beans are ready to cook or eat freshly sprouted when the sprout is about 1 inch long.

To cook the sprouted beans, cover them with water and boil for 5 minutes. Allow to rest for a further 5 minutes in the cooking water; then drain. Boiling does cause the loss of a minute amount of nutrient; however, the amount is insignificant relative to the nutrient cache released by soaking, which remains largely within the bean.

OTHER BEANS

For kidney, lima, and black beans, rinse the beans three to four times each day. These beans are ready for cooking (do not eat them uncooked) when the sprout is ¼ inch long—after about three days of soaking. Boil kidney beans for 10 minutes before lowering the heat. You can also sprout garbanzo beans (chickpeas), then boil them after sprouting. Fava beans are good for sprouting as well. Soak and rinse them for two to four days, until the sprout is ¼ inch long. Cook them before eating. We especially like soup made with sprouted fava beans; see the Sprouted Fava Bean Soup recipe on page 146.

Lentils

To get started, consider how long you will sprout. For cooked recipes, use a shorter sprout (3 days). If you are adding lentil sprouts to a raw recipe, such as a sandwich or a salad, you will want a longer sprout (5 days). To sprout 2 cups of lentils: For a shorter sprout use a standard mason jar; the longer sprout will take a lot of room, so be sure to use a large 1-gallon glass jar or bowl for 2 cups of lentils.

Grains

Souring, or lightly fermenting grains, is the method of choice for making grains safest for bones and overall health and also the method of choice for preparing soybeans (which are a legume, not a grain). To make a traditional ferment, people introduce bacteria to act on the foods. Many Asian ferments use a bacterial culture from mold growing on raw or cooked grains. In some cultures people would chew some raw grain and spit it out into a pot, knowing intuitively that the enzymes and bacteria in saliva would break down the grain during fermentation. Other ferments relied on gathering wild yeast, which were used for local sourdoughs. Most grain ferments take a few days to develop.

In traditional cultures, grains and legumes were often fermented together. In this way, the reduction in phytic acid is much greater—sometimes complete. Indian cooking relies heavily on this principle: The addition of sprouted chickpeas to sprouted grain flour reduces phytic acid 100 percent. Yeast and aspergillus are known to produce phytase, which is why yeast is often used with grains, and aspergillus is the fermentation enzyme used most often in Asian cooking for preparation of beans and grains.

SOAKING AND FERMENTING GRAINS

Traditionally, grains are soaked, ground, and allowed to sour ferment for a period that ranges from 12 hours to several days. If grains and wild yeast are left to sit together, the grains ferment naturally. This symbiotic relationship is greatly beneficial for humans. Fermenting whole-grain flour neutralizes the phytic acid and does such a good job of breaking down the grain itself that many people who suffer from gluten intolerance have no trouble eating sourdough bread with flour that has been prepared in the traditional way with a starter (flour that has been fermented and left to develop in the fridge).

While soaking before cooking reduces toxins and anti-nutrients, grinding and fermenting multiply the benefits many times over. Grinding greatly increases the surface area of the grains and breaks up their cellular structure, releasing enzymes. As for fermenting, which begins when you add a starter, lactic acid bacteria rapidly acidify the batter.

Why is acidifying the batter beneficial? The phytase in the grain is optimally active at a pH of between 4.5 and 5.5, which is mildly acidic. For that reason the Weston Price Foundation recommends soaking grains in an acidic medium before cooking.

Millet, rice, and oats don't contain much phytase, so they require a longer fermentation time or the addition of high-phytase grains. Whole raw buckwheat, wheat, and especially rye contain a large amount of phytase, so when this phytase is activated the grain becomes much more digestible and nutritious.

Fermentation also substantially reduces levels of lectins; cooking reduces the levels even more.

Grains do not contain a full complement of amino acids, so traditional cultures combined grains with legumes to create a complete protein. It is interesting to note that bacterial fermentation produces the amino acid lysine, often increasing its concentration manyfold, increasing the grains contribution toward a complete protein.

Refined grains are neither a natural nor a nutritious food. In the refining process, the bran and germ are removed from the whole grain, which removes the fiber and most of the vitamins and minerals. More and more, producers further refine the grains by bleaching and bromating them. Bromating means adding potassium bromate to flour. This readies the flour for baking much faster than the traditional method, which is exposing flour to oxygen. For more about natural grains and flours, see chapter 22.

Since the early 1990s, when scientists found that potassium bromate caused cancer in animals, the additive has been banned in many countries including many EU countries, Canada, Peru, and China. The FDA has not banned the additive, claiming that most of it degrades to potassium bromide, which has not been shown to cause cancer, so potassium bromate residue may remain. Nevertheless California requires a label on any package of bromated flour warning that the product contains a known carcinogen.

Poorly prepared and over-refined grains with all the vitamins and minerals either removed or constrained provided little of the benefit of the natural properly prepared grain, so after removing the natural goodness companies now enrich their grain products with synthetic vitamins. Go figure.

SPROUTING GRAINS

Traditional grain preparation techniques are similar to bean preparation. You sprout the whole grain then use as is or dry it again in a dehydrator before grinding it into flour. You can then soak milled whole-grain flour in an acidic medium such as buttermilk, whey, yogurt, lemon juice, or vinegar before cooking to further enhance the benefits.

Sprouting grains neutralizes the phytic acid and thereby increases the availability of nutrients. Sprouted wheat contains four times the amount of niacin, nearly twice the amount of vitamin B_6 and folate, five times the amount of vitamin C, and more protein.

A Note on Wheat and Gluten

It isn't unusual or surprising to learn from Americans that they cannot digest wheat at home, yet when they're abroad, eating wheat doesn't bother them at all. US food production has been so severely compromised that many foods, such as wheat, are no longer in harmony with the human body.

There are agricultural and processing practices that we believe explain this US wheat-intolerance phenomenon. Some producers spray a well-known herbicide on the wheat crop just before harvesting. This pesticide forces the wheat to sprout (probably a reaction to the threat of imminent death) and rapidly increases yield. Some food producers use this pesticide-laden wheat in their products, adding extra gluten and preservatives to it as well.

Some wheat producers bleach and bromate flour. The adulterated remains of one or more of these processes become the standard wheat product you find on a supermarket shelf, and the wheat that becomes commercial packaged bread and even freshly baked store bread. Needless to say this poor proxy for wheat, which in natural form has been part of the human diet since Paleolithic times, is no longer tolerated by many human bodies. It is also not surprising that more and more people report gluten intolerance. Some people truly are gluten-intolerant, just as there are always a few people intolerant of practically any natural substance found in food. But we suspect that many who report wheat or gluten intolerance are actually intolerant of or allergic to the toxic chemicals and artificial ingredients that make their way into the grain unannounced and disguised as whole wheat.

When Laura's patients report unpleasant reactions to wheat, she encourages them to sprout organic wheat berries, dry them in a dehydrator or low-temperature oven, and grind them into flour before baking. If their reactions are to the adulterants rather than the wheat itself, this fixes the problem.

Greens for Bone Health

Low-Oxalate Greens

Alfalfa sprouts
Arugula
Bok choy
Broccoli rabe/rapini
Cabbage (napa, purple,
    green, savoy)
Collard greens
Cornsalad
Creasy/American cress
    (boiled)
Dino kale, also called
    lacinato or Tuscan
    kale (boiled)
Lettuce (iceberg, Bibb)
Lettuce (romaine, butter,
    Boston)
Mustard greens (if boiled
    for 5 minutes)
Pea greens
Turnip greens (boiled)

Medium-Oxalate Greens

Belgian endive or chicory
Broccoli (steamed)
Broccoli rabe/rapini
    (steamed)
Brussels sprouts
    (steamed or boiled)
Collard greens
    (boiled or steamed)
Curly kale
Dandelion greens
    (raw or boiled)

Fennel (raw or boiled)
Grape leaves
Green onions (green part)
Mustard greens (steamed)
Shallots
Turnip greens (steamed)
Watercress
    (raw or boiled)

*Greens to Eat
Braised or Steamed*

Belgian endive
    (light heat only)
Bok choy
Broccoli
Broccoli rabe
Brussels sprouts
Cabbages (all types)
Collard greens
Curly kale
Dino kale
Fennel
Mustard greens
Pea greens
Turnip greens
Watercress (light heat only)

Greens to Eat Boiled

Broccoli
Broccoli rabe
Brussels sprouts
Cabbages (all types)
Collard greens
Curly kale

Dandelion greens
Dino kale
Fennel
Mustard greens
Pea greens
Turnip greens
Watercress (in soups)

Greens to Eat Raw

Alfalfa sprouts
American cress
Arugula
Belgian endive
Bok choy
Broccoli
Cabbages (all types)
Curly kale
Dandelion greens
Fennel (leaves especially)
Lettuces (all types)
Watercress

Greens to Ferment

All cabbages
Bok choy
Broccoli
Broccoli rabe/rapini
Collard greens
Dino kale
Fennel (bulb)
Grape leaves
Kohlrabi
Mustard greens
Turnip greens

Managing Oxalic Acid

Like phytic acid, oxalic acid is primed to bind with minerals—or in this case with one mineral, calcium. Once bound, it forms a calcium salt that the body then excretes. To lessen the amount of oxalic acid in greens, you can boil them and pour off the cooking water. As for the other foods that contain oxalic acid, such as beets and buckwheat, you just have to limit the amount of them that you eat.

If you like chocolate, you'll be happy to know that chocolate is a special case. Cocoa beans have one of the highest phytic acid levels in the plant kingdom and also contain oxalic acid—before using them producers ferment cocoa beans that weakens the anti-nutrients.

Some people are intolerant of oxalates. If that's you, good substitutes for spinach are dino kale (cooked), turnip greens (cooked), and romaine lettuce (raw). Refer to the "Greens for Bone Health" sidebar on page 52 for information on natural oxalate levels in greens and the best way to prepare and eat them.

Note that oxalate levels vary depending on how the greens are prepared. For example, boiled mustard greens are low in oxalates, but steamed mustard greens have moderate levels. In the lists, foods are listed in order from those with the highest calcium content to lowest—because for bone health, we want to not only minimize the amount of oxalate, but also make the most of calcium-rich foods. All oxalate values in these lists are from the Autism Oxalate Project or the oxalate testing program[2] lists provided by the Vulvar Pain Foundation, whose work is concerned with women's ailments.

The "Greens for Bone Health" sidebar lists vegetables that are high in minerals and other nutrients required for bone health yet relatively low in oxalates. High-oxalate greens such as spinach, raw dandelion greens, and raw mustard greens do have a high calcium content but have a very low fractional absorption rate.

You may notice that mustard greens appear twice—as low oxalate and medium oxalate. Both are correct; the level of oxalate depends upon how you cook the green—steamed (cooked above the steaming water) or boiled in the water.

Vinegar Wisdom

For thousands of years people have used vinegar to preserve food, maintain health, and enhance food as a condiment. Vinegar contains acetic acid, which helps to release calcium and minerals from leafy greens and promotes mineral absorption.

Vinegar forms in two stages. First it ferments to alcohol, and then—with the help of a collagen-and-bacteria substance called mother, which makes enzymes—the liquid turns to vinegar. Vinegar was reportedly so named by a French winemaker who tasted a brew left too long in the barrel and said, ooh, *vin aigre*—bitter wine.

One of the lost nuggets of healthy-eating wisdom is vinegar on greens. By adding just a small amount (we recommend apple cider vinegar), you can release some of the minerals locked up in leafy greens.

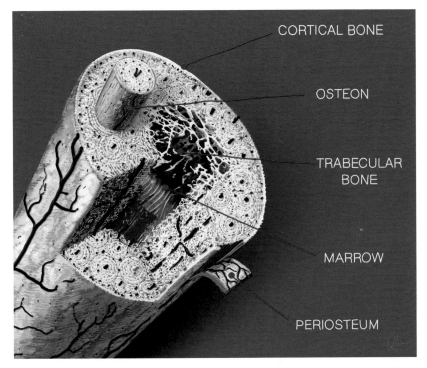

Figure 1. The bone matrix. Trabecular bone is a collagen scaffold dense with calcium phosphate crystals. *Illustration by Daniel Auber*

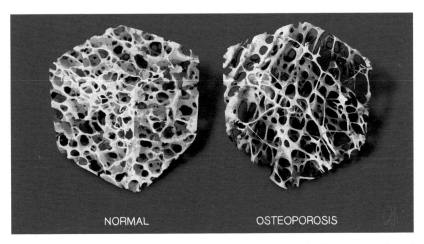

Figure 2. Normal trabecular bone (*left*) has a dense network of collagen strengthened by thick layers of mineral deposits. The collagen scaffold is irregular—thereby allowing the bone to resist impact from every possible angle. Osteoporotic bone (*right*) has lost much of the mineral deposits and scaffolds have become weak. As they weaken, so does the ability of bone to withstand impact. *Illustration by Daniel Auber*

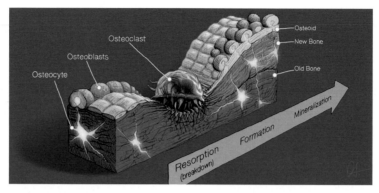

Figure 3. The process of bone remodeling happens in stages. The osteoclasts break down bone, then the osteoblasts secrete the collagen matrix called osteoid. Last, the osteoclasts mineralize the matrix, forming the hydroxyapatite and cementing it into the osteoid. Osteocytes communicate information about stress on the bone, signaling the breakdown or formation of bone. *Illustration by Daniel Auber*

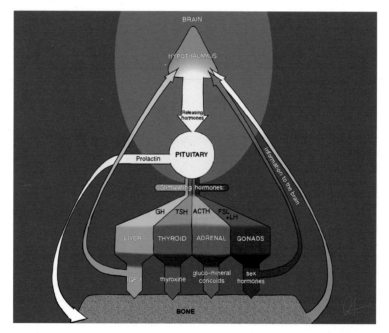

Figure 4. The brain signals the release of hormones that interact with bone. The hypothalamus releases signals that tell the pituitary to produce hormones to stimulate either bone growth or bone breakdown, depending on what information is being fed back to the brain from the body. Growth hormone stimulates bone formation, as does IGF-1; sex hormones stimulate bone growth and inhibit bone breakdown. Thyroid and adrenal hormones also affect bone turnover. Prolactin enhances the entire process of bone turnover. *Illustration by Daniel Auber*

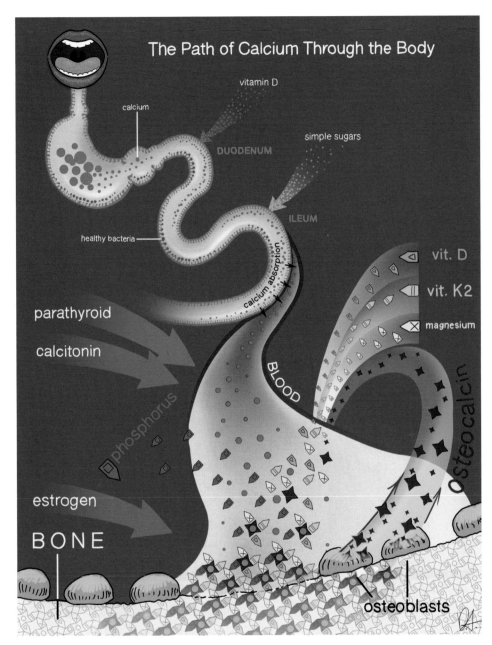

Figure 5. Calcium absorption in the duodenum requires the presence of vitamin D_3. Vitamin D is not required in the ileum, although absorption is increased if there is a simple sugar present. After that, hormones regulate the path of calcium through the body. Osteocalcin, a hormone produced by osteoblasts, helps to move absorbed calcium into bone instead of into soft tissue. Osteocalcin is activated in the presence of vitamin D_3, vitamin K_2, and magnesium. PTH and calcitonin regulate the larger scope of calcium in the blood. Estrogen helps regulate the osteoblasts and osteoclasts. *Illustration by Daniel Auber*

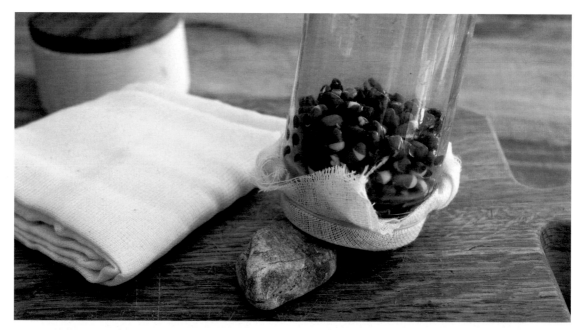

Figure 6. Sprouting pulses, beans, seeds, and nuts increases protein and nutrient content and availability. For instructions, see "Sprouting Beans" on page 48.

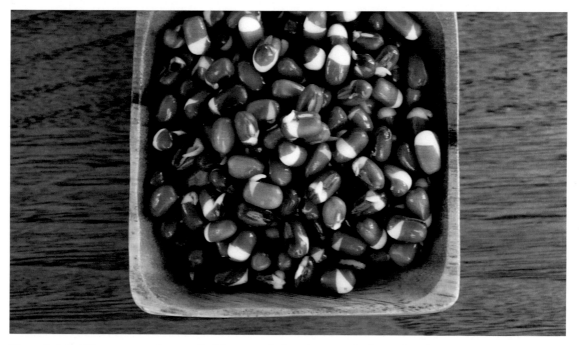

Figure 7. Adzuki beans are ready to eat freshly sprouted when the sprout is about 1 inch long.

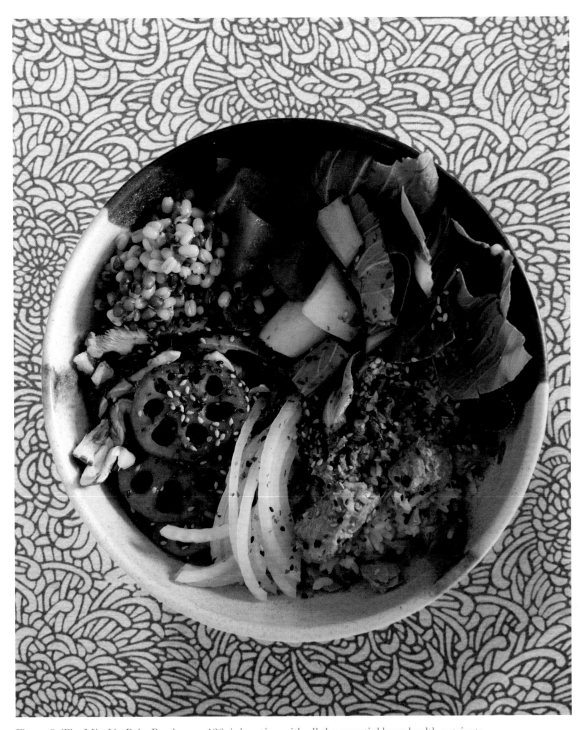

Figure 8. The Mix-Up Poke Bowl, page 126, is bursting with all the essential bone health nutrients.

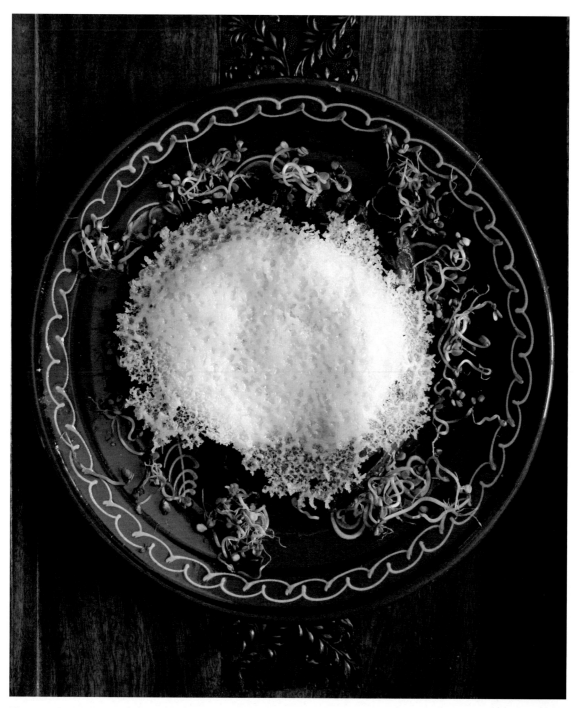

Figure 9. Upside-Down Savoyarde Eggs, page 138, are a great start to the day with key nutrients for proper calcium transport.

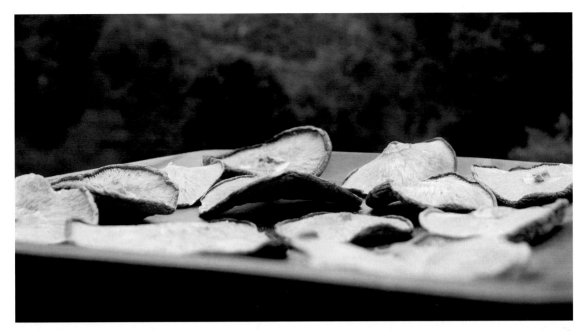

Figure 10. Sunned mushrooms produce prodigious vitamin D, which can supplement natural sources. For instructions, see "Sunning Mushrooms" on page 129.

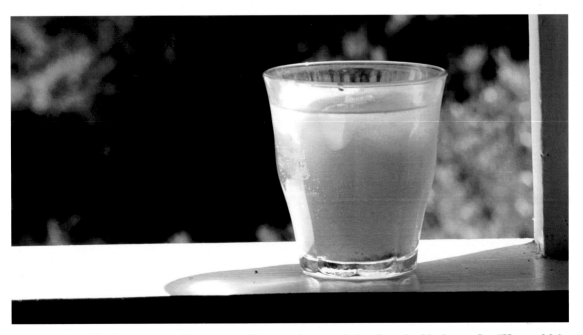

Figure 11. Bone shrubs are an excellent source of base nutrients needed to foster healthy bones. See "How to Make Shrub" on page 131.

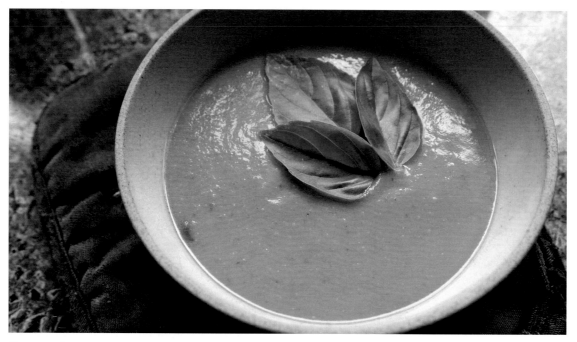

Figure 12. Butternut Squash and Natto Powder Soup, page 145.

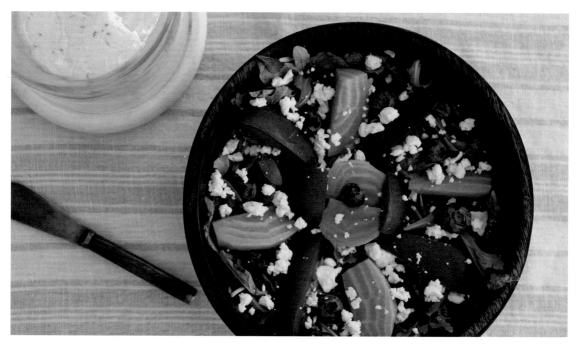

Figure 13. Colorful Arugula Salad with Fresh Lemon Dressing, page 151.

CHAPTER 5

Gut Bugs Can Be a Bone's Best Friends

Ailing gut (gut dysbiosis) is on the rise in the United States. According to the National Institute of Health, nearly one-third of the population has a digestive complaint. In a healthy gut, the lining of the intestine is intact, food is digested efficiently, and the vitamins and minerals in the food you eat can be absorbed properly into the bloodstream. A compromised gut has a pitted lining or even leaks as the junctions between the cells loosen. Molecules that are not supposed to pass can pass through the lining, foods don't get properly broken down, and vitamins and minerals may not get absorbed. Where you are in the continuum from healthy to unhealthy gut turns on the relative health of your gut bacteria. Healthy gut bugs ferment foods and produce compounds that keep the intestinal lining intact and healthy, produce hormones, and play a huge part in immunity. And all of this has implications for bone health.

Gut bugs are part of the total microorganism population that inhabits your body's skin, mouth, gut, organs, and individual cells. Together, these bacteria, fungi, and archaea (organisms that have no nuclei) number about 100 trillion, which is 10 times the number of a human body's cells. Most of these organisms are part of the bacterial colony (which scientists call the gut flora) in the long, winding gut. Lately they've (justifiably) enjoyed a lot of press because they influence illness, recovery, inflammation, and longevity.

In fact they play such an important role that doctors have begun to treat some gut illness with fecal transplants from healthy donors. Meanwhile geneticists have mapped the genome of many species of bacteria that come and go in the gut flora, and nutritionists are working hard to learn what foods influence desirable colonies.

But don't forget: This invisible teeming microenvironment, a powerful force for good or ill,

> ## Important Actions of Good Gut Bacteria
>
> The beneficial bacteria in the gut serve many functions. These bacteria:
>
> - Synthesize vitamins so they can be utilized properly by the body.
> - Change which genes are active in gut cells.
> - Keep harmful bacteria from spreading in the body.
> - Help prevent infections.
> - Help digest food efficiently.
> - May help prevent colon cancer.

needs to eat. And what your gut bugs eat determines their own health outcomes.

Gut Bugs, Prebiotics, and Probiotics

We can promote the health of our gut bacteria in two ways: by feeding them what they need in order to reproduce normally and thrive; and by introducing other bacteria that enrich the environment for the indigenous populations.

Prebiotics

Prebiotics are preeminent among foods that nourish lower-gut bacteria, which in turn can positively influence calcium absorption. Prebiotics are carbohydrates that humans can't digest but specific populations of highly beneficial resident gut bacteria can. Prebiotics remain in the gut after the foods that contain them are digested, yet they almost certainly do not raise blood sugar. Because healthy gut bugs are central to human health, we advise consuming prebiotics daily. The largest group of prebiotics are called oligosaccharides, and within the oligosaccharides, oligofructose and inulin are the most studied. Scientists across many disciplines are working to identify even more prebiotic sources.

These foods contain prebiotics:[1]

Artichokes
Asparagus
Bananas
Beer (unpasteurized)
Chocolate
Cold cooked rice
Dark, leafy vegetables such as
    spinach and kale
Garlic
Honey
Jicama
Leeks
Legumes, such as red kidney beans
    and lentils, sprouted and/or soaked
Maple syrup
Onions
Red wine
Tomatoes
Whole grains, fermented and/or
    sprouted (barley, rye, oats,
    flaxseed, and other grains)

Here's how that works. Feeding the good bacteria with prebiotics positively affects mineral absorption. When the healthy bacteria are fed properly, bacterial production of short-chain fatty acids (acetate, propionate, and butyrate) increases. Short-chain fatty acids (SCFAs) are the great benefit of healthy gut bacteria—and even in the presence of antibiotics, they assist in all aspects of healthy gut function, stabilizing the intestinal flora and ecology. Butyrate specifically nourishes all layers of the gut lining, thereby expanding the population of healthy flora and creating a more stable, more robust absorption surface. A well-fed healthier gut population degrades phytic acid—which has the effect of improving the release of minerals from plant-based food we consume, and therefore our ability to absorb them.

Most directly, however, the short-chain fatty acids increase the presence of proteins, called calbindins, that are necessary for calcium absorption. Without calbindins we would have a hard time absorbing the calcium even in the presence of vitamin D.

Short-chain fatty acids also help in bone stability by facilitating and increasing the release of bone-modulating factors such as phytoestrogens from foods (see "What About Phytoestrogens" on page 75).

Probiotics

Probiotics are bacteria that coexist with humans or that you consume through fermented food or in supplements. These bacteria do not naturally grow in the human gut, but their presence helps to improve the environment for the locals. They beef up the numbers of good bugs, help with digestion, and help to destroy pathogens. Probiotics, like those in yogurt, don't live permanently in the human gut;[2] you have to eat them every day. However, if you eat them regularly, they do provide a good environment in which your own human-derived bacteria can thrive.

Fermented foods have been making news for very good reason: They boost the number of probiotic bacteria available to join indigenous gut populations in maintaining human health.

Fermenting foods mimics the process of digestion that takes place naturally when the gut bacterial community—known as the biome—enjoys optimal health.

To ferment, you set bacteria to the job of transforming carbohydrates or sugars to alcohol and on to organic acids. Think apples to apple cider to apple cider vinegar. Think yogurt, a cultured milk. Or soak grains overnight, or set freshly made butter on the counter, exposed, overnight. Bacteria begin to break down the food to create a culture, and when we eat it the culture acts as a probiotic.

Consuming raw fermented food provides bacterial reinforcements that improve your gut's ability to manage the many and varied functions it performs.

These fermented foods contain good quantities of probiotics

(listed beginning with those most likely to be familiar as sources of beneficial bacteria):

Yogurt, provided it contains live, active cultures (read the label to be sure)

Buttermilk, uncooked only

Sourdough bread

Soft cheese, either aged or containing raw (unpasteurized) milk

Cultured butter and cultured cottage cheese

Miso (a Japanese paste of fermented soybeans)

Kombucha (a fermented tea-type drink made from a mushroom starter)

Tempeh (an Indonesian fermented soybean patty)

Sauerkraut, labeled as containing live cultures and not pasteurized (read the label)

Kimchi (a Korean dish of fermented and pickled cabbage)

Pickles

Food Combining

Daniel P. Reid has studied and written extensively about Traditional Chinese Medicine and ancient Taoist approaches to health. The following information is adapted from his book *The Tao of Health, Sex, and Longevity*.

The classic Western dinner is meat, potato, and veg—protein, carb, and plant. Dietary recommendations support that tradition, but is that a good plan for digestion and nutrition? In other words, does it matter which foods or food groups you eat together?

It does. Each food type stimulates only one digestive enzyme. If it's a free-for-all with digestive enzymes competing for energy and space, you compromise optimal digestion. Here's a bit of the background on food combining and enzymes. It's a complex story. We do not spare the science. We do include some practical suggestions for ideal combinations.

Protein is digested only with the secretion of pepsin, and pepsin can only fully digest the protein in an acidic environment. But carbohydrates/starches require ptyalin and other *alkaline* secretions, which begin in the mouth, and require an alkaline environment to fully digest. So eating potato with meat means that acid and alkaline substances are secreted simultaneously, each weakening the other's ability to do its job. Lack of complete digestion allows the food to sit in the gut. So ideally, you should consume protein and starch separately.

Although you would think acidic foods would go well with protein, acidic foods also inhibit the proper digestion of protein. That's because highly acidic foods will inhibit the secretion of hydrochloric acid (stomach acid), thereby slowing down protein digestion. Starches and acids also do not combine well, as the starches' digestion begins in the mouth—the presence of acid will inhibit the salivary secretion, and the starch will get to the stomach without the important initial digestive enzymes from the mouth.

Fat is said to inhibit the secretion of gastric juices, delaying digestion of protein. Eat a lot of raw vegetables with a fatty steak; that will help.

Sugars also inhibit gastric secretions. They digest in the small intestine, not in the mouth or stomach. Eat sugar with other foods and you can trap the whole lot in the stomach, where it sits and ferments.

The takeaway, for starters, is that all foods go better with raw and fermented vegetables, as the intact enzymes in raw vegetables help everything digest well. So if you have a steak for dinner, have an arugula salad with it—and save the potato for the next day's lunch.

If foods rich in probiotics are not readily available, you may wish to consider probiotic supplementation. You will certainly wish to consider probiotic supplementation if you have taken a course of antibiotics to combat infection, because the antibiotics will kill many among your beneficial gut bugs. As always when considering supplements, speak with your healthcare provider.

Ferment Vegetables for Bone and Gut Health

Almost any raw vegetable—carrots, cucumbers, peppers, cabbage—can easily be turned into a natural probiotic. To keep your gut flora healthy and fighting fit, eat fermented vegetables several times a week at least. To ferment, a food sits in a liquid—it may be water or a culture like buttermilk or whey left over from making soymilk—until the bacteria that naturally reside on the surfaces of the food digest some of the sugars. Along the way nutrients are released and pectin hardens, which leaves the vegetable crisp and the liquid rich with welcome nutrients and bacteria friendly to your gut. The fermentation process weakens phytic acid in the vegetable, so minerals and trace elements are readily absorbed. Another word for "fermented" is *cultured*. Both mean that bacteria act on the original substance.

You are probably familiar with pickles and sauerkraut—American as baseball and backyard barbecue. If you've been to Britain you'll know that pickled onions accompany many a sandwich. In Korea, kimchi—fermented napa cabbage or daikon radish—is traditional as a part of lunch or dinner. In the springtime, people ferment garlic scapes in black peppercorns and dill. Throughout traditional diets, fermented foods play a part, daily.

It's possible to ferment just about any raw vegetable, as well as hard-cooked eggs, fish (think pickled herring with onions or sour cream), garbanzo beans, and grains. There are two popular methods: in salt (which makes a brine), or with starter.

The simple way to ferment a vegetable is to fully submerge it in a salt solution—brine. Before refrigeration, preserving food in brine was common. It is reliable because in the presence of salt, bacteria that naturally live on the surface of vegetables thrive, but pathogens and mold die off.

Adding a Starter Culture

If you want to speed up fermentation, add bacteria—in the form of a bacterial starter—to the brine. For quick ferments aiming to break down phytic acids and activate phytase in order to release nutrients, starters are the key. Some people use whey and some use bacteria specific to soil. The resulting tastes are different, so it is a matter of trial and error to find the method you like best.

WHEY

Whey is a starter commonly used for lactobacillus fermentation. Whey is the liquid that remains after you add an acid medium to milk to make yogurt. The acid makes the milk curdle, which leaves curd (solid) and whey (remaining liquid). Another type of whey is the liquid that remains after you coagulate soymilk to obtain curd for making tofu or fermented bean curd dishes such as natto or tempeh.

Whichever is your whey of choice, strain it and keep it very fresh in a cold fridge until you add it to the vegetables, or you will taste the whey flavor in your fermented product. Adding a pinch of salt along with whey helps with flavor.

You can make your own whey (see "How to Make Soymilk" on page 246), or you can find whey (and a host of other starter cultures) at Cultures for Health (culturesforhealth.com).

SOIL-BASED STARTER

The strain of lactobacillus involved in whey or other dairy ferments breaks down milk and dairy products. However, because vegetables' properties are different from those of dairy foods, some say it makes more sense to use soil-based bacteria to ferment vegetables.

Here is a list of soil-based bacteria used in starters for fermented foods:[3]

Lactobacillus brevis
Lactobacillus plantarum
Leuconostoc mesenteroides
Pediococcus acidilactici

These bacteria naturally exist symbiotically with organically grown vegetables. Cultures for Health (see resources, page 267) has done solid research on pairing vegetables with the most appropriate bacteria. The company sells a vegetable ferment starter kit we like.

When it comes to taste, timing, and vegetable texture, experiment to find the starter you like best. You'll find our basic recipe for Fermented Vegetables on page 236.

Gut Bacteria Communicate with the Brain

Collectively, the thousands of gut microorganism species are nothing less than the first-line defenders of health and well-being. Their principal jobs are maintaining immunity, protecting intestinal wall integrity—the barrier between the external environment and the body's interior—and managing digestion and absorption. Successful execution of these jobs spins off into defense against pathogens, maintenance of healthy brain and organ system function, and feelings of well-being. Disrupted gut health shows correlations with all major chronic illnesses, and scientists are illuminating the details on a daily basis.

For instance, it is established that gut bacteria both produce and respond to the same neurochemicals that the brain uses to regulate mood and cognition. Such neurochemicals—including serotonin and melatonin—probably allow the brain to attune its behavior to the feedback it receives from the army of bacteria in the gut. An example? The gut produces much more serotonin than the brain—about 95 percent of the body's production. Serotonin can influence mood, appetite, memory, sleep, and possibly sexual desire. This is one reason why a healthy gut has such a positive effect on mood.

Gut bacteria appear to communicate with the brain via the vagus nerve. This may seem surprising because most people think of nerves as simple instruments of signal relay. But the vagus nerve, a cranial nerve bundle (it originates in the brain), plays a part in many aspects of health including but not limited to inflammation, breathing, heart rhythm, and memory making.

Animal studies show that tweaking the balance of beneficial and disease-causing bacteria in the gut can alter brain chemistry and increase boldness or anxiety. The brain can exert a powerful influence on gut bacteria. Even mild stress can tip the microbial balance in the gut, making the host more vulnerable to infectious disease and triggering a cascade of molecular reactions that feed back to the central nervous system. The presence of the healthy bacteria and their by-products of digestion helps promote positive genetic response—turning on beneficial genes and turning off detrimental ones.

Unfortunately pesticides, air pollution, pharmaceuticals, processed foods, preservatives and dyes, the chemicals produced by stressed animals, heavy metals in water, and other unnatural substances that enter a gut divert bacterial resources to damage control. These unnatural substances sometimes so overwhelm the bacterial populations that they cannot effectively eliminate toxins and pathogens and keep the gut wall intact.

Biotics and Diversity

In nature, a key to strength is diversity. Diversity of gut bugs appears to correlate closely with health. The more varied and diverse species of healthy bacteria lining and working in your gut, the better protected you are from disease, the better you are at digesting your food and the more successful you are at making the molecules you need to keep your body running.

Equally important is a plentiful population of each type of beneficial bug. An ailing population will have a hard time producing enough of the key short-chain fatty acids that your gut needs to perform its functions as a barrier and as an ab-, sorptive surface, even if you feed them properly.

Many of us Americans are impaired or even severely impaired in gut bug diversity and population, and this state is no doubt related to the terrifying rise in the incidence of chronic disease. Luckily it is possible to rebuild the population—and this is where probiotics and prebiotics come into play. Many of the recipes in this book contain *synbiotics*, which are foods that contain both probiotics and prebiotics. Such powerhouse foods provide both the beneficial bacteria themselves and the food they need to sustain themselves within our guts. We also note that although it contains no probiotics, bone broth is one of the most potent remedies we can prepare to heal an ailing gut. See "Bone Broth" on page 141.

It's beyond the scope of this book to provide in-depth information on gut health—we've provided only an introduction here, because gut health is the foundation on which you can then build bone health. To learn more about gut health, we recommend *Gut and Psychology Syndrome* by Natasha Campbell-McBride and *The Heal Your Gut Cookbook* by Hilary Boynton and Mary Brackett.

CHAPTER 6

Considering Supplements

When we started developing bone health recipes, we didn't have a cookbook in mind. But the more we learned, the more we realized that no single nutrient or supplement could ensure healthy bones and that some artificial interventions such as some prescription drugs could provide short-term solutions but could have potentially deleterious longer-term consequences. So we proceeded apace developing recipes that would provide nutrients in the right setting and combinations for ongoing bone mineralization.

The National Health and Nutrition Examination Survey (NHANES) is data collected by the government reporting on nutrition in the United States. The Environmental Working Group (EWG), a non-profit organization dedicated to helping people live healthier lives, interpreted the NHANES data. It seemed imperative, especially in light of the 2011 NHANES data (the most recent available), which shows that in our land of plenty, deficiency is rife: 95 percent of us over the age 19 are deficient in vitamin D; 61 percent are

deficient in magnesium; 49 percent in calcium; and 43 percent in vitamin C.

From the EWG report:

Some American adults get too little vitamin D, vitamin E, magnesium, calcium, vitamin A and vitamin C. More than 40 percent of adults have dietary intakes of vitamin A, C, D and E, calcium and magnesium below the average requirement.

Some Americans get too much Vitamin A while others get too little. On one side, more than half of American adults and American teenagers have low dietary vitamin A intake. On the other side, at least 13 percent of children 8 and younger ingest vitamin A in amounts exceeding the tolerable upper intake level set by the Institute of Medicine.

We note that the NHANES data includes neither vitamin K₂ nor trace minerals though both are key to bone health.

The US Dietary Guidelines Advisory Committee (DGAC) also interpreted the NHANES data and found that independent of where the food is prepared or obtained, overall the US diet does not meet recommendations for fruit, vegetables, dairy, or whole grains, yet does exceed recommendations, leading to overconsumption, for sodium and saturated fat as well as refined grains, solid fats, and added sugars.[1]

A key piece of the bone health puzzle is nutrient levels—in other words, what nutrients are present in your body and in what amounts. It is important to know what nutrients you have in good supply and what you are lacking, and it is important to make sure you are eating and/or supplementing to meet the requirements for healthy bone growth.

In the course of researching the ideal nutrient levels for bone health, we found that our recommendations often differed from those of the Dietary Guidelines Advisory Committee. On page 65 we provide the committee recommendations from 2016 for a female 51 years old or older, and then ours, complete with research. This RDA information could form a starting point for a conversation with your healthcare provider.

The Recommended Dietary Allowances (RDAs)

The United States RDAs were initially computed during World War II in order to keep armed forces, and civilians, from deficiency. These are not necessarily optimal levels; they do not reflect intakes known to reduce or prevent chronic illness. Unfortunately it is often assumed that these are the gold standard for health and the upper safe levels of intake. This does not appear to be the case.

Additionally, standards for nutrient intake can vary significantly by country. The EU's

> ### The Epidemic of Chronic Disease
>
> As this book went to print, the 2015–2020 US Government dietary guidelines were released. Here is the second sentence: "Today, about half of all American adults—117 million people—have one or more preventable, chronic diseases, many of which are related to poor quality eating patterns and physical inactivity." The Committee lists poor bone health among the top five chronic conditions facing the United States. The guidelines focus on the idea that nutrition and health are intimately related, and the easiest way to address the epidemic of chronic illness in the United States is through changing dietary eating patterns.

recommended daily allowance for calcium is 800 mg per day. The UK's is 700 mg a day; Japan's, 600 mg a day; and India's, also 600 mg a day.[2]

Ratios, Not Measures

Our nutrient intake recommendations differ from those of the dietary committee, because research for the prevention of disease is showing that optimal levels are often higher than those the committee prescribes. Also, for some nutrients, we offer a range of values rather than a set amount, because the concept of ratio is so important. For example, if you take a calcium supplement and your dietary calcium is 1,200 mg or even higher, you will need to have higher amounts of vitamin K_2. Calcium is proportionally the largest

2015 Recommended RDAs from the Dietary Guidelines Advisory Committee	Our Nutrient Intake Recommendations
Calcium: 1,200 mg	Calcium: 800–1,000 mg[3]
Vitamin D_3: 600 iu	Vitamin D_3: 5,000 iu[4]
Magnesium: 320 mg	Magnesium: 600–1,000 mg[5]
Phosphorus: 700 mg	Phosphorus: 700–1,000 mg
Protein: 46 g	Vitamin K_2: 80–300 mcg[6]
Vitamin A: 700 mg	Protein: 50–150 g[7]
Vitamin C: 75 mg	Vitamin A (retinol): 10,000–15,000 iu
Zinc: 8 mg	Vitamin C: 400–600 mg[8]
Copper: 900 mcg	Zinc: ≥10 mg
Manganese: 1.8 mg	Copper: ≥2.5 mg
	Silicon: ≥40 mg
	Boron: ≥3 mg
	Manganese: ≥2 mg
	Strontium: <5 mg
	Phytoestrogen: ≥50 mg

component of bone matrix—but as discussed in chapter 1, it is very important to understand the results of too much supplementation. It is also important to note the calcium-to-magnesium ratio. There is increasing evidence suggesting that magnesium intake should potentially be equal to or possibly even higher than calcium. Data about diets in countries with traditionally low osteoporosis rates may support this idea, and updates will be posted on the Medicine Through Food website. Also, note that ideal protein intake can vary enormously depending on your age, your weight, and how active you are. Assuming that you exercise regularly for at least 40 minutes at a stretch and vigorously enough to work up a sweat, Laura recommends more protein rather than less—at least 25 percent of your calories from protein—in order to build muscle and bone.

These recommendations apply only if you are getting the proper balance of all nutrients. For example, some people will experience vitamin D toxicity when taking 2,000 iu per day of vitamin D if their magnesium and vitamin A intakes are too low. On the flip side, too much vitamin A without the right levels of vitamin D can result in increased risk of hip fracture. These recommendations also do not include therapeutic doses, which could be recommended by your healthcare provider if you are found to be deficient in any nutrient. It's important to consult a healthcare provider to determine your baseline levels and together work out a plan that's right for you.

> ## The Vitamin Answer to the Common Cold?
>
> In a 1941 study, Irwin G. Spiesman, an MD who had reviewed early literature on the beneficial effects of cod liver oil and specifically on the concurrent administration of vitamins A and D in higher-than-usual doses, decided to systematically test the impact of high vitamin A with high vitamin D to see if either substance, or the combination, could prevent the common cold. The combination proved effective, and only the combination prevented toxicity of the other. The ratios are all-important.

Supplementing Your Diet

The basic nutrient content of what you eat is only one part of the digestion/absorption/nourishment equation; the other is balance and ratio.

As we explained in chapter 5, if the gut microflora are in balance and the gut lining is healthy, when you eat whole food you absorb the nutrients properly. But across the board whole foods are not regularly a lifestyle choice; fads bait people with watered-down, misleading, and often incorrect information about nutrition; and processed foods are a tempting convenience. Thus many people end up out of nutritional balance. Although relying on whole foods is ultimately the goal if possible, along the way many people need assistance from supplements—especially those who are deeply deficient to begin with.

A first step in assessing your need for vitamin and/or mineral supplementation could be speaking with your doctor or health provider about a nutrition evaluation.

A nutrition evaluation reports information about the levels of vitamins in your body. It does not specifically reveal the status of your bone health; rather it offers you and your healthcare provider a high-level look at how well your body is absorbing nutrients. This laboratory test, along with the worksheets you'll fill out as part of creating a Personal Nutrition Plan (see chapter 9), provides a rich picture suggesting needs for changes to diet and possibly supplementation. The test is ordinarily ordered by a healthcare provider, and so a nutrition evaluation is a great way to start the conversation about diet as a way to protect your bone (and overall) health.

Supplements Can Serve Two Purposes

Supplements can be a top-up when you don't or can't consume recommended daily amounts of vitamins, minerals, enzymes, and other substances for gut health that in concert foster mineral absorption, transport, and deposition in the bone. For example, if you do not want to consume natto or eggs from pastured chickens, which are the traditional sources of vitamin K_2, you might prefer to take K_2 in pill form to supplement the K_2 in the Gouda cheese and dark-meat pasture-raised poultry that you eat.

The second purpose of supplements is to be therapeutic—to correct a deficiency. If you are vitamin D–deficient, your doctor might recommend a very high dose for a short time period. If you have osteoporosis, your doctor may prescribe a therapeutic dose of vitamin K_2 drops. Although therapeutic doses of vitamin D and K_2 have been researched and appear to be safe as well as useful in bone and cardiovascular health, therapeutic supplementation should always be prescribed by a qualified healthcare practitioner.

Generally, the most effective supplements are natural, not synthetic; that is, derived from whole food and not from the chemistry lab. Here is some general information about supplementing key nutrients for bone health.

Supplemental Calcium: Start Slowly, Be Cautious

The idea that calcium supplementation could magically fix bone loss became popular in medical circles first and then became an overnight consumer marketing success. However, worrisome studies show that taking high levels of calcium puts a person at risk of higher all-cause and cardiovascular death rates (except deaths from stroke). In one study[9] the association of calcium intake and all-cause and cardiovascular mortality was especially strong when the study participant had a high level of calcium from diet combined with calcium supplementation. In this study there was no mention of vitamin D, vitamin K_2, or other minerals, nutrients, or trace elements.

The highest death rate was among women who have sufficient calcium in the diet and on top of that take supplements. Too much of a good thing can be dangerous, so the saying goes, and it is certainly apt here. There is no such thing as a magic pill for bone health.

The highest intakes of calcium (more than 1,400 mg per day) were associated with higher all-cause risk for death (after adjustment for age, total energy, vitamin D, and calcium supplement intake, as well as other dietary, physical, and demographic factors) as compared with intakes of 600 to 1,000 mg a day, and women with the highest intake of calcium (more than 1,400 mg per day) and who used supplement tablets had an all-cause risk for death 2.5 times higher than women who had similar total intakes but were not taking a supplement.

The study authors explain that serum calcium levels "are under tight homeostatic control" and do not normally correlate with the amount of calcium intake. However, low or very high intakes override this control.

MILK ALKALI SYNDROME

Milk alkali syndrome, a side effect of consuming too much calcium, is reappearing these days with unfortunate consequences.

Recently a patient told Laura she was afraid to take vitamin D with calcium. That seemed odd, because it's widely advertised, rightly so, that vitamin D promotes calcium absorption in the gut and helps the body keep calcium and phosphate available for bone mineralization. Then she told Laura that her grandfather had suffered from ulcers and doctors had warned him off calcium and vitamin D.

Hearing that, her worry suddenly made sense. One of the now discarded treatments for ulcers was milk and cream mixed with sodium bicarbonate that would neutralize stomach acid and protect the stomach. Unfortunately some patients who followed this treatment developed a life-threatening condition called milk alkali syndrome, which is characterized by high blood calcium, high blood pH, kidney dysfunction, and calcifications of the cornea, lung, and lymph nodes. Someone with this bit of family history might easily fear that vitamin D would promote too much calcium absorption.

This ulcer treatment was left behind but the syndrome is reappearing, largely because people are taking more calcium than the body can process at one time, and they are not taking it with the nutrients that prepare calcium for transport to bone. The excess calcium is excreted or deposited to joints or vessels or—in extreme cases—to additional sites like the eye and lung.

Many people are advised to take calcium supplements but are not advised that a human body cannot process more than 500 mg of calcium at any one time. Also, they are not told that they need the supporting cast of critical nutrients we talk about so prominently in this book in order for their bodies to use the calcium properly. One of Helen's doctors advised her to just pop some Tums—a highly processed calcium carbonate acid indigestion remedy. But taking Tums combined with calcium supplements combined with vitamin D–assisted absorption can send the body's calcium load sky-high.

People who consume more than 2,000 mg per day of elemental calcium and who combine high-dose calcium with vitamin D to increase its absorption are those most at risk of milk alkali syndrome.

Note: With the addition of vitamin K_2, the aberrant calcifications would be inhibited, and so milk alkali syndrome would most likely also be inhibited.

HOW TO TAKE CALCIUM

The body's inability to process more than 500 mcg of calcium at one time is evidence of the body's tight rein on calcium levels. The bottom line? Calcium alone—no matter what form it's in—will not improve bone density, and overdosing can be as dangerous to your future health as breaking one of your bones. Do not increase your calcium intake without first talking with your doctor, and take calcium with vitamins D_3 and

K_2 only in the proper ratios. Do track how much calcium you get via diet as one step in finding out whether you need more from food or supplementation, and if so how much. Consume calcium from food sources over the day rather than in one meal—and if you are taking a calcium supplement, take it with meals. If you feel you need supplementation, start with 400 mg per day, which gives you a good base but still leaves room for natural sources from food.

Here's the most important point lost in the heat of the calcium supplement craze. We do need calcium to make strong bones, and calcium is widely available in the Western diet, so ordinarily people can easily get enough calcium through food. Yet when it comes to the vitamins and nutrients that support proper calcium function, that's another matter, because those vitamins and nutrients are not nearly as readily available from food. Clearly it is not more calcium supplementation we need; instead, we should focus on those key nutrients, harder to come by in diet, that assist the calcium in absorption and transport: vitamin D, vitamin K_2, magnesium, and trace minerals.

Calcium Insufficiency

People who eat very little or who have a nutritionally impoverished diet may not obtain enough calcium from food. They need calcium supplementation (see "How to Make the Supplement" on page 244 for instructions on making a calcium supplement yourself). The degree of need should be based on lab test results assessed by your healthcare provider.

Supplemental Vitamin D

Sunlight is the best source of vitamin D. But with so much of life indoors, exposure is not what it used to be and many people are deficient. Vitamin D deficiency can be serious because this vitamin is central to calcium absorption, cardiovascular health, DNA integrity, and proper function of the immune system. A deficiency can lead to unwelcome conditions such as depression and hypertension.

It has been generally noted that populations in higher latitudes (who suffer what is called a "vitamin D winter," where there is a lack of sunlight) have higher rates of osteoporosis. Age can affect how your skin transforms the sun's ultraviolet rays into vitamin D. Skin can make more vitamin D when it is warm than when it is cold. Darker skin requires more exposure to sun than lighter skin.

Gut health is also important for vitamin D absorption. Liver and kidney function are very important as well, because some liver disease can affect vitamin D absorption, and levels decline with decline of kidney function.

As always vitamin D is operating in a complex, interactive system of interdependent parts that must work together for good health.

Laura recommends 5,000 iu daily to her patients (sometimes 5,000 iu every other day), but blood levels will be the final arbiter. It is important to have your vitamin D levels tested, because assimilation is based on so many factors that levels vary greatly from person to person.

Easily the least expensive and best way to get this supplement is to make it yourself—by exposing the majority of your skin to the sun for 20 minutes a day. This is safest when you top up your vitamin C because vitamin C can protect your skin from most damage for up to 20 minutes. It is not advised to sit in the sun any longer than 20 minutes as too much exposure will destroy the protective vitamin C and leave your skin open to damage.

As with vitamin K_2, vitamin D is more difficult to obtain from diet than calcium, and it will probably take time for you to work the right balance of food and sunlight to meet your vitamin D needs.

Sunned mushrooms provide the body with a combination of the D_2 form (ergocalciferol) and D_3 form (cholecalciferol) of vitamin D, while animal products provide more of the D_3 form. Supplements should be D_3.

Optimal Vitamin D Levels?

At this writing, the medical community is still debating the optimal levels of vitamin D. The Vitamin D Council recommends total intake from all sources at around 7,000 iu per day, and researchers have recently challenged the National Academy of Sciences Institute of Medicine in their RDA calculations of 600 iu per day, which the researchers convincingly argue are about 10 times lower than they need to be.

An ideal blood level of vitamin D appears to be about 50 nanometers per milliliter.[10] Lower than 35 nanometers per milliliter and it appears your body will not store any vitamin D in tissues, and below 32 nanometers per milliliter appears to increase fracture risk. It is believed that modern humans get about 2,000 mg per day from food and sunlight, which leaves 3,000 to 5,000 iu (depending on your vitamin D blood level) to be found elsewhere.

Scientists confirm that D_3 lasts longer in the body than D_2 and is the form your body uses most readily—and that D_3 is more efficient—you need about three times the amount of D_2 to equal D_3's effectiveness. It has been reported that supplementing with isolated D_2 could potentially be harmful, so always choose to supplement with D_3. It is unknown whether there is any detriment from ingesting natural forms of D_2 such as in mushrooms, but based on the scientific information currently available, Laura has concluded that consuming D_2 from natural sources such as mushrooms and alfalfa shoots is safe as long as this is combined with vitamin D in the D_3 form from the sun, fish, fish eggs, and cod liver oil.

For her patients who require both K_2 and D_3 supplementation, Laura recommends that they take a Thorne Research product that combines K_2 (MK4) and D_3 in conjunction with Jarrow's MK7 supplement, which is derived from natto. If testing shows you are deficient in vitamin D—or bone mass decline and/or atherosclerosis or heart disease suggests a need for K_2/MK4 and MK7 supplementation—you may wish to discuss these supplements with your healthcare provider.

Cod liver oil is an excellent source of vitamin D, but much supplemental fish oil is processed, deodorized, and preserved, corrupting not only the product but the vitamin D:vitamin A ratio. There are a few good sources, and fish oil supplementation is recommended for all. For information on sources of cod liver oil, see resources on page 266.

Supplemental Vitamin K_2

In 1939 during a cholesterol study a Danish scientist, Henrik Dam, inferred the existence of what he later called vitamin K. Subsequently research confirmed the existence of vitamin K and the many processes made safe by this newly discovered vitamin. Ongoing research has turned up new K forms and subsets and important K_2 functions including several on which bone health depends. The research shows that among Westerners, key proteins[11]—proteins that assist in both forming bone and inhibiting calcium deposition in cartilage and artery walls[12]—are insufficiently activated.

What's key here is that analyzing forms of K_2 and aiming to understand metabolic functions of each is a new science. Under the K_2 umbrella are several forms collectively called menaquinones. For bone health, we are concerned with menaquinones 4 and 7, commonly called MK4 and MK7. Both appear to help to clear calcium from arteries and joints, protect bone sheath flexibility, and deposit calcium in bone matrix.

Our bodies make very little K_2, so unless you eat the Japanese fermented bean called natto it can be challenging to get as much of this essential vitamin as we need from food. Natto is the major source, with Gouda cheese, pastured poultry dark meat, pastured eggs, natural milk, and some other foods in lesser quantities being a distant second (see table 10.1. Bone's Favorite Foods on page 116).

Because it is difficult for the typical Westerner to obtain vitamin K_2 from the diet, Laura recommends MK4 and MK7 supplementation to her patients of all ages who do not consume natto. Laura refers to research on high (therapeutic) doses[13] that shows, at this writing, no adverse effects—vitamin K_2 is not stored in quantity in the liver, so toxicity is not a problem. For some patients, she recommends high levels (thousands of micrograms) daily to correct long-standing bone loss or severe atherosclerosis, as well as other compelling conditions. In general however, even low-dose (50–150 mcg) supplementation improves bone metabolism.[14]

We remind again that you should make all therapeutic dose decisions, including even the choice to take supplemental K_2, in partnership with a healthcare provider and always in the context of overall mineral intake: amounts of calcium, vitamin D, magnesium, and vitamin A. As with all nutrients, the most effective are those from whole food/natural sources. The best MK7 once-daily supplements are derived from natto (see "Natto, Because We Must" on page 235 for instructions on making your own). MK4 is more abundant in the diet naturally (though still not really abundant), but has a shorter half-life in the body. It is not yet clear which is most effective in bone health.

Supplemental Magnesium

Sorting out how to nourish a body for optimal health is a fascinating task that nonetheless does turn up some frustrating dilemmas, and magnesium is one of them. Magnesium is absolutely essential to bone health, and magnesium deficiency is complicit in osteoporosis, cardiovascular disease, fibromyalgia, Alzheimer's, anxiety, and diabetes among other conditions and illnesses. Ninety-five percent of the magnesium we absorb from food is absorbed in the small intestine—the remaining 5 percent is absorbed in the large intestine—but more than half of the magnesium we ingest is not absorbed at all. Furthermore, compromised gut flora or a problem with the gut lining—or deleterious intestinal conditions such as Crohn's disease, irritable bowel syndrome (IBS), and inflammatory bowel disease (IBD)—may reduce magnesium absorption even more.

The bottom line here? Magnesium is not made by the body, is not readily absorbed, and

upward of 60 percent of the US population appears to be deficient.

Luckily, magnesium is also absorbed efficiently through the skin, so an excellent way to boost magnesium absorption is by taking a bath or using a spray.

MAKING A MAGNESIUM SPRAY

A bath with Epsom salts (magnesium sulfate) was a common remedy for pain and stress long before its contribution to magnesium absorption made it a star. Simply add a cup of Epsom salts to your bathwater a few times a week.

Magnesium chloride is much more bioavailable than magnesium sulfate, and you can make your own magnesium spray using magnesium chloride. Boil equal parts magnesium chloride salts (readily available in many forms) and water, allow it to cool, and decant it into a pump spray bottle. The result is a suspension rather than a solution, and the liquid feels oily. Spray it on your belly, arms, and legs. It can tingle. Leave it on for 20 minutes. Wipe off gently with a soft towel, and then take a shower.

Magnesium oxide is not a candidate for making a spray, because its bioavailability is only 4 percent.

You can also buy commercial magnesium oil. The one we use contains magnesium from the Zechstein Sea bed, which is principally deep beneath a stretch of northern Europe. It contains magnesium salts that formed about 250 million years ago, and the sea is deep enough so the bed has remained uncontaminated. These salts provide the most highly bioavailable magnesium you can find (see resources on page 266).

If you have been deficient for a while, you may choose supplementation, at least when you are setting out to remedy the deficiency as part of your bone health regimen. We recommend only magnesium baths or spray, not supplements in pill form—stomach upset is a common complaint with magnesium pills.

And a final note on magnesium: B_6 activates magnesium. You'll need to keep up with B_6/B-complex vitamins, and the levels you require will depend upon your personal nutrient profile. (Information about working with your healthcare provider to obtain a nutrition evaluation is set out in chapter 9.)

Supplemental Vitamin A

The 2016 US dietary guidelines show that a large portion of the US population is deficient in vitamin A. This vitamin is common in foods that are good for bone health, so as your diet shifts toward bone health you will almost surely consume enough. These foods are high in vitamin A: sweet potatoes, carrots, winter squash, dried apricots, cantaloupe, fish, liver, and tropical fruits. Too much vitamin A without enough vitamin D can stop vitamin D from converting to its active form, so it is best to avoid vitamin A in stand-alone supplements. The best source, and the only one you will most likely need, is simply natural food. Vitamin A is an important part of the production of Gla, proteins that helps keep calcium from depositing in the soft tissues/arteries.

Supplemental Phosphorus

Phosphate is essential because it is part of bone matrix crystal. However, here nature is very generous. Phosphorus is found in almost all foods, bioavailability is very high, and phosphorus deficiency is extremely rare, so phosphorus supplementation is rarely required. Nevertheless, some foods interfere with phosphorus absorption, and you need to prepare them properly in order to ensure peaceful

---

Sweet Potato

In certain parts of Central America and Africa, sweet potatoes are named *Cilera Abana*—protector of children. We think of them as a protector of bones. Sweet potatoes contain abundant precursors of vitamin A. Prepared correctly one medium-sized sweet potato can yield up to 500 times the standard RDA; and, because of the vitamin's structure in sweet potatoes, there is little danger of an imbalance unless you are consuming a whole sweet potato every day and there is not enough vitamin D in your daily diet.

Be sure to consume sweet potatoes with ghee—or organic or raw butter if you haven't any ghee—which allows the fat-soluble vitamins, including vitamin A, to be absorbed.

---

coexistence. Phytic acid in grains, legumes, seeds, and nuts traps phosphorus and makes it much less available. Soaking, sprouting, and fermenting help to tame phytic acid (see chapter 4).

Commercial sodas are very high in phosphorus. When you drink a commercial soda, this high dose of phosphorus stimulates the parathyroid gland, which triggers the body to remove excess phosphorus. This trigger also signals the bones to release calcium. This is a short-lived spike, but watch out: Each one adds up.

Supplemental Protein/Collagen

If you don't eat much meat or if you are an athlete in training or pregnant, you may be lacking in essential amino acids (those your body can't manufacture on its own) that help form the complex proteins your body uses for growth and repair. If you are trying to help your bones you need a good supply of collagen as much as you need calcium, for the scaffold must be strong to support the mineral deposition. An ideal protein supplement will provide a good balance of essential amino acids, be lower in methionine, and higher in glycine. Collagen peptides—amino acids that make up collagen—fulfill these requirements perfectly especially for bone health. People living a Paleo lifestyle (which includes eating a lot of meat) can balance out the high intake of methionine in muscle meat by supplementing with collagen peptides. Anyone wishing to increase bone strength can benefit from collagen, in either powder or gelatin form. And note that it may be important to increase vitamin C intake as well as trace minerals when taking a collagen supplement for purposes of building bone.

Supplemental Enzymes

A nutrient profile analysis can show nutrient deficiency, but the shortage may derive from lack of enzymes to digest the food—or from gut health issues—rather than insufficient intake of the nutrient itself.

If your diet does not include raw natural foods regularly then you are relying completely on your body to create and build enough enzymes to break down everything you ingest. In these cases supplementing with digestive enzymes can be very helpful. Speak with your healthcare provider about whether you require supplements and, if so, how much.

Supplemental Trimethylglycine

Trimethylglycine (TMG) is a methyl donor. These substances help our systems transform nutrients into forms usable by our bodies (explained in detail in chapter 3). A modern diet high in processed foods can be deficient in methyl donors. Supplementing with trimethylglycine can give your body the assistance it needs in order to carry out the foundational transformations that lead to health.

TMG, also called betaine, can be helpful for people transitioning from a diet high in processed foods to a whole-foods diet. You can find betaine plus natural digestive enzymes as a single supplement. The combination helps your body get the most nutrition from your food and convert it to forms your body can use.

Supplemental Silicon

Silicon is the second most abundant element in the earth's crust. It is abundantly present in plants—especially in cereals and grasses—and in seafood, particularly mussels. Silicon exists principally in the form of silica.

A growing body of scientific literature[15] reports that silicon plays an essential role in bone formation and maintenance. Silicon improves bone matrix quality and facilitates bone mineralization. Increased intake of bioavailable silicon has been associated with increased bone mineral density. Silicon supplementation in animals and humans has been shown to increase bone mineral density and improve bone strength.

Average daily dietary intake of silicon among European and North American populations is 20 to 50 mg daily; daily intake is higher in China and India (140 to 200 mg a day), where grains, fruits, and vegetables form a larger part of the diet. This higher intake of silicon, combined with the lower intake of calcium that characterizes a typical Asian diet, is notable in light of the historically lower incidence of hip fractures in China and India compared with many Western countries.

Diets containing more than 40 mg per day of silicon have been positively associated with increased femoral bone mineral density compared with dietary intake of less than 14 mg a day. In a North American study, none of the postmenopausal women achieved 40 mg a day of dietary silicon intake.

Horsetail, an herb, contains very high levels of silicon, and it is central to our Bone-Building Calcium-Rich Vinegar recipe (see page 231).

An important note: Some research[16] indicates that silicon works to assist bones only in the presence of estrogen. If you are postmenopausal, silicon may not help improve your bone density unless your diet contains a good level of phytoestrogens—plant estrogens—which are abundant in some herbs and beans. This illustrates the importance of natural sources—something you may have noticed we mention every chance we get. For more in-depth information on phytoestrogens, see chapter 7.

Supplemental Trace Minerals

Modern farming practices along with soil erosion deplete minerals from the soil. Because of this trend, modern diets often don't include sufficient trace minerals that in tiny amounts contribute to good health, including bone health, even when diets include lots of fresh, whole foods.

Mineral salts such as Himalayan salts contain all the essential trace minerals in the right balance, so Himalayan salt is a good choice for table salt. See the "Salt" sidebar on page 39.

Traditional medicines included Shilajit (in Sanskrit: "invincible rock"), high in humic and

---

Strontium

There's another cautionary note in the calcium supplement story: strontium. Some people choose strontium as an osteoporosis remedy. In some countries strontium ranelate is sold as a supplement. We do not recommend high doses of strontium as a treatment for osteoporosis. Here's why.

Scientists seem to agree that bodies and bones need strontium. It increases bone mass by stimulating osteoblasts—which make new bone—and inhibiting osteoclasts, which break down bone. On the face of it, all well and good. However, supplementing with strontium increases calcium but not magnesium retention, and it has the potential to lower stomach acid levels, insulin, and white blood cells, as well as depleting important trace minerals. High doses of strontium appear to increase cortical bone thickness, but in so doing strontium decreases bone tensile strength—flexibility.

---

fulvic acids.[17] It is present in a tar-like substance that seeps through the cracks between rocks in the mountains in and around Tibet. Shilajit contains all the trace minerals needed for bone health—and overall health. Trace minerals are key for all steps of the bone building process, and their presence is essential—see the resources on page 265.

CHAPTER 7

Phytoestrogens, Cholesterol, and Bone Loss Pharmaceuticals

When we speak about natural foods and bone health, audience members raise important questions. We recommend soy; people ask about phytoestrogens. We recommend saturated fat; people ask about cholesterol and heart disease. And of course people want to know about bone loss pharmaceuticals.

How do we respond? There are no absolutes. When it comes to safety and efficacy of phytoestrogens, it depends on factors including but not limited to diet, stage of life, and health history. Cholesterol is vital to health, not the villain it was once thought to be. And while there are good reasons to avoid bone loss drugs, a small percentage of people with bone loss may benefit by taking them.

To understand why there are no one-size-fits-all guidelines, it is useful to understand how phytoestrogens, cholesterol, and bone loss pharmaceuticals operate in the body.

What About Phytoestrogens?

Phytoestrogens—isoflavones, lignans, and coumestans—are plant compounds that act like weak estrogen in the human body. To a greater or lesser degree phytoestrogens are present in many plant-based foods: seeds, beans, nuts, grains, and leafy greens. These foods are widely promoted for their health benefits. One of the most famous isoflavones is resveratrol, which exists naturally in grapes and red wine. The traditional plant-based foods that contain phytoestrogens we hear most about are soybeans and soy products such as miso and tofu.

Phytoestrogens, and soy, have been controversial. Hormones are natural; they trigger essential metabolic function. Many plant hormones are structurally similar to the human form, so once in the body they behave as our own do. The concern has been that phytoestrogen together with natural human estrogen could be overload, resulting in too much estrogen in the body, which could cause or exacerbate reproductive cancers.

Research shows that phytoestrogens can help trigger the same beneficial effects as our own estrogen, with the results being healthier, stronger bones.[1] Some ask: Should we eat phytoestrogens to help our bones, or avoid them to avoid cancer? This is a big topic, but it has been well researched and the answers, for most of us, are now clear.

Many doctors counsel strict moderation or even avoidance of high-phytoestrogen foods, like soy, for premenopausal women, because natural estrogen levels are already at peak and there is a connection between estrogen and reproductive cancers. Although, this recommendation was certainly prudent at one point in time. The American Cancer Society reports that the initial studies on soy and reproductive cancers were done on rodents, and that rodents metabolize soy differently from humans. Further, and vital to any assessment of the connection between plant estrogen and illness, the initial studies on soy and reproductive cancers were done with isolated soy protein rather than with whole intact or fermented soybeans.[3] Take note: Most studies done in the United States are done with soy isolates—parts of the soybean separated out, such as soy protein powder—and genetically modified isolates at that, which have not been properly prepared or fermented for human consumption.

We now know that phytoestrogens actually help to lower the incidence of reproductive cancer in most women.[2] Japanese studies that use properly prepared soy foods indicate that consuming 50 g of soy phytoestrogens a day is protective for breast cancer.[4] This means having a glass of soymilk a day. Those Asian women who consumed more than that, two glasses or two to three bowls of miso soup per day, had increased protection against breast cancers.

The American Cancer Society goes on to report that where women (principally in Asian countries) consume up to four servings of soy a day, incidence of breast cancer—and recurrence—are lower by between 25 and 50 percent. Yet studies done previously in the United States often showed either no effect or just a slightly protective effect. One of the reasons is likely due to the nature of the soy isolates used. Another reason is that Asian women begin to eat soy earlier in life, and this appears to confer benefit. Perhaps most significant, it appears that particular bacterial species in the human gut are able to convert soy phytoestrogens into forms usable by our bodies, but more than half the people in the US lack these bacteria.

Fortunately, gut bacterial populations adjust in response to dietary intake. It has been shown that changing your diet over the course of two days affects the type of bacteria you have in your gut.[5] It's that fast. We can assume that regular soy intake will induce the correct bacteria.

The Long Island Breast Cancer Study Project,[6] a group of studies conducted over 10 years starting in 1993, showed that soy intake had a positive impact on breast cancer and recurrence, which is a confirmation of most contemporary studies showing a decreased risk of recurrence.[7]

Studies in the West also clearly confirm decreased low-density lipoprotein (LDL) and cholesterol as well as lower cardiovascular disease when properly prepared soy is part of a good diet.[8]

A Deeper Look

Let's take a closer look at the science of phytoestrogens, and why it makes sense that they are protective.

Receptors are docking stations on cell surfaces for compounds such as hormones, enzymes, and other substances that interact with the cell and trigger metabolic activity. For example, humans have receptor sites on brain cells for a naturally occurring form of diazepam, but plants do not have any receptor sites for this substance. Human cells also have receptor sites for hormones, including estrogens. Once a compound is docked, interaction begins. Since plant estrogens are molecularly similar to human estrogen, they can also bind to our cells' estrogen receptors. Humans have two different types of estrogen receptors—alpha and beta. Estrogen receptor positive breast cancers express the alpha receptor, as the alpha receptor triggers cell division and tumor growth. Phytoestrogens tend to bind to the beta receptors. Estrogen beta receptors appear to have anti-proliferative, anti-tumor effects, therefore opposing the cell-proliferation actions of alpha receptors in reproductive tissue.

It actually appears that plant estrogen can safely stand in for human estrogen to bind with receptors and trigger an increase in bone-building activity without raising the risk of reproductive cancers.

In the human gut, two plant estrogens, genistein and daidzein, are fermented by the presence of specific bacteria and become equol, which is a nonsteroidal estrogen. Equol can exist in two forms, (S)-equol and (R)-equol. Soy daidzein converts to S-equol, which preferentially activates estrogen receptor type beta.

It is reported that S-equol may have beneficial effects on the incidence of prostate cancer, bone health, skin health, and physiological changes during menopause, including reducing severity and frequency of hot flashes and stiffness in the neck and shoulder. Other benefits may be realized in treating male pattern baldness, acne, and other problems because it functions as a DHT (dihydrotestosterone) blocker.

Even when phytoestrogens do bind to alpha receptors, in doing so they block the binding of

Soy Sprouts

Sprouting soybeans increases the phytoestrogen component thousands of times. This is surely why it was used medicinally in ancient times.

In the third century AD, soy sprouts were called *dadou huang chüan*, "soybean yellow curls," as well as *huang chuan p'i*, "sprouts curl skins," by the Medical Prescription Books (Fang Shu). They were given to women after childbirth "to purify their milk and increase their strength" (translated by Ch'i-chün Wu, 1848).

During the Ming dynasty (1368–1662), Ming Chen-i wrote a rhythmic prose piece (Fu) titled "Tou-ya Fu," or "Soy Sprout Poem." Here is the translation by Wu (1848):

We have other things which are like the frozen flesh of jadelike mixture. The seed does not enter the foul earth. The root needs no support to hold this plant erect. The golden sprouts are one inch long. The pearly kernels are doubly prolific. There are some variegated green or blue, but none vermilion or crimson. In the white dragon's hair the spring silkworms hibernate. These words are quite true and really, the soybean deserves this description.

the more potent endogenous estrogen, and this can prove beneficial for women who are genetically predisposed to breast cancer.

The ability of plant estrogens to mimic human estrogen looks to improve overall and bone health at all stages, and especially among postmenopausal women and men by standing in for the body's estrogen, which declines in later life. Plant estrogens may shift the bone mineralization balance toward renewed growth by triggering the death of bone breakdown cells, just as human estrogen does.

Consuming Soy

Because soy acts as a powerful medicine, there are different recommendations for different stages of life. There appears to be a small subset of women who have a negative response to the benefits of these phytoestrogens, though the reasons are unknown.

We do not endorse and we do discourage the use of soy supplements, soy protein supplements, or any isolated soy supplements in any form.

CHILDREN, PREMENOPAUSAL WOMEN, AND MEN

We do not recommend, in fact we strongly disapprove of, soy formula (or any formula for that matter) for infants, or a soy-heavy diet for developing children. Apart from any other issue, high levels of phytohormones can interfere with normal development.

However, it appears that incorporation of properly prepared soy products from a young age—for example, properly prepared soy twice a week—increases the protective benefit, lowering the risk over a lifetime of reproductive cancers. Generally, though, each human system is unique. Each person must use this medicinal food as it works with their own unique metabolism.

We also caution against extremely high soy consumption by premenopausal women. The weaker estrogenic effect of soy phytoestrogens can lessen the impact of our own human estrogen if it fills up the receptors.

The same goes for men—high consumption can lower sperm count. However, normal consumption (tofu for dinner twice a week, soymilk occasionally, edamame with sushi) will not affect your manliness; in fact, it appears to protect against prostate cancer.[9]

POSTMENOPAUSAL WOMEN

Phytoestrogens are a great addition to a postmenopausal woman's diet. As estrogen declines, phytoestrogen can stand in, helping the system trigger a more robust bone breakdown/rebuild process. The presence of the weak estrogen has also been associated with decreased symptom severity in menopause.

Soy sprouts are perfect for menopausal and postmenopausal women. Sprouts' high phytoestrogen content makes getting enough phytoestrogen much easier. However, this must be a steady and slow intake, increasing over a couple of years.

Laura advises Helen to eat properly prepared, fermented soybean foods at minimum three times per week, daily if possible, with some soy sprouts thrown in.

People sometimes ask us about the wisdom of consuming soy if one has the BRCA mutation. There is much confusion about this, even in the medical community. BRCA1 and 2 are tumor suppressor genes, functioning to repair broken DNA. Mutations in these genes cause them to malfunction, and increase the risk of breast and ovarian cancer. Only about 5 percent of breast cancer arises from these mutations, but these

---

Exercise, Estrogen, and Bone Density

The positive effects of exercise on bone density are undisputed, and impact exercise is an integral and necessary part of building bone mass. The effects of exercise on bone can be amplified in the presence of estrogen (or phytoestrogen). Here's how it works.

Pressure on a bone is called mechanical stress. When you walk, run, jump, dance, play tennis, lift weights, or do Qi Gong, yoga, or pilates, you are putting mechanical pressure on your bones. The pressure causes hydroxyapatite, the bone mineral crystals, to emit little currents of electricity, called the piezoelectric effect, which in turn kick osteoblasts into action to build bone. (If you need a refresher on bone structure, refer back to chapter 1.)

The most abundant cell type in bones are osteocytes. These worn-out osteoblasts no longer build bone but do take on another important function. They become incorporated into the bone matrix, forming a network and extensions (called osteocyte processes) that connect with other osteocytes and with active osteoblasts on the surface of the bone. The osteocyte network senses mechanical force—compression, stretch, impact—on bone. It transmits a signal through the osteocyte network to influence the activity of osteoblasts and osteoclasts. Osteocyte death increases after estrogen loss and/or lack of exercise for long periods. When there's no stress upon them, your bones behave as if they don't need as much mineral crystal, and bone formation is suspended. Or, even worse, osteocytes signal osteoclasts to tear done bone.

Exercise also offers another benefit for bones: It stimulates the thyroid to produce calcitonin, which puts the brakes on osteoclast activity, thereby slowing bone breakdown. Moreover, exercise that induces sweating is the only known way to generate new mitochondria—our body's power generators.

---

genes appear to be suppressed by the tumors in the remaining 95 percent of breast cancers. In all cases properly prepared soy intake appears to be beneficial. In the case of suppressed genes this intake appears to actually reactivate the suppressed genes, thereby reinstating the protective properties of the BRCA genes.[10]

What About Cholesterol?

Cholesterol is a fat-like compound though it is not a fat. Over the past 50 years, there have been hundreds of scientific studies on the role of cholesterol in the body, and prevailing opinions about the role of cholesterol in human health have undergone a dramatic change. Once considered a villain that caused heart disease, cholesterol is now being acknowledged as necessary and important for human health. Cholesterol makes up 50 percent of all cell membranes of all tissues. It is the precursor to all sex hormones. Cholesterol promotes myelin and synapse formation for a baby's brain growth. Cholesterol maintains the intestinal wall and is actually an antioxidant that protects against damage. Cholesterol is so highly prized that your liver recycles it.

The UV(B) rays of the sun interact with cholesterol to produce the vitamin D_3 our bones need—if your cholesterol is too low, this all-important step of vitamin D production will not happen.

The ingredients in some of our bone health recipes include butter, eggs, and full-fat milk and cream from pastured animals. That's because natural fat from pastured animals and eggs from pastured hens contribute to an overall healthy diet, which must contain healthy fats such as natural saturated fats, and cholesterol.

So what regulates cholesterol levels and what part do dietary cholesterol and dietary fat play in blood cholesterol levels? Cholesterol is manufactured in your liver, which produces about 75 percent of the cholesterol a human body uses. Furthermore the body naturally controls cholesterol levels. In general the more cholesterol you eat the less your liver produces. If you eat a lot of cholesterol, your liver will produce less.

The level of cholesterol manufactured in the liver differs from person to person, thanks principally to genetics. It appears that there are broadly two types of people, in terms of cholesterol. Most people are normal responders. This means that for about 75 percent of the population, eating cholesterol will not significantly affect their blood levels. Statistically, this is probably you.

In some rare cases natural cholesterol levels are very high, a condition Helen endures. It's called familial hypercholesterolemia. If you have this condition your bloodstream can end up overloaded with cholesterol, and that excess can raise the risk for heart disease. But these conditions are rare. For most people, the cholesterol they eat does not significantly affect their blood cholesterol, and even if it does this is not the determining factor for arterial plaque or heart disease.

Heart disease appears to occur in relation to the *oxidation* of small dense LDL particles rather than cholesterol numbers per se. If there are more LDL particles in the bloodstream, there is a higher chance one will lodge in the artery wall, but high cholesterol by itself is not a cause. The *condition* of your LDL particles is more telling than your cholesterol numbers. Small dense oxidized LDL particles plus high levels of inflammation are most likely the culprits. And generally speaking, higher intakes of refined carbohydrates and fructose appear to cause much more damage than eating cholesterol and fats in a balanced natural foods diet.

The Framingham,[11] San Francisco, Albany, and Honolulu cohort studies are large-scale, long-term studies on heart disease. They have shown that: total cholesterol is not a predictor of future heart disease; LDL cholesterol is a "marginal risk factor"; and HDL ("good" cholesterol—higher levels are protective) cholesterol is a fourfold better predictor of risk than LDL cholesterol and the only reliable predictor of risk for people over 50. It was shown that saturated fat raises HDL cholesterol (a good thing) while carbohydrates lower it. It was shown that saturated fat and total fat were positively associated with longevity.[12]

This drastic change in viewpoint has been surprising and unsettling to many people. After being told for so long to cut back on cholesterol, it's hard to break the habit—but there are tasty ways to reintroduce it to your diet. We encourage you to explore this new information and to discuss the details with your healthcare provider.

What About Fats?

Fats have a legacy of bad press, but people are adjusting to the news that natural fats have a central role in a healthful diet. While recommendations on dietary fats have shifted over the years, it is established now that for good health, the human body depends in part on all natural fats, including saturated fat and cholesterol. Except in some cases of genetic variant, dietary fats are not the enemy. The big problem is the oxidation of the fat.

Monounsaturated and Polyunsaturated

Fats are chains of molecules. All oils are fats. Each type of fat contains a different combination of molecules, and the molecules themselves have different numbers of binding sites (bonds). Those with more binding sites are called polyunsaturated fats, and they can combine more easily with molecules outside the chain. If the molecules combine with oxygen, that creates a state called oxidation. If we eat oxidized fats they raise the risk of inflammation, and as explained in chapter 2 inflammation is a major factor in many serious health problems.

The molecules that make up monounsaturated fats have one (mono) bond, so they tend to remain relatively intact. The molecules in a polyunsaturated chain have several (poly) bonds. So polyunsaturated fats have many more opportunities to bond with oxygen—to oxidize. This is one reason monounsaturated fats, found in olive oil, avocado oil, and nut oils among others, are considered better for you. They are less likely to oxidize; they are more likely to remain intact and not cause inflammation. Oils that are predominantly monounsaturated—olive oil is one—increase calcium absorption.

Omega-3 and omega-6 are polyunsaturated chains. Humans don't manufacture the precursors,

Your ApoE Profile and the Management of Lipids

Everyone needs to consume some saturated fat and cholesterol, but there is no hard-and-fast rule about how much saturated fat is okay in a person's diet, because in part it depends on which genetic variants you have of the ApoE gene.[13]

ApoE is a protein that is a component of lipoproteins, the particles that transport cholesterol and fats throughout the body. The gene that codes for these proteins is your ApoE gene. There are three variants of the gene, and each one affects fat transport differently.

The three ApoE variations are 2, 3, and 4. You inherited one variant from each parent, so your combination might be 2/3, 4/4, or 3/3, for example. The dietary recommendations for the different groups are still very much being researched, and no concrete results have been generally accepted as of yet. The 4 genotype is least efficient at managing fat, and appears to raise the risk of Alzheimer's and heart disease.

Although the science is still evolving, Laura advises all her patients to take a blood test to learn their ApoE variant to have some idea of how their body is processing lipids.

but they are essential precursors to the manufacture of certain fatty acids and to the manufacture of hormones, all of which are involved in immune function, blood clotting, and cell growth among dozens of other functions including bone formation. An in-depth discussion of omega fatty acids is beyond the scope of this book, but another reason many polyunsaturated fats (such as safflower oil, corn oil, and other vegetable oils) are *not* recommended is because their ratios of omega-3 to omega-6 fatty acids are not optimal.

Did we forget about saturated fat? Not at all. We just wanted to keep the best news for last. In this context saturated means the same thing it does when a piece of paper towel cannot absorb any more water. The molecules in saturated fat are fully bonded with hydrogen. The chain is a closed set; the fat is stable without potential to bond with oxygen. In this natural state saturated fat should not cause inflammation. The brain depends on saturated fat. Saturated fat is necessary for cell membranes, hormone production, and fuel production, and a moderate intake actually appears to *lower* cholesterol.[14]

Trans Fat

Trans fats are synthetic. Industry created them to mimic the action of saturated fat when the margarine craze started. By adding hydrogen to vegetable oils, the fat would remain solid and in the fridge and the margarine would look like butter. And it increased margarine's shelf life.

It worked and from there the industry went wild. Nothing was sacred. Want to use inexpensive oil maybe from genetically modified seed instead of real butter? At room temperature all those packaged foods would melt, so use trans fats. And what about shelf life? Use chemicals to press the oils out; use chemicals to preserve them. Even the

health food industry jumped on board. Fish oil is a polyunsaturated fat, so it tends to oxidize. To create a long shelf life, many producers add

Omega Fatty Acids and DHA

The story of the omegas—omega-3, omega-6, omega-9—is a complex one; in fact, too intricate to tell in full here. But the takeaway? It's the omega-3 to omega-6 ratio that is of concern to us here. The omegas have to exist in a certain ratio for the body to function properly. Scientists are closing in on the desirable ratio, which currently stands at between 1:1 and 5:1, omega-6 to omega-3. Problems result when the omegas are seriously or continuously out of balance. High levels of omega-6 are pro-inflammatory, and Western diets sometimes have a ratio up to 60:1. Corn oil, ubiquitous in packaged foods, is about 49:0.

DHA and EPA are the long-chain omega-3 fatty acids, and DHA is believed to be the one that confers more benefit to human health. They are found only in seafood and algae. ALA is the plant version of omega-3, for example in flax- and hemp seeds, and the body can convert ALA to the more beneficial forms DHA and EPA. However, it appears that only a very small percentage of ALA actually gets converted. And it only happens in the presence of zinc and iron. DHA appears to be not only beneficial for bone health, but essential to overall health. See "Supplemental Vitamin D" on page 69 for more on fish oil.

preservatives. If you consume fish oil, confirm that your brand is free of preservatives and deodorizers, which some add because the oil goes rancid (oxidizes) easily and deodorizers mask the smell. If possible, instead of consuming fish oil as a supplement, eat natural foods that are rich in saturated fats: fatty fish such as wild salmon, mackerel, and sardines, and also walnuts and flaxseeds.

Trans fats are an entirely unnatural substance that causes widespread inflammation. Trans fats contribute to insulin resistance and inflammation and have no place in a bone-healthy (or any other) diet. We consider them the enemy. To their credit, and with our admiration and thanks, UK supermarket chains Sainsbury's and Morrisons have voluntarily discontinued the sale of any products containing trans fats. Would that all the food stores and restaurants would follow suit.

Our Recommendations

We recommend cooking with olive oil, coconut oil, and grass-fed ghee. Nut oils, such as peanut oil, avocado oil, and rice bran oil, are also good for occasional use. Fresh chicken, duck, and goose fat are also great and delicious for cooking occasionally.

Extra-virgin olive oil is ideal for salads and general light cooking. The smoke point is around 350°F (177°C), so we don't recommend using it for high-heat cooking. Refined (non-virgin) olive oil has a higher smoke point, around 465°F (241°C), so can be used for higher-heat cooking.

Nut oils can also be used for high-heat cooking. Peanut oil has a smoke point of 450°F (232°C), and so do rice bran oils. The omega ratios of these oils are not as favorable as olive oil, so we recommend using them occasionally rather than regularly.

Coconut oil is one of the few fats in our diet consisting of medium-chain fatty acids. The human body can metabolize coconut oil without the action of enzymes produced by the pancreas. It is easily and readily digested, even by people who have had their gallbladders removed. It contains lauric acid, which helps protect against pathogenic microbes. Coconut oil is almost completely saturated, so it will not oxidize in high heat. Coconut oil has been studied for use against loss of bone density and has shown very promising results.[15]

Ghee is essentially the butter oil that remains after you clarify butter to remove the milk solids. It is a staple in Indian cooking and has a very high smoke point (450°F) due to the removal of the milk solids, so is an excellent choice for high-heat cooking. Ordinarily it does not trigger milk allergies because the milk solids are removed. It is also rich in butyrate (see chapter 5), which suppresses inflammation in the gut. Perhaps this is the reason it is considered a divine food in Ayurvedic (Indian) medicine. (See "How to Make Ghee" on page 243.)

What About Pharmaceuticals?

When it comes to bone loss, Western medicine's pharmaceuticals of choice are widely prescribed. You may know them as Fosamax, Reclast, Actonel, or Boniva, to name a few. We will explain the pharmacology—mechanisms of action—here, because that will equip you to make informed judgment should you find yourself with bone loss and a recommendation to take drugs. (You may wish to review chapter 1 before reading on here.)

Bisphosphonates

Western medicine offers several different approaches to the treatment of bone loss. The most widely prescribed pharmaceuticals are bisphosphonates, which are substances that promote the death of osteoclasts, the cells that dissolve bone. The longest serving among the bisphosphonates is Fosamax. Although these drugs do slow bone loss and can be useful in some cases, their mechanism of action reveals serious flaws and potential risk to the patient.

Bisphosphonates were developed in the 19th century to soften water that was laden with minerals. (The water was used in orange grove irrigation systems.) Looking for possible treatments for bone loss, scientists at Merck & Co. experimented with these bisphosphonates. In 1995, the FDA approved Fosamax (alendronate), the first of the nitrogenous bisphosphonates. The others followed.

BISPHOSPHONATE MECHANISM OF ACTION

Bisphosphonates attach to the hydroxyapatite binding sites on calcium/bony surfaces, especially those undergoing active resorption (breakdown). There are two classes of bisphosphonates: nitrogenous and non-nitrogenous. Presently the newer version, nitrogenous, are prescribed more often because they have proven more effective at reducing fractures.

After binding to hydroxyapatite, nitrogenous bisphosphonates (Fosamax, Actonel, Aclasta, Boniva, Reclast, Nerixia, Aredia, APD) are absorbed into osteoclasts, causing them to die.

In large-scale trials, Fosamax and Reclast appear to decrease risk of fracture by about 10 percent.[16] Among those trial participants taking Fosamax, slightly more than 10 percent suffered fracture during the first three years compared with 21 percent on placebo. There were similar results with the Reclast trial.

We explain the effects this way. Since it takes time for the drug to attach to the bone, during the first few months bone turnover proceeds as it did before the start of therapy. Then as the drug takes effect, breakdown stops suddenly and over the next six months bone formation continues, unopposed. This is the positive window of bisphosphonate use. However, at the end of six months bone formation slows until it virtually stops. After two years, less than 1 percent of the bone surface shows any bone formation. And it appears that once absorbed bisphosphonates remain at the site of action for at least 10 years. Whatever gains a person taking these drugs makes in the six-month window may be the only gains (although sometimes doses are doubled at year 2 to attempt to increase the gains), because the suppression of not only bone breakdown but also suppression of bone building will continue well beyond the therapeutic period.

This suggests that even if you are attempting to increase bone density in other ways, your attempts may be stunted by the presence of the drug. This has yet to be studied.

Thus, the basic mechanism of action of bisphosphonates is to decrease or halt the breakdown of bone, as long as the drug remains absorbed in the bone. Unfortunately, because the processes of building and breaking down are inextriably linked, the mechanism also severely cripples bone building.

COMMON ADVERSE EFFECTS

Upset stomach and inflammation and erosion of the esophagus are the principal problems with oral dosing of bisphosphonates. People who take intravenous doses may develop flu-like symptoms. Bisphosphonates given intravenously are also correlated with osteonecrosis of the jaw, in which the jawbone—typically the lower jawbone—deteriorates. Over 50 percent of these cases occur in women who have recently had dental surgery.

The FDA also lists severe bone, joint, and muscle pain and atrial fibrillation among the side effects most often reported by patients who take bisphosphonates.

BISPHOSPHONATES IN THE LONG TERM

In 2012 the FDA recommended a reassessment by physicians treating osteoporotic patients with bisphosphonates, recommending that treatment be reassessed after three to five years of therapy to determine whether the patient should continue treatment.

It was suggested that women who are taking bisphosphonates with a diagnosis of osteopenia or just slight density loss are unlikely to benefit from long-term use. They should "probably stop taking the drugs after about three years," the researchers said. Women with osteoporosis seem to be in a gray area: Depending on their risk factors, taking bisphosphonates may or may not be recommended for more than three to five years. Unfortunately no matter which group you are in, after you stop taking the drug, when it has fully cleared from the bones, bone loss will continue. The FDA recommendation that a majority of women stop after three to five years leaves a large question—as the drug leaves the bone, the bone will start to lose density again. What then?

Bisphosphonates have proven successful in the long term in one circumstance. It seems that among patients who are in clear and present danger of vertebral fracture, in certain circumstances bisphosphonates can minimize the risk if the patients take the drug beyond the ordinary three-to-five-year suggested limit. However, the risk of other bisphosphonate fracture among women increases progressively with the duration of use.

According to a report in the *New England Journal of Medicine*, via the *New York Times*:[17]

There is not much evidence beyond vertebral fractures . . . We [the journal article authors] believe that if a patient's femoral neck is seen as low mineral density (clear osteoporosis) remaining after 3–5 years of treatment, these patients are at the highest risk for vertebral fractures and might benefit from continued bisphosphonate use, as would be patients who have already suffered a vertebral fracture. All other patients would be unlikely to benefit from continued treatment.

So where does this leave us on the pharmaceutical front? For most women, there are no additional recommendations after the first three years. As of this writing there are no drugs on offer, and there are no further recommendations for stopping bone loss.

Bisphosphonate therapy can be useful in severe cases where other options to strengthen bone are limited or absent. Keeping what bone there is in place is a better option than letting more and more bone deteriorate without attempting to replace the weak bone with stronger bone.

For most of us, however, there is no reason not to try to build stronger, better bone via diet and exercise even while using bisphosphonates. It is clear that bisphosphonate effectiveness is improved by taking the proper levels of calcium and vitamin D (and, we would add, vitamin K_2).

There is also now enough evidence to show that vitamin K_2 alone plus bisphosphonate therapy increases bone mineral density.[18] NASA has also shown—in space—that exercise plus bisphosphonate therapy increases bone density over bisphosphonate therapy alone.

Finally, it must be noted that large-scale studies have demonstrated that women have an increased risk for what is termed bisphosphonate fracture, also designated *atypical* fracture, in the femur. Bone fractures are most common in the shaft of the bone. Since hip fracture is not a typical bisphosphonate outcome and hip fracture can lead to death, the medical community concludes that bisphosphonates are the lesser of two evils. The logic here is that preventing hip fracture is a greater good that outweighs the increased risk of femoral fracture.

LAURA'S RECOMMENDATIONS

There is a place for the use of bisphosphonates. If you have serious bone loss and cannot use—or choose not to use—nutrition, supplementation, and exercise to counteract bone loss, then slowing down the bone loss by taking pharmaceuticals is a reasonable option.

There will also be cases of long-term progression of bone loss that are difficult to stop in time, as it takes time to put the brakes on the bone loss process. Nutritional and exercise interventions can and should be started, but if the risk of fracture is very high the interventions might take too long to kick in. If this is you and you are interested in and able to use some degree of natural approach to strengthening bones, then combining the two—nutrition and exercise for bone health plus bisphosphonates—could be a good plan.

If you are suffering from osteopenia or mild bone loss, or are interested in strengthening bones and/or building bone reserves, then a long-term diet, nutrition, and exercise approach should be all you need to maintain your bone mass even into older age.

We cannot say yet whether following a bone health diet might counteract the long-lasting negative effects of bisphosphonates or whether the drug will vanquish even the most diligent of nutrition efforts. But it is clear from the limited studies done on basic supplementation that any healthful additions to the bisphosphonate therapy show better results.

Other Drugs Prescribed for Osteoporosis

Prolia (denosumab) has a similar mechanism to bisphosphonates although it is a monoclonal antibody, which is a clone of a human immune molecule. The mechanism of action is inhibition of osteoclast formation, which slows or diminishes the breakdown of bone but does not initiate healthy bone formation. This drug is prescribed solely for patients at high risk of fracture, because the drug increases the risk of infection.

Forteo (teriparatide) is a genetically recombined form of human parathyroid hormone. PTH acts in the body to release calcium from the bones when your body needs calcium. However, when Forteo is taken intermittently it actually stimulates bone formation. It is usually prescribed only for patients at serious risk of fracture, as it carries a black-box warning for bone cancer. An FDA black-box warning—literally a box around a warning on the label—warns of serious/potentially deadly side effects. It is the strongest FDA warning.

Forteo is the only FDA-approved pharmaceutical that actually stimulates new bone formation. However, the risk is potentially perilous.

Evista (raloxifene) is a selective estrogen receptor modulator, meaning it acts in estrogen receptors of select tissues, mimicking estrogen. The FDA document reads: "Serious and life-threatening side effects can occur while taking Evista. These include blood clots and dying from stroke." Anytime you interfere with hormone cycles you potentially introduce serious side effects; in this case they are potentially deadly.

For patients who cannot take other medication doctors sometimes prescribe hormone therapy such as estrogen/progesterone and testosterone for men.

Miacalcin/Calcimar (calcitonin) is a hormone that occurs naturally in the body and helps regulate calcium levels and bone turnover. The pharmaceutical version, which is a synthetic form of salmon calcitonin, was approved in the 1970s as a drug that inhibits bone breakdown. The European Medicines Agency has banned the use of calcitonin for osteoporosis, citing increased cancer risk. Health Canada has also stopped recommending the drug. The FDA reviewed its recommendations on the drug in 2013 and although they state that "a meta-analysis of 21 randomized, controlled clinical trials with calcitonin-salmon (nasal spray and investigational oral forms) suggests an increased risk of malignancies in calcitonin-salmon treated patients compared to placebo-treated patients," they continue to allow the drug because they found "no conclusive evidence between the use of these products and cancer."

Cathepsin K, trade name Odanacatib, is currently (2016) seeking regulatory approval. The drug works to inhibit an enzyme involved in bone resorption. It was developed by Merck and is predicted to generate $1 billion annually by the year 2020. It is unknown how altering the function of the enzyme will affect other systems in the body in the long term.

GLP-2 (glucagon-like peptide 2). GLP is a natural hormone that the body releases in response to food intake. Bone resorption peaks at night, and administering this hormone before bed appears to reduce bone breakdown. However, it does not stimulate bone formation. Still in clinical trials at the writing of this book, it helps stop the bone loss associated with rapid weight loss.

Abaloparatide is an investigational new drug. It's a synthetic PTH-related protein similar to Forteo and no doubt carries similar risks.

CHAPTER 8

Speaking with Your Doctor

Before Laura had developed the bone-health nutrition regime and when osteoporosis had become severe, one of Helen's doctors fired her as a patient because she refused to take pharmaceuticals. He is a superbly educated, kind, and caring medical professional. He never became angry, demanding, dismissive, or disrespectful; he did become extremely frustrated because he was worried about Helen, and said so. The gist of this doctor's argument was: I don't want you to succumb to a fractured hip. I do want you to live out your life in the best possible health and well-being. I know that the pharmaceuticals available to treat bone loss are less than perfect and even that they can cause problems, but we have no alternatives, and fracture is a greater risk than the side effects. How can I help you if you won't help yourself? Please; just take the drugs.

This was a philosophical difference between a dedicated physician and an admiring patient, each committed to the same goal yet unable to agree on a path, and it left both Helen and her trusted physician feeling sad. However, if either

had known about nutrition evaluation, Helen and her doctor would have had an objective analysis as the basis for making decisions rather than the emotional contest of well-intentioned wills.

A nutrition evaluation is a blood test for nutrients in circulation in the body. If you undergo a nutrition evaluation and it shows that you do not have a full complement of nutrients required for bone growth, then a cautious, reasonable first step is to address that situation through food. After all, if eating foods rich in the nutrient combinations that keep bones flexible and healthy will do the trick, then you avoid any need to risk taking pharmaceuticals.

Unfortunately some physicians will smile indulgently if a patient asks about a nutrition evaluation or about trying food as a means of improving bone health, clearly humoring the patient while holding the certain conviction the patient will be back soon asking for the pharmaceuticals. And in our experience this is not a matter of the physician's age or gender, because a great deal of a doctor's attitude depends on the dogma, traditions, history, and even location of the medical school he or she attended and how doctrinaire the medical school dean was. And of course personal background plays a role.

So if you introduce nutrition and diet as route to bone health and you receive what seems a dismissive or patronizing—or even arrogant or haughty—response from your doctor, we encourage you to step back and consider the possible reasons for that response before formulating your own. Almost always your doctor feels responsible for protecting your health and well-being and has invested immeasurable time, energy, passion, and probably money in order to learn how to do so. Approving an unknown approach could leave the doctor on shaky ground. And a few physicians might sense a challenge to the foundational assumptions on which they've based their entire professional lives.

Since you can't know what's behind an emotional response without a lot more information, try to remain serene, tolerant, nonjudgmental—and to the extent possible, not intimidated. This is very important because you need your doctor's support in finding the most natural path to bone health, and in monitoring your progress. Without that support you could proceed on your own but most likely at very great expense. And even if you can procure a nutrition evaluation without a doctor's order, how would you find a doctor to interpret the results, work with you on a nutrition plan, and monitor your progress? Best to spend time up front speaking with a doctor you trust or seeking one who understands and accepts the wisdom of trying food first.

Ground Rules and Important Questions

Introducing the subject of nonpharmaceutical approaches to bone health may be tricky. We cannot provide you with a script, because each patient–doctor relationship is unique and complex. That said, we can offer you a few suggestions.

First, before you start a conversation with your doctor, be sure you are conversant with the key ideas: bone turnover, bone flexibility versus bone density, causes of bone density decline, medicine through food. Be able to explain what these phrases mean and how the processes work in your body.

Let the doctor know that should a nutrition evaluation show the need for high levels of one or more supplements, you would want her or him to supervise administration and monitor effects.

Hold to the belief that the benefit of talking with your doctor about bone health goes two ways. Should your doctor see possibilities for another mode of treatment that is also safe and effective, he or she will become engaged with you and later others will benefit. It is a fair exchange every way around.

The hallmark of education in any discipline or field of practice is knowing what the central questions are. Medical education rarely includes lectures, readings, or discussion about medicine through food—that is, the potential for our bodies to heal themselves if we provide high-quality nutrition by eating the right kinds and combinations of natural foods. Without such training, how would a busy physician know the core concepts, the research, or the current thinking in this field? Best if you raise the questions and then in discussion explore together for answers.

You may be surprised to find that your doctor is in fact well aware of the questions but lacks sufficient detail to be confident about addressing bone health through nutrition. Here are some questions and statements you might use to start a conversation:

- I've learned lately that calcium and vitamin D actually rely on a cast of other nutrients, vitamins, and enzymes—along with good gut health—in order to be properly absorbed and travel to bones. Could we consider a nutrition evaluation to get a baseline profile of the vital nutrients in circulation for me? Then we'd know how much I need to take in through food and what supplementation you would advise.

- I've learned lately about how bones grow and what happens to bone turnover when hormones decline. It seems that food, and especially properly prepared plant-based foods, can supplement hormones in a safe way; and adding exercise to the regimen increases these benefits. Can we talk about this as a possible approach to bone density loss?

- I've been avoiding saturated fats and cholestrol for years. Now, as a way to protect my bones, I want to add whole foods that contain saturated fats back into my diet. I'd like to explain my thinking and have your take on it.

- I'd like to include in my diet all the nutrients required for making bone, instead of just calcium and vitamin D, and then have another DEXA scan [a test that measures bone density] in two years to see whether this nutritional adjustment influences density. I've sketched out a treatment plan and would like to have your views on how I could improve my chances of success.

Be Prepared with Answers

Your doctor will almost certainly have questions in response to any or all of the conversation starters suggested above. As you plan for a discussion with

him or her about food as medicine for bone health, prepare yourself to answer questions like these:

- Why do you need a nutrition evaluation? We already know you've lost bone density. You need more calcium and pharmaceuticals.
- What's wrong with taking calcium supplements? You need them.
- What makes you think food could ever be powerful enough to change the status of bone health?
- I haven't seen any scientific evidence that people your age can prevent/stop bone loss by what they eat. Why would you proceed without scientific evidence when the risks associated with bone loss are proven?
- You have osteoporosis; don't you realize how serious this is? You need pharmaceuticals, not more food.

If you anticipate these kinds of questions, formulate your responses in advance, and remain confident, you will feel—and be—equal in the conversation. Your preparedness will engender respect, and your doctor may well feel—and become—a partner in a new approach to protecting bone health.

Calcium Dairy-Free

If you have known intolerances or allergies to dairy products or choose not to consume any animal-based food, your doctor may wonder how you can meet the bone health nutritional requirements. After all, for so many years milk (and dairy generally) was the gold standard insurance against calcium deficiency. Your doctor may be a firm believer that dairy is indispensable. If you do not consume dairy, it is best if you are prepared to address your doctor's double concern that you wish to avoid pharmaceuticals and dairy. Here, then, is some information about traditional plant-based diets that supply all the nutrients and enzymes necessary for bone health, including the calcium.

Choose calcium-rich plants. Decidedly, relying on plants for calcium takes a bit of planning. The greens listed here are higher in calcium than most other vegetables. We've included the percent of our bone health RDA of calcium that 1 cup of these greens supply:

Collards, cooked: 36 percent
Kale, raw: 14 percent
Turnip greens, cooked: 10 percent
Arugula, raw: 4 percent
Broccoli raab (rapini): 6 percent
Mustard greens, cooked; 15 percent

Notice that we include information about whether the calcium is available from the cooked or from the raw vegetables. Preparing the vegetables correctly helps to weaken oxalic acid, one of two chemicals in plant-based foods that bind with calcium and other mineral nutrients, rendering the nutrients unavailable for digestion. For a fuller discussion of oxalic acid and other anti-nutrients in plant-based foods, see chapter 4.

Provide support for mineral absorption. Be sure that your diet plus supplementation supplies the recommended dietary requirements for vitamins D_3 and K_2, magnesium, trace minerals, and enzymes that support mineral absorption and transport.

Combine cooked and raw greens. Everyone who relies on diet to prevent and treat bone loss wonders whether—and if so, how long—to cook greens.

Raw plants naturally contain enzymes that catalyze digestion, but cooking can destroy those enzymes. Yet boiling greens helps reduce the anti-nutrients that trap minerals. What's a savvy cook to do?

For maximum mineral absorption, boil greens for 3 or 4 minutes to break down some anti-nutrient defenses; then drain away the cooking water. But don't cook *all* of the vegetable portion you're going to serve. Set aside a bit of the raw. Then chop and mix the raw with the cooked. Eating them together will provide plenty of bioavailable nutrients and a helping of the vegetable's helpful enzymes, too.

And, as Helen's grandmother and her generation used to tell their children—and grandchildren: *Put a little vinegar on your greens*—raw and cooked. Before processed foods were so readily available, homemakers seemed to know intuitively that vinegar releases minerals from the leaves, which makes the stored calcium and other minerals much more available for absorption.

We encourage readers on dairy-free diets to make bone vinegars and use vinegar (see "Vinegar Wisdom" on page 53) on cooked and raw greens.

Include molasses. Include 1 tablespoon of unsulfured blackstrap molasses in your daily diet. But watch out. Unsulfured blackstrap molasses can differ dramatically in quality. One tablespoon of Plantation brand supplies 20 percent of daily calcium requirement and 20 percent daily potassium requirement, and it has just 42 calories. In 1 tablespoon of most other brands—including some brands of organic molasses—you'll find only 10 percent of your daily calcium requirement and one-third more calories. Poor-quality molasses products contain just 4 percent of daily calcium requirements, little of the other minerals, 70 calories, and some sodium to boot.

Make your own supplements. You can make your own nondairy calcium supplements using eggshells and your own bone-building vinegar. This will supply a great supplemental boost of all the ingredients for bone health.

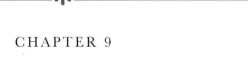

CHAPTER 9

Launch a Plan and Start Cooking

You may recall that Helen was astounded when she learned that little of the calcium in the calcium-rich foods she was eating had reached her bones. Preventing and arresting bone loss was more complex than just consuming foods containing the individual nutrients; her ultimate success depended on consuming foods containing specific nutrient groups—and on the form of the foods containing them.

That's where our recipes come in. Virtually all of them supply nutrient groups required for bone health and specify using foods in the form that supports nutrient absorption and transport. But does it matter *which* of the recipes you choose? Does it matter *how often* you include them in meal planning?

We'd like to say no, it doesn't matter—but nature isn't that indulgent. We want you to keep your bones healthy for the fullness of your life. So here's what we recommend. If you're younger than about 50, and you don't smoke or overindulge in alcohol and you aren't taking medicines that compromise your metabolic processes, it's fine to informally start trying out our recipes as you wish. But if you are in midlife, if you smoke, if you have a history of drinking alcohol to excess, or if you have been diagnosed with osteopenia or osteoporosis—or if, for any reason, your goal is to systematically prevent or treat osteopenia or osteoporosis—we advise taking a more methodical approach.

Toward that end, we have created a set of worksheets you may choose to use as you begin to introduce ingredients and combine foods to cook for bone health. All of the worksheets are in the appendix of this book, and you may download any or all from www.medicinethroughfood.com. Since each journey is individual—Helen followed her program over a two-year period—these worksheets are tools that help you create your path and measure your progress.

As you become familiar with the foods and nutrient combinations that promote bone health and then identify which you will require for your own Personal Nutrition Plan, please keep two things in mind: There are no one-size-fits-all plans, and there is never a time constraint. We invite you to move ahead at your own pace and in your own time, and enjoy the journey.

A Quick Start Guide

We've set out the journey to bone health in three phases. In Phase One, you will identify your nutrient gaps, if any, and identify foods, food combinations, and recipes that can help to close the gap. In Phase Two, you will create your Personal Nutrition Plan and begin to incorporate ingredients and recipes into your thinking, shopping, and cooking. In Phase Three, over a period of two years, you will close your nutrient gaps and strengthen your bones.

During the first fifteen months of her own personal journey toward bone health, Helen found it extremely useful to keep all of her notes, worksheets, recipes, and other tidbits of information in a journal. A notebook with dividers and pockets can be especially useful for this purpose, because you can organize the worksheets and reference documents in the pockets and add pages of notes over time. Or you can clip or staple worksheets to blank pages. The goal is to keep track of your progress and of the ingredients, food combinations, and recipes that make the most potent contribution to your bone health.

Table 9.1. One-Day RDA Calculation

Daily Meal	Vitamin D₃ 5,000 iu or 125 mcg	Calcium 800–1,000 mg	Phosphorus 700 mg	Vitamin A 10,000–15,000 iu (as retinol) or 700 mcg
Breakfast				
Breakfast Salad	150 mcg	600 mg	4,000 mg	100 mcg
with 2 poached eggs	100 mcg	...	...	...
Snack				
Trail mix, ½ cup	...	...	...	500 mcg
Lunch				
The Mix-Up Poke Bowl	24,000 iu	400 mg	300 mg	...
with sunned mushrooms	...	74 mg	...	...
canned salmon + adzuki bean	...	130 mg	...	...
Dinner				
Fava + Pork Sliders with yogurt	...	110 mg	50 mg	...
Fresh Mint Salad + ½ cup green beans	...	...	...	...

In this sample of a one-day RDA calculation, you'll notice that in the case of some highly nutritious bone-friendly plant-based foods, some nutrient values are above the upper limits of the recommended dietary allowance. However, many vitamins in plant-based foods undergo a conversion process that almost always leaves the vitamin supply within the recommended range upon digestion.

Phase One:
Document Your Starting Point

Your significant task in phase one is to take a Nutrition Evaluation test to determine your baseline nutrient profile. Recall that this is a simple blood test your doctor can order that shows how much of the baseline bone health RDA your diet is supplying. (See chapter 6 for more about RDAs.)

Ideally you want to know your levels for these nutrients: calcium, phosphorus, magnesium, vitamin D, vitamin C, vitamin A, vitamin B_1, vitamin B_2, vitamin B_3, vitamin B_6, vitamin B_{12}, folate (vitamin B_9), and trace minerals including zinc, copper, manganese, boron, iron, silica, and sulfur. If you have or suspect you are at risk of osteopenia or osteoporosis, you can discuss with your doctor whether you should take additional tests.

Later in this chapter, we discuss in detail how you can use testing as part of your plan to strengthen your bones: see "More About Testing" on page 101.

Phase Two: Gather Information

Phase Two includes several steps, and in this phase you'll be doing the bulk of the work required to incorporate food for bone health into your lifestyle.

Step 1. Compare your personal nutrient profile with our recommended RDA for maintaining strong bones and preventing bone loss. You can find this list in the "Our Nutrient Intake Recommendations" sidebar on page 65. With this information in hand you can identify the gap between nutrients your body already has in

Magnesium 600–1,000 mg	Vitamin K_2 80–300 mcg	Vitamin C	Protein 50–150 g	Trace Minerals	Probiotic	Phytoestrogen >50 mg
...	...	...	...	...	...	...
100 mg	14 mcg	...	...	...	...	...
...	...	...	...	...	variable amount	...
240 mg	...	...	23 g	...	...	...
...	...	...	17g	...	...	...
...	...	...	variable amount	...	...	...
100 mg	10 mcg	...	23 g	...	variable amount	variable amount
...	14 mcg	...	...	...	...	...

sufficient supply and those of which your body needs more for optimal bone building.

Step 2. Make a master list of what you buy, what you like to eat, what you like to cook—and how much, if at all, you rely on prepared foods. You may use the worksheet "My Food Preferences" on page 253 for this task. Please don't be anxious about writing down this information; this is not a record for the food police. You needn't show any of your worksheets to anyone. Rather, this worksheet provides an objective look at the bone health benefit you are receiving from what you eat.

Step 3. Take notes on your food consumption over the course of one week. What did you eat this week? What did you cook? You can use the worksheet "What I Ate This Week" on page 254 to record this information. Or you can simply make notes on plain paper in a journal. If you do so, be sure to make note of the dates for each week.

Step 4. Table 9.1, One-Day RDA Calculation, is a nutrient analysis of a day's meals. In this step of Phase Two, you will make your own analysis of the nutrient content of one day's worth of what you eat. The "One-Day RDA Calculation" worksheet on page 258 is a blank version of the chart that you can use to record your own data and make calculations. And once again, the purpose is to produce information you can use to make decisions about how and under what circumstances you may tweak your eating habits.

Step 5. This is a continuation of step 4. You'll keep tabulating one-day RDA calculations, and then you'll compile those once a week for four weeks. There are worksheets to help you with these calculations, too, which we explain in more detail later in the chapter.

Step 6. It is very likely that some or even most of the food you eat is supplying nutrients essential for bone health, yet the Western diet usually leaves some gaps. This step is a gap analysis—time to take an objective look at nutrients you are getting from your food and those you need to supply—through your diet and perhaps via some supplements. You can use the "Gap Analysis" worksheet on page 260 to help with this analysis.

Phase Three: Launch Your Personal Nutrition Plan

During Phase Three eating for bone health will gradually become a state of mind and ultimately a natural part of the way you practice the art of food preparation. For example, you will remember to enjoy that cube of Gouda all on its own instead of putting it on a cracker and to snack on a square or two of 70 percent to 90 percent organic dark chocolate during the day. When you have a salad or prepare dinner greens, you will remember to add a teaspoon of vinegar to the vegetables on your plate. And it will become a habit to spray a bit of magnesium oil on your arms and legs twenty minutes before you take a shower. You will become mindful of the bad effects of processed foods on your bones, and you'll replace packaged meals with dishes you create from scratch. You'll be mindful of saving money by eliminating processed food may allow you to include small amounts of pastured meat in your diet and excited when you top that fish dish with sesame seeds, knowing it will make a difference to your bones.

With your RDA calculations worksheets and your gap analysis worksheet for reference, use the "Personal Nutrition Plan" worksheet on page 261 to set out a strategy for creating a Personal Nutrition Plan for bone health. You may wish to structure your own plan, and your goals may be as broad or narrow as you wish: identify the most cost-effective source of organic greens: make bone vinegar and use it on greens; or set a goal that is wider in scope, such as create a plan to gradually replace processed food with fresh food.

Then use the "Bone Health Improvement Goals and Action Plans" worksheet on page 262 to set individual goals, create action plans to meet each goal, and keep notes on progress toward your goals. These goals will help you improve your bone health one step at a time. Remember, too, that your goals aren't set in stone, and you may find yourself revising them from time to time.

Here's an example of a goal and an action plan.

Goal: Increase the availability of calcium in the food I prepare.

Actions: Learn which greens to eat raw, steamed, and boiled (see page 52). Prepare three greens this week and use one teaspoon of vinegar on each serving.

Keep it simple! Other examples of goals include:

Improve my mineral absorption.
Learn to sprout grains.
Learn to ferment vegetables.
Reduce my intake of phytates and oxalates.

"Bone Health Plan and Progress Checklist," on page 263, is a checklist of actions that promote bone health. You may peruse the list and undertake whatever seems interesting and feasible, and you may skip around on the list, checking off items as you complete them in whatever order you wish. For example, you discover that you love drinking bone shrub and find it easy to drink bone shrub every day, so you might tick that box long before you are making four bone health meals four time, a week or have a second nutrition evaluation. In total, though, once you have

ticked all the boxes—again, give yourself two years to do so—you will be keeping your bones healthy naturally and perhaps every now and again having the pleasure of creating your own recipes. There will always be an opportunity to create a prototype and share it on the Medicine Through Food website; members of the community will be able to test and refine with you as you go along.

One Size Does Not Fit All

There is no one-size-fits-all plan. Many factors shape your bone health and nutritional needs: your stage of life; the state of your health including but not limited to bone health; conditions or illnesses you have that might suggest a modified RDA; whether you smoke; how much alcohol you drink; what you like to eat; and your healthcare provider's advice. Thus a premenopausal woman and a man who smokes may be the same age, but their nutritional needs may vary. Identical twin sisters may have different nutritional needs if one eats natural foods and the other a preponderance of prepared foods, or if one has had chemotherapy or a hysterectomy.

And we emphasize the value of intuition and the wisdom of the body. Often the most nutritious food is seasonal—your season, not another country's season—and you will digest most readily fresh food tuned to your environmental cycle. And your body may suggest where you begin eating for bone health and how you progress. Trust it. The bone health foods that you choose intuitively as your starting point are most likely the right ones for your body.

With your Personal Nutrition Plan at hand, and the knowledge you will gain over time about the nutritional profile of various foods, the bulk of your efforts over the following year to two

Eating with the Seasons

Left alone to make choices, children naturally choose foods that help to maintain a balance of nutrients for optimal health—and they often choose foods that are in season. Daoshing Ni, a doctor of Traditional Chinese Medicine and the founder of Yo San University, Marina del Rey, California, and the Tao of Wellness in Santa Monica, California, explains why eating with the seasons is nutritionally beneficial. Following his explanation, we set out the research on children's choices that demonstrate the wisdom of the body in naturally redressing deficiency by diet.

Daoshing Ni writes:

As earth goes around the sun, the length of days and degree of heat changes with the seasons and influences which plants grow to their maximum nutrient potential. Across the year seasons create ecological diversity that naturally provides the wide variety of nutrients essential to plant and animal—including our—life.

Strawberries, asparagus, cherries, peas, radishes, fava beans, apricots, artichokes, rhubarb, and mushrooms are in season during Spring. Summer brings us fruits that are sweet and plentiful: peaches, watermelon, plums, basil, figs, tomatoes, eggplant, zucchini, summer squash, and blueberries. Lighter carbohydrates and fibers from these vegetables and fruits are gentle on our digestive system and allow it to absorb and assimilate nutrients more easily in these two warmer seasons. Autumn
brings us cooler temperatures and sweet potatoes, kale, butternut squash, pears, pumpkin, apples, fennels, broccoli, grapes, cranberries, leeks, and walnuts. Warm soups, meats, and grains are natural sustenance in winter, especially if you live in a cold region where few plants grow.

So as you consider your Personal Nutrition Plan and develop a picture of the nutrients your food provides, please rely as much as possible on natural—and seasonal—foods.

Each food has a place in the diet in its own time, and foods align with the body's needs in climate and season. The body's natural inclination for health is demonstrated in a unique research study called The Wisdom of the Body study.

The Wisdom of the Body

In June 1939 Clara Marie Davis, an Illinois MD, told the Canadian Medical Association Section that, given a chance, just-weaned babies aged 6 to 11 months will choose the foods their bodies need. This wasn't speculation or presumption; Dr. Davis had run just such an experiment. She had provided a wide array of locally available natural animal- and plant-based foods—nothing canned, herbed, spiced, or otherwise adulterated—to a group of children. The foods were presented cooked and raw with sea salt as one of the choices.

Specific food choices varied among the children (because individual metabolic and biochemistry profiles vary), but all the children proved healthier—lean, strong, robust, cheerful, no constipation, few colds, virtually no major illnesses—than the control group whose diets were designed by nutrition experts of the time. Furthermore, during an epidemic the self-nourished children became less ill and recovered more quickly than the control group.

Dr. Davis's research became known as the Wisdom of the Body study, and though critics complained that her papers were thin on statistics and her samples were too small, many people knew she was right. Today people are visiting the study with renewed appreciation, especially because Dr. Davis said that gut health and pH balance influence health.

years will be to plan and use ingredients, dishes, and full meals most likely to strengthen your bones. Your Gap Analysis worksheet and your Personal Nutrition Plan will help you and your healthcare provider decide whether you need to take supplements as well and develop a strategy for gradually replacing supplements with food.

Summing Up

Tailoring a Personal Nutrition Plan for bone health is straightforward. First, by reading this book you'll become familiar with the various nutrient-rich foods and combinations that add up to a day's worth of minerals, vitamins, enzymes, and trace elements required for maintaining bone health. We'll help you put that new knowledge into action, slowly and gradually over a period of about two years, with the instructions in this chapter and some worksheets (included at the back of this book and available on our website). You can photocopy these worksheets; download them and print them at www.medicinethroughfood.com; or fill them out directly on your computer. Creating your route does take a bit of up-front planning. For most people, that planning will pay valuable dividends in fracture risk reduction.

Notice we said two years. That's an estimate. There's no set time frame for implementing a Personal Nutrition Plan. You can start with an intensive plunge or you can incorporate bone health food slowly over time. Aiming to achieve a Personal Nutrition Plan gradually over two years makes it likely that incorporating bone health will become a natural part of your lifestyle.

So please, don't rush. Research shows that if you develop new habits steadily over time, they are likely to endure. And your patience will be rewarded. Over time, your complete bone health nutrition profile will emerge in your Food Journal. It won't be long before you know instinctively what kinds of delicious dishes will satisfy your palate, that of friends and family, and everyone's bones.

Now let's briefly recap the tasks involved in creating a Food Journal and Personal Nutrition Plan.

Obtain a nutrition evaluation. Just by taking a simple blood test, you can receive a lab report that tells you how much of each bone health nutrient is present and accounted for in your system. The results will fall along a continuum. You may find that your status quo way of eating is meeting all your nutrient needs. Or you may learn that you lack some trace minerals you can easily fold into your diet, or that you need to begin cooking for bone health in earnest immediately. If you have osteoporosis, there are additional tests your doctor can order to provide more detailed information about your bone metabolism, such as rate of breakdown versus bone building. We discuss these tests in more detail below.

Keep notes about what you eat. Remember, this isn't a list for the food police; rather, it is valuable data that will reveal the source of nutrients in your diet. You can write your notes on plain paper or use the worksheets included in the appendix.

Do a gap analysis. This helps you determine what's sufficient and what's missing in your diet's bone health nutrients. When you know what's missing, you'll have an idea about which foods to incorporate, which recipes might be most helpful, and how often to cook for bones. For this step, we've provided worksheets you can use to track your progress with bone health cooking to close the gap. The worksheets cover a full two-year period, though you may choose to move into bone health cooking more quickly.

Get cooking! Use the recipes exclusively or use them as tools and as a jumping-off point for learning about ingredients, food preparation, and combinations that support bone health. Then you might like to experiment, widen your horizons, create recipes, and watch out for recipes online or in print that seem just right for bone health. We hope you will share them with us on the Medicine Through Food website.

Getting Started

This plan is purposely designed so that you can tailor it to meet your own needs and lifestyle. On average, new habits take hold over two years. For practicality, we've set out benchmarks in the worksheets as Year 1 and Year 2, but starting points vary widely so all are fully flexible and you can feel free to set your own time lines. Try your hand, see what feels right, and progress at your own pace.

Naturally the shape of your plan will reflect your age and stage, your health history, eating habits and patterns, allergies, your experience with supplements, your healthcare provider's approach to medicine, and your approach to change. Along the way we hope you'll post your questions, suggestions, caveats, and successes on the book's website.

So please, get ready to get started but also, get ready to start slowly. The Chinese philosopher Lao-tzu, who reportedly lived in the 7th century BC, wrote in Tao Te Ching that "a journey of a thousand miles begins with a single step." He was a wise person. If you take your time, one step at a time, you'll enjoy the journey and measure the miles in peace of mind, knowing you're taking care of yourself in the happiest, safest, most satisfying way possible. It will take time before the big picture of foods and nutrients, exercise and supplementation runs in the background as you shop, prepare, cook, season, and choose foods that feed your gut bacteria and your bones.

Also, before setting out to cook for bone health—and perhaps before inviting other people including your doctor and your family to learn, understand, support, and join you—it is best if you address uncertainties you may have. If they hover in the background, you risk giving yourself mixed messages or doing what you think you should do, but then abandoning the project because you feel confused or unsettled by unanswered questions.

Thus, as your very first step, we invite you to take some time to reflect. List your concerns and your ideas for addressing them. Here are some concerns that Laura's patients and the people who have attended our bone health presentations have expressed to us, along with our suggestions about how to address them.

Concern: Does your approach conflict with my doctor's advice?

Suggestion: Review chapter 8, *Speaking with Your Doctor*. Then discuss your ideas with your doctor or healthcare provider.

Concern: Is it safe to both cook for bone health *and* take the pharmaceuticals my doctor has prescribed?

Suggestion: Yes, research supports the idea that nutrition improves the effects of bone health pharmaceuticals. We recommend that you do a baseline nutrition evaluation now, and then another one 6 or 12 months from now, depending on how much cooking for bone health you introduce. Keep your healthcare provider involved at every stage.

Concern: What is the relationship between natural food and bone health?

Suggestion: In general, natural food supplies nutrients plus digestive enzymes. You'll find a fuller discussion of this relationship in chapters 3 and 4.

Concern: Bone health cooking includes full-fat dairy, grass-fed marbled meat, and plant-based foods that supply plant hormones. This directly contradicts the advice we've been given over the years about fat, meat, and plant hormones. Which advice is right?

Suggestion: Consider this. Science and medicine are evolutionary. As medical technologists refine research tools and improve the ability to gather data at the cellular and molecular levels, facts help scientists

modify assumptions and advice, wh[...] change over time. Helen has three chil[...] With each pregnancy, she received differe[...] advice about vitamins and about weight gain. Closer to home, the advice about bone health pharmaceuticals has changed dramatically from automatic prescription to extreme caution and time limits.

So yes, advice changes with findings. Scientific method is about making a hypothesis, testing the hypothesis, and learning from the results. That is how medical science aims to help people live longer lives in better health, and why we rigorously review valid, reliable new data as a possible source of better recommendations.

But even more strongly we invite you to consider the reason we propose choosing and preparing natural food: the multitude of unsettling legitimate concerns about processed foods fade away. You no longer have to worry about chemicals in the food, which ones do or don't cause illness and disease and if so in what amounts, and whether the studies are unbiased and conclusive.

More About Testing

As you're launching your Food Journal, speak with your doctor about the nutrition evaluation, a simple blood test that shows levels of nutrients present in your system. The test results will fall along a continuum. You may find that what you naturally enjoy eating is keeping your bones healthy, or that you lack some trace minerals you can easily fold in, or that you need to begin cooking for bone health in earnest immediately. If you have osteoporosis there are additional tests your doctor can order to provide more specific

...ne metabolism such as ... bone building. We de-...below.

...our personal nutrient ...d Journal they are a ...mation, not a report ...judgment implied or made in assessing the patterns that emerge. You need to know what nutrients you're getting from the food you eat so you can decide what you might need to alter for bone health. After all, cooking to naturally prevent and treat bone loss isn't common knowledge, and few people are routinely educated in the ancient arts of preparing foods to foster a healthy gut and mineral absorption. That's part of why there's so much perilous bone loss among seemingly healthy people, and it's part of the reason we wrote this book.

While there are recommended daily allowances for a few minerals and vitamins that promote bone health—typically calcium, vitamin D, and magnesium—the overall RDA for preventing and treating bone density loss is broader, incorporating additional vitamins and minerals as discussed in chapter 6.

What to Test For?

Ideally, a nutrition evaluation should include your levels for these nutrients: calcium, phosphorus, magnesium, vitamin D, vitamin C, vitamin A, vitamin B_1, vitamin B_2, vitamin B_3, vitamin B_6, vitamin B_{12}, folate (vitamin B_9), and trace minerals. At the writing of this book no test specific to vitamin K_2 is available.

Additionally, testing for fatty acids, carbohydrate metabolism, liver function, digestive health/gut flora, and antioxidant function are going to help you see a fuller picture of your overall body function.

Bone Density Tests and Other Tests

As explained in chapter 1, bones are constantly undergoing both formation of new cells and resorption of old cells (bone turnover). There are three types of tests that provide important and different information about how well your bones are keeping up with balanced turnover.

DEXA (OR DXA) SCANS: START EARLY

The DEXA scan (also known as a DXA scan) is the most widely used bone density test in the United States. The results are called T scores. Using enhanced X-ray technology, DEXA measures the density of your bone compared with the density of an average healthy young person who has peak bone mass. Typically physicians recommend the test for women 65-plus whose estrogen, and often bone density, has declined. If the test shows osteopenia or osteoporosis, doctors typically recommend a DEXA scan every two years.

Estrogen plays a central role in bone health right from puberty, and menopause typically begins well before age 65. Therefore, if DEXA is the scan of choice, Laura suggests having a DEXA scan before age 65, while there is still time to strengthen bone that shows very little loss—or to get started on a bone health diet for those whose bones suggest significant dietary deficiency. Scanning when the bones are already osteoporotic turns many doctors and patients toward pharmaceutical treatment—though at this writing the bisphosphonate treatment period is just three to five years. After that it's back to square one (see chapter 7 for more about pharmaceuticals).

Estrogen plays a vital role in creating bone able to resist aging. Age of menopause is strongly genetically linked, so absent other factors such as health problems and severe medications, in most cases you will reach menopause within a few years one way or another at the age your mother did. If the age of first DEXA scan were lowered to, for example, five years before a woman's menopausal transition, then there would be ample time to strengthen bone against future loss and reduce the chance of relying on pharmaceuticals. Preventive scanning would no doubt save a great deal of money worldwide.

FRAX—FRACTURE RISK ASSESSMENT

The WHO fracture risk assessment tool FRAX appears to be better than lumbar spine and femoral neck T scores (DEXA scans) for assessing fracture risk. The FRAX tool considers bone density, but it is not limited to this, and repeatedly performs better than bone density alone.

See the resources section to learn about an online tool that can assist with fracture assessment. You can discuss this with your doctor.

MARKERS OF BONE RESORPTION

Tests that measure markers of bone turnover balance are extremely useful as a baseline, especially if you have a first test done before you start a program to strengthen your bones naturally. Then results from annual repeats of the test will give you an idea how effective your bone health strategies are. Depending on your age, health status, and other variables such as estrogen levels, exercise, and what you eat, these tests can be a great window into the functioning of your body and how the steps you take are affecting it. There are several types of these sensitive tests, which your doctor can order to understand more about how your bone tissue is functioning.

Osteocalcin (serum N-terminal). Osteocalcin, also known as bone gla protein (BGLAP), is a bone-specific protein that has proven to be a sensitive and specific marker of osteoblast activity. Activated osteocalcin requires the presence of both vitamins D_3 and K_2.

Alkaline phosphatase (bone-specific). Alkaline phosphatase in serum has been used for more than 50 years to monitor bone metabolism, and it is still the keystone marker. Alkaline phosphatase, an enzyme, attaches to the surface of osteoblasts.

Hydroxyproline-containing peptides. Urinary hydroxyproline values rise after menopause and fall when antiresorptive drugs such as hormones or bisphosphonates are taken. They will also fall as turnover trends toward creating bone density.

Propeptide type 1 collagen. Type 1 collagen peptides in the blood are a marker of bone formation.

CTX. Elevated levels indicate increased bone resorption. They will drop as your bone breakdown stops.

Anti-Mullerian Hormone Test. As of this writing there is a new test reported that helps predict whether a woman will lose bone faster than average. Ideally the test is taken in early menopause transition, when there is still ample estrogen present and bone building effects will still be strong.

Keep a Food Journal

Keep a Food Journal. In it document the ordinary day-to-day patterns of shopping, cooking, and eating that make up your food life. Accuracy is essential. No one will judge your choices. In fact, no one sees these pages except you, unless you invite someone else to review them with you.

Your Food Journal will help you discover how much of each vital nutrient you are already getting from what you eat. Here's why that matters: You'll find out how much of your diet already supplies nutrients required for bone health, and what aspects of your diet you need to tweak. You may be pleasantly surprised to find that much of your diet already supplies nutrients required for bone health. Or, more like Helen, you may be chagrined to find that your healthy eating habits are actually skewed toward bone loss. Perhaps your busy life has called you to convenience, take-out, and packaged food that may mean your diet is poor-to-impoverished in bone health nutrients. But once you know your personal baseline, whatever it is, then you can make a realistic plan.

Your Food Journal can be the foundation on which you fashion meals that include the right mixes and balances of bone health nutrients in your daily meals. For example, you can calculate how much calcium you need, which foods you'd like to include that supply the calcium you need, which foods are good companions for the calcium-rich foods, and which recipes will supply sufficient calcium to reduce the amount of calcium you take by supplementation or enable you to leave out calcium supplements altogether. You can calculate how much vitamin D you need and how much of each food will supply it—and what supplementation if any you or your healthcare provider wish to include. You can even chart a gradual shift from supplements to nutrition as choosing the right foods becomes second nature.

The first Food Journal pages can be "My Food Preferences" and "What I Ate This Week" (see pages 255–257). Or you can simply choose a favorite notebook and record the information in your own style. What's important is creating an accurate picture of your food profile and, from there, making a realistic plan to redress deficits. You may make adjustments monthly, weekly, or daily. Any time frame is good. What matters is that in your own time you begin to incorporate cooking for bone health into your daily life.

Note: The amount of calcium you require depends on your age, your bone health status, and how much you consume. Keep in mind that the human body can process no more than 500 mg of calcium at a time, so depending on your supplement needs you will have to take it twice or three times a day, ideally with meals. From your journal you will develop a profile that suggests whether or not you need calcium supplementation. However, as a starting point Laura recommends calcium supplementation of no more than 400 mg per day. This gives you a good base but still leaves the room for natural sources in food.

Flesh Out Your Plan

Once you have spoken with your doctor about results of your nutritional evaluation and other tests she or he may have ordered, you're ready to fully launch your Personal Nutrition Plan. Read on for more guidance on how to implement the plan over time. We'll say again too, that the timing of your plan will be as personal as your food choices. Please feel free to tweak the timings to suit the realities of your lifestyle and personal or family needs.

Use the Nutrient Calculations Worksheet

An important step will be to calculate the nutrients you're getting from the food you currently eat. The "One-Day RDA Calculation" worksheet on page 258 is the form you can use. Before you try to fill out the worksheet, though, take a look at table 9.1, which is a completed example of the worksheet, using recipes from this book. The RDAs for bone health, set out in table 9.1 are, you may recall from chapter 6, slightly different from the USDA general RDA recommendations. The RDAs for each meal of the day show in the columns.

As we prepared this example, we included the three usual meals, breakfast, lunch, and dinner, plus one snack (though most people will have more than one snack during the day).

We measured all the major bone health nutrients: calcium, phosphorus, magnesium, vitamin K_2, vitamin D, and protein.

With the exception of vitamin K_2, the bone health chef who filled out this example requires no additional supplementation—at least not based on this one day of eating. All other nutrients are covered—no calcium pills needed.

Keep in mind that if you are already showing osteopenia or osteoporosis then therapeutic doses of nutrients may be advised by your healthcare provider. If this is the case, the One-Day RDA calculation will be a guide for the additional nutrients, not the ones you are taking therapeutically.

Fill in Your Own Data

Now that you've studied the example, it's time to try filling out a worksheet yourself. But first, we want to point out that it's beyond the scope of this book to provide nutritional information about all the foods that you might choose to eat. This exercise in filling out a one-day profile is a way for you to get started finding out whether what you like to eat is also kind to your bones. After you've spent time with this book learning about our world of bone health nutrition and food—and then after you've filled out your first few profiles with what you usually eat in a

day—you'll discover whether there's a nutrition gap you choose to address. From there, over time you can review foods you like and foods you decide to add.

There are websites that will be useful as you are building the profile of what you eat, outside of the recipes in this book, including NutritionData.self .com, Nutrition.gov, and Healthaliciousness.com. These sites contain complete nutrition information for many foods, and will help you understand the nutrition of the foods you are choosing.

Year One: First Month

Once you have a sense of your patterns and habits, it's time to take a closer look. One way to do that is through a gap analysis. The example earlier in this chapter showed the result only from a single day of eating; for a more valid picture of your nutrient intake, you need to look at your intake over time. This will show you what's sufficient and what's missing in bone health nutrients. When you know what's missing, you'll have an idea about which foods to incorporate, which recipes might be most helpful, and how often to cook for bones. Check the "Gap Analysis" worksheet on page 260, which you can use for notes about which nutrients you are lacking, what foods you can add to your shopping list to supply those nutrients, and which recipes you'll try making.

At this stage, you may want to use the recipes in this book exclusively, preparing them exactly according to the written instructions. Once you gain confidence, we encourage you to also use our recipes as a jumping-off point for learning about ingredients, food preparation, and combinations that support bone health. Take your time. Find some recipes that appeal to you and study them. Taking the time to study recipes will reinforce everything you've learned so far about the intersection of food, healthy digestion, and bone metabolism. Which greens should be steamed before eating? Which combinations of food provide the highest nutrient levels? Then you might like to experiment, widen your horizons, create recipes, and seek out recipes online or in books and magazines that seem just right for bone health. We hope you will share your best creations on the Medicine Through Food website.

Year 1: First Six Months

At this point you will have an excellent idea of your nutrition status, what you are consuming, and what you need to supplement. It is time to start your journal. Incorporate new bone friendly whole foods each month for six months—and join the online bone health cookbook community at the book's website: www.medicinethroughfood.com.

Refer also to the "Bone Health Plan and Progress Checklist" on page 263. You can copy this page and use it as a checklist as you accomplish tasks and try new things.

So here's the next step. At some time in each month for six months running—at this stage aim not to skip months—introduce at least four new bone-friendly foods to your meal plans. Then, when you have woven in all the Bone's Favorite Foods—the list is on page 116—dip into our recipes to find more bone-healthy ingredients and fold some of those into your meal planning, too. Here's another chance to be creative. You might find it fun to pair up foods in new ways, to create recipes and share and partake in recipes at the book's website. For example you might decide to add organic chicken thighs to Mexican beans or thigh meat to enchiladas. You might like to note in your journal the reasons each food you add is a bone health choice. Now it's time to consider

recipes rather than single ingredients, and here's where *The Healthy Bones Nutrition Plan and Cookbook* community comes into play. You might find it fun to share ideas, food pairings, and recipes.

Year 1: Second Six Months

During the second six months, you increase the effectiveness of your bone health efforts.

At this point, depending on how much you have done in the first six months, you may want to obtain a second nutrition evaluation, though you can wait until the end of the first year.

The instructions for this phase are simple, crisp, and clear:

- Four bone health meals four times a week.
- After clearance from your healthcare provider, exercise each day you include a bone health meal.
- If you haven't already, make your bone health vinegar and drink your bone shrub daily.

Year 2: First Six Months

Here you may begin to see your efforts pay off. If you did not after the first six months, have a second nutrition evaluation.

We also advise you to eliminate processed foods from your diet. To the degree you balance nutrients, your body will shift the messages it sends and you'll want to eat differently. You won't crave sugar. Interesting salads, marbled meat, steamed vegetables, soups, and fruits will appeal to you; you'll search them out and even turn to them if you tend to overeat when you're stressed.

This isn't bone health magic. Rather, it's allowing the body's natural needs to express themselves. Processed foods and unhealthy ingredients upset the apple cart. When you take

Sample Transition Plan

Here is an example transition plan that may
be useful as you move from more familiar
foods to those that may be less familiar.

Year 1	Transition	Year 2 (especially if you have osteopenia or osteoporosis)
Apple cider vinegar on salads.	Apple cider vinegar or aged balsamic vinegar on lightly boiled greens.	Bone vinegar shrub every day and a teaspoon of vinegar on all greens.
One tofu recipe each month.	Miso soup.	Natto powder or natto.
Find a source of pastured eggs.	Find a source of raw milk Gouda.	If you can obtain raw milk, make butter at home.
Learn which foods are prebiotic and probiotic and include some of each at least once each week.	Include prebiotic foods twice each week. Include probiotic foods twice each week.	Ferment your own vegetables.
Include mushrooms in at least two meals each week.	Except for maitake, sun your own mushrooms.	Create one or more mushroom recipes and consider sharing them on the Medicine Through Food website.
Use organic sugar exclusively.	Include some maple syrup in your cooking.	Except on occasion, use molasses as your only sweetener.
Include fish in your meals at least twice each week.	Unless you have restrictions due to hypercholesteremia, include seafood in your meals at least twice each week.	Include fish eggs in your diet twice each week.
Choose breads made with sprouted wheat or other sprouted grain flour.	Make your own Ezekiel bread.	Limit your bread consumption to sourdough, rye, and Ezekiel, all preferably homemade.
Add chicken drumsticks to your menu.	Add chicken livers to your menu.	Add all the gizzards to your menu.
Try soaking and sprouting beans.	Trying soaking Brazil nuts.	Try soaking and sprouting seeds.

those disruptors you find out what foods your body needs. This is the Wisdom of the Body, as described earlier in this chapter.

Year 2: Second Six Months

After 18 months you will be used to shopping and cooking for bone health. At this stage you'll have the space and understanding to sprout your beans, and maybe even seeds and nuts.

New projects to try include: Fermenting your flours, or sprouting, drying, grinding, and fermenting your own grains for flour, if it interests you. If not make sure to use sprouted flour in your cooking.

Your body should be stronger now. Perhaps you can incorporate a new exercise routine—maybe there's a class or a sport you've always wanted to try.

At the end of two years, your final nutrition evaluation should be done. If you suffer from osteopenia or osteoporosis, a set of bone turnover tests should be repeated.

If you have osteopenia or osteoporosis, have successfully completed two years, meet your daily dietary RDAs, yet still show bone mineral density loss on scan, we recommend that you supplement daily with:

- Bone vinegar shrub
- Vitamins K_2 and MK7

- Collagen powder
- Vitamin C
- Daily exercise
- Cod liver oil

Also strongly consider these guidelines:

- Avoid all processed food.
- Sprout grains, and try sprouting seeds, nuts, and beans.
- Make a sourdough bread starter and bake your own sourdough bread.
- Choose to eat sourdough, Ezekiel, and rye breads.
- Consider starting a backyard garden or putting up a small greenhouse to grow your own organic greens and herbs.

We are excited for each and every person who will keep bones healthy by cooking for bone health, and we wish everyone great pleasure in shopping, cooking, and enjoying the foods you prepare and the fruits of your labor.

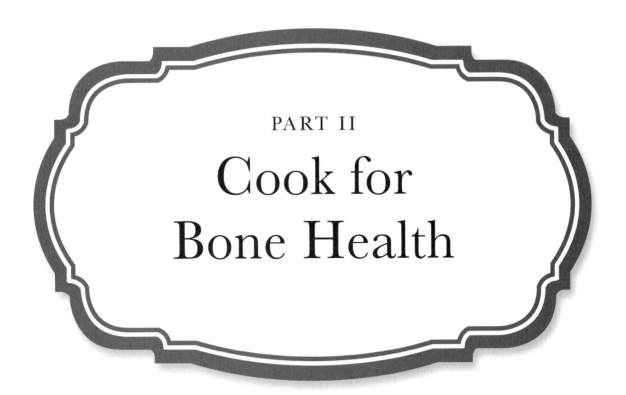

PART II

Cook for Bone Health

Cooking has fallen so far from favor that Planet Earth is clogged from the ocean bottoms up with the paper, hardened plastic, tin, and Styrofoam used to package processed food and drink. Human health is slowly, steadily declining due to the effects of consuming the preservatives, artificial coloring, endocrine disruptors, and other chemicals that are part of the processed, packaged, fast-food deal. It is so much nicer to choose fresh ingredients and prepare them at leisure in order to offer yourself, and perhaps family and friends, food that is delicious, nourishing, and lovely to behold—with no hidden chemicals.

All well and good, you say, but who has the time to cook from scratch? We want to make a case for finding the time.

Here is our opening argument. If you were to pour into one of your drinking glasses all the chemicals used to prepare, preserve, and store a week's worth of processed food, along with the chemicals used to manufacture that food's packaging—including some known and suspected carcinogens—would you drink the contents yourself or offer it to your children? Of course not. And yet if you eat processed foods, you're consuming these chemicals, even though usually you can't see or taste them unless they are weighty with artificial flavors.

Even so-called fresh food may have an invisible chemical component. Once, Helen noticed that all the supermarket chickens looked alike, so she called the chain's consumer line and asked if the chickens were treated in some way. Yes, she was told. In order to eliminate germs, they said—and okay, to increase shelf life—all our chickens are washed in Clorox bleach. Bleach? Oh no. Let me out of here.

Another time Laura noticed that a head of organic lettuce in her fridge (purchased from a different supermarket chain) was still fresh as a daisy 10 days after she bought it. She called the supermarket. Sure enough, they spray the leaf produce with a cocktail of artificial chemicals guaranteed to preserve original color for two weeks, with not a sign of brown edges. And yes, they apply that spray to all the produce—even the organic stuff.

That's our cooking-to-avoid-toxins argument. Now we'd like to let you in on a not-so-secret secret—the joy of cooking that scientists say can release endorphins, which are hormones that bind with opiate receptors in the brain, spinal cord, and gastrointestinal tract to erase feelings of pain, induce calm, and reduce inflammation.

The first moment of cooking pleasure is opening unbleached paper wrapping around fresh food, and gently rinsing, washing, or wiping food that has been allowed to grow or roam naturally. Let's say you are looking at a chicken. You know that this bird you're preparing to eat has enjoyed its life roaming free—enjoyed the hum of pecking at worms and seeds in the natural cycle of things—and that it will be deliciously rich in authentic poultry flavor—something that will surprise and delight many consumers.

This is the pleasure of being in harmony with your food—with nature—a pleasure that opens the five senses and releases a deep sense of well-being. Chopping *herbes fines*, jointing poultry, rubbing beef with garlic cloves you've halved and left to stand for 10 minutes, creating vegetable chunks from zucchini, peeling broccoli stalks, and blanching green beans—all these and the dozens of tiny tasks associated with preparing ingredients for dishes you will cook in your cooking space will steadily release endorphins that relax your body and prime you for optimal digestion.

Perhaps you agree that creating meals from natural whole foods is more pleasurable than opening boxes, cans, and pre-mixes but you still have a holdout: It's too expensive.

We disagree. By weight and volume, processed food is expensive and poor value for money. You pay for all the labor it takes to process, preserve, and package what's on the shelf, and then what you buy doesn't offer good nutritional value. Processed, previously heated foods interfere with gut bug health and force digestion too soon, leaving you undernourished and also hungry much sooner than you would be had you eaten whole foods. Furthermore, with processed foods it's one step forward and at least one step back in terms of nutrition. Since processing destroys so many natural nutrients and digestive enzymes, it's hard to know how much of a processed food to eat in order to stay within a desirable body mass index, stay healthy, and keep your gut bugs healthy, too.

This isn't pie in the sky. We are not wealthy, and yet, for the sake of our health, we and our spouses made a commitment to eat organically grown fruit, prepare organically grown vegetables, and eat hormone-free meat—treating ourselves to organic, pasture-raised meat and poultry when we can. By reducing the amount of animal protein we buy, and by preparing it at home so it is scrumptious and we can savor every bite, we find that within our budget we can easily afford organic plant-based foods. Organic greens need so little dressing up except for ½ teaspoon of apple cider vinegar and/or some butter or ghee, there's lots of time to dream up salads and side dishes that have brought vegetables and salads front and center on our families' most-requested lists.

So if you're new to cooking, picture yourself in the center of your cooking space. Maybe it's a hot plate and maybe it's a chef's cooking theater; no matter, it's your cooking space. Then feel the space boundaries opening out until you can stretch yourself and know there's plenty of room to maneuver. With a sharp knife, a cutting board, and some heavy-bottomed pans to work with, you're ready to set out ingredients and take great pleasure in the preparation.

What follows is the cookbook per se. We've organized the recipes by parts of meals in American—and in fact most Western—households. But there are no rules about when you eat the things you like. Laura has The Mix-Up Poke Bowl at breakfast. Sides can be snacks, salads can be main stage; no matter. What does matter here is counting up the nutrients you're consuming and measuring your totals against what you need for your own bone health profile.

The Finishing Touch

Whether you are dining alone or among others, take the time to create a pretty plate with whatever you have in the fridge. That sprig of parsley or dill is rich with calcium, the olive rich with healthful oil, that touch of roe will feed your bones as little else can, and—not to spoil the mood—that tasty cornichon is just what your gut bacteria crave. A dessert spoon of fig jam can cheer up a wedge of Gouda; a small mound of chopped red or yellow bell pepper or a curly bright-green lettuce leaf can brighten up the most mundane of sandwiches.

Then set the table with a tablecloth or a place mat, a napkin in a pretty ring if you have one, and the condiments (if any) to accompany the dishes you will enjoy. If it's dinnertime, light a small candle. Then take a moment to take pleasure in the welcoming site of your table.

Fractional Absorption

Thousands of web pages detail the amount of calcium in this or that plant or dairy food but rarely mention that you may be able to absorb and/or use only a fraction of the calcium. That's why nutritionists speak of fractional absorption rather than absolute content when calculating a food's calcium benefit. They measure the amount of the nutrient that is bioavailable, which means free to be absorbed and able to most efficiently be used by the body.

The reasons for fractional absorption differ with the food. For example, in plants there are chemicals that bind with phosphorus and calcium—in fact with all minerals—and keep them locked up during digestion so they are not free to be absorbed into circulation. Or the food itself may not contain the companion nutrients required for transporting the calcium into circulation.

Consider spinach. It is very rich in calcium, but fractional calcium absorption is just 5 percent. That's because the compound that binds with minerals is abundant in spinach and also because the nutrients required to transport calcium aren't present. So for bone health, kale is a better choice. Kale is relatively low in chemicals that bond with minerals, and it includes calcium's partner nutrients phosphorus and magnesium. So you can absorb a lot of the calcium in kale— even more than from pasteurized milk.

Bioavailability also matters when you are considering sources of nutrients other than calcium and companion minerals. For example, if you want more omega-3 fatty acids in your diet, does it matter whether the source is ground flaxseed or a fish? It does.

Flaxseed and fish both contain omega-3, but human bodies much more readily absorb and process fish oil, so your body is able to use the omega-3 from a fish or from fish oil quite easily. Not so when it comes to plants. Our bodies have to work harder to absorb and use plant compounds, so you may need 10 measures of flaxseed oil to 1 measure of fish oil. Next, the body needs to transform the nutrients into usable forms, and fish oil versions of omega-3 are much more efficiently transformed by the body than is the flax version of omega-3.

Fractional absorption rates are very useful when planning daily requirements because they suggest how much will be absorbed and how much your body will be able to use—and that, in turn, suggests how much of a food you need to eat to obtain a certain percent of the target nutrient total for the day, and also which foods are the most efficient sources of a given nutrient.

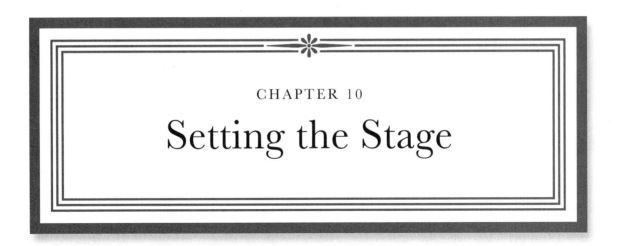

CHAPTER 10

Setting the Stage

As you begin your cooking-for-bone-health journey, we hope that some practical information—guidelines on diet for bone health, a list of bones' favorite foods, tips on stocking the pantry and the fridge, and advice on choosing bone-friendly ingredients—may prove useful. We hope you will choose organic ingredients for all your cooking whenever possible.

Eleven Dragons: Guiding Principles for Bone Health

Nine Dragons is a scroll almost certainly by 13th-century Chinese artist Chen Rong, a painter famous for his depiction of dragons. The scroll's nine reptiles, symbols of fertility, are forces of nature that permeate Taoist philosophy. They direct humans to live in harmony with nature. Likewise our Eleven Dragons are principles of cooking for bone health that are rooted in and arise from patterns of the natural world.

Keep these guidelines in mind as you develop your Personal Nutrition Plan (see chapter 9). Return to them often. Over time they will prove invaluable as you nurture your intuition and build the habits of cooking for bones. Notice that vitamin K_2, coconut oil, phytoestrogens, and exercise can each independently be agents for bone density growth.

1. Achieve the right ratios. Balance vitamin and mineral intakes, especially calcium, vitamin D, and vitamin K_2. Vitamin K_2 alone will increase bone strength.
2. Learn the facts about fats. Coconut oil increases bone strength, while trans fats will damage your arteries and bones. You can eat coconut oil out of the jar by the spoonful or use it in cooking.
3. Drink bone shrub (the recipe is on page 130) and /or nettle infusion (the recipe is on page 126) every day. Bone-strengthening herbs

alone increase bone density, and the additional benefits are enormous.

4. Consume phytoestrogens. Phytoestrogens alone increase bone density.

5. Nurture and protect gut bacteria. They are a key to long-term bone health.

6. Exercise. Exercise alone will increase bone strength.

7. Manage anti-nutrients. Know which foods hide anti-nutrients and take action to weaken their chokehold on phosphorus and other minerals.

8. If you drink soda, make your own. Drinking commercial sodas will damage your bones.

9. Consider raw dairy. State law differs; investigate to learn about possibilities.

10. Consume vegetables. Aim for several cooked and one raw vegetable dish a day.

11. Be realistic and be prepared. It takes two years to change a lifestyle. The benefits will last a lifetime.

Bone's Favorite Foods

In part 1, we reported that foods in natural form store vitamins, minerals, nutrients, and enzymes. These team up to support the healthy function of cells including the cells that make up DNA. Bone's favorite foods are especially rich in the nutrients that keep bones strong and keep new bone growing. Not only are these foods rich in at least one key nutrient and live enzymes, but when eaten in the right form, all are easily digested. In the presence of a normally healthy gut, virtually all are well absorbed and used. For example, omega 3 from wild unprocessed fish is 100 percent available while omega 3 from flaxseed is less so.

Table 10.1. Bone's Favorite Foods, on page 116, includes our Recommended Dietary Allowance—the amounts we recommend to sustain bone health and treat bone loss—for each nutrient in the group of nutrients that work together to support bone health. It also provides general guidance about how much of each nutrient, on average, one serving provides. Once you've reviewed the list, you'll find yourself more aware of these foods when you're shopping—the way a new word you learn seems to pop up often when you hadn't noticed it before. You'll become confident to use these foods as you work with your Personal Nutrition Plan, track your nutrient intake, and start following your inspiration to create recipes of your own.

Stock the Pantry

The pantry will be a joyful place when you've stocked it for bone health cookery. Start with lots of fresh herbs from your garden, windowsill, or greenhouse that you've dried and stored in bags or glass containers and organic apple cider vinegar. Later we'll speak about foraging for herbs to make bone vinegar. Here's our list of foods to keep on hand in the pantry and fridge. You'll be using them regularly as your bone health cooking repertoire expands.

In the Pantry

Almonds: sprouted by you and then dehydrated or purchased sprouted; dried almonds

Apricots: dried, unsulfured

Beans, fava: dried or sprouted

Beans, garbanzo: dried or sprouted

Beans, mung: dried or sprouted

Beans, white: dried unsprouted, or dried already sprouted

Berries, goji

Chocolate, dark: 85 percent cocoa

Cocoa powder

Coconut manna, organic

Cornstarch

Flour, rye: organic sprouted

Flour, unbleached all-purpose: sprouted organic

Fruit, dried: including dates, figs, prunes, and
raisins (oil-free)

Garlic

Ghee

Lentils

Molasses, blackstrap unsulfured:
Plantation brand

Mulberries

Mushrooms, sunned, dried (the vitamin D
endures for up to one year)

Oil, avocado

Oil, coconut, organic

Oil, walnut

Onions, all types

Pecans, sprouted

Seeds: including chia, hemp, pumpkin,
sesame, and squash

Soy sauce, organic

Tomatoes, sun-dried

Vinegar, aged balsamic

In the Fridge

Butter, cultured

Cheese, cream

Cheese, Gouda

Eggs (from pasture-raised chickens)

Kimchi and or other pickled vegetables

Pepperoni, made of beef and pork

Sourdough starter

Soymilk: homemade or purchased (Eden brand)

Tahini

Tofu: homemade or purchased unfortified

Vegetables, fresh: including bok choy,
cabbage, collard greens, and kale

Shopping and Storage Advice

Capillaries absorb pesticides; pesticides cling to the outside of fruit. Even bananas absorb pesticides through their tough skin. Antibiotics and hormones remain in animal flesh even when the flesh has been baked, broiled, or boiled, and the effects of ingesting these substances over the long term are largely undocumented. How genes in a genetically modified plant interact with animals and humans is largely unknown, and what's known is unwelcome news. So whenever possible think organic and buy organically grown plants, organic pastured meat, and eggs from pastured hens.

Labels and Packaging

It bears repeating that cheaper ingredients dominate prepared food and that some of the most noxious ingredients don't show. But don't ignore what legislators do allow you to see: Food labels are important! Chocolate is a prime example. Many brands contain more sugar than cocoa powder and more hydrogenated fat than cocoa butter. So chocolate can be either an important source of magnesium, antioxidants, polyphenols, omega fatty acids, and beneficial fats, or it can be a perilous glut of empty calories that sap energy and jeopardize arterial health. Whatever you buy, we encourage you to read labels carefully.

Bisphenol-A (BPA) is an endocrine disruptor.[1] In tiny amounts it acts to disrupt fetal development, and in larger amounts it disrupts hormone balance and almost certainly promotes serious endocrine disorders. Unfortunately bisphenol-S (BPS), the substitute, is proving equally hazardous in similar and the same ways. So avoid prepared foods or food wrapped in hardened plastic. Store food in glass storage containers until

Table 10.1. Bone's Favorite Foods

Source	Quantity of Nutrient Provided	Notes
For calcium (RDA 800–1,000 mg per day)		
Almonds, 1 cup	40% of RDA	Soak, sprout, and dehydrate before eating—or buy sprouted almonds.
Bok choy, 1 cup	70 mg	Good eaten raw.
Savoy cabbage, 1 cup	50 mg	Good eaten raw.
Broccoli raab/rapini/broccolini, 1 cup	60 mg	Good eaten raw; relatively low in oxalic acid.
Sardines, salmon (with bones) canned, per serving	115 mg	Many canned sardines proudly announce bones-free—which is not good for your bones! Read the label.
Collard greens, 1 cup	175 mg	
Milk, yogurt, mozzarella cheese, 1 cup	100 mg	100 mg is the amount that will be absorbed; the actual amount present is 350 mg.
Turnip greens, 1 cup	100 mg	Boil for 5 minutes to release oxalic acid. Add a splash of apple cider vinegar to release calcium.
For magnesium (RDA 600–1,000 mg per day)		
Dark chocolate, 70% minimum, 1 cup	440 mg	
Pumpkin and squash seeds, ½ cup	325 mg	
Soybeans, 1 cup	150 mg	Soybeans must be properly prepared, and the process is complex. See "Soymilk and Tofu" on page 246.
Swiss chard and spinach, 1 cup	160 mg	Boil for at least 3 minutes.
White beans (cannellini beans), French beans, 1 cup	90 mg	
For phosphorus (RDA 700–1,000 mg)		
Beans and lentils, 1 cup	450 mg	Sprouted.
Brazil nuts, 1 cup	964 mg	
Pork chop, 1 chop	550 mg	Any cuts of pork or beef are a good source.
Pumpkin and squash seeds, 1 cup	1550 mg	
Romano cheese, 1 ounce	215 mg	
Salmon, 1 fillet	1000 mg	Choose wild when possible, Farming practices vary; farmed salmon can be low in nutrients.
For boron (RDA ≥3 mg)		
Almonds	Trace	Should be sprouted.
Avocado	Trace	
Bananas	Trace	
Beans	Trace	Should be sprouted.

Chickpeas	Trace	Should be sprouted and cooked.
Oranges	Trace	
Pears	Trace	
Walnuts	Trace	
For silica (RDA ≥40 mg)		
Beer	Trace	
Horsetail	Trace	An herb.
Jerusalem artichoke	Trace	
Millet	Trace	
Oats	Trace	Must be properly prepared; see page 137.
For vitamin D (RDA 5,000 iu)		
Cod liver oil, 1 teaspoon	500 iu	
Fish roe (fish eggs), 1 tablespoon	Up to 8,000 iu	Often sold in supermarkets in small jars labeled as fish eggs. You don't have to buy the expensive kind to get the bone health benefit.
Maitake mushrooms, 1 cup	1,200 iu	Also called Hen of the Woods; not the same as Chicken Mushrooms.
Pastured egg yolk, from 1 egg	50 iu	
Salmon/oily fish/swordfish, mackerel, smoked salmon, per serving	600 iu	
Shiitake, portobello, and other mushrooms, sunned for 2 days, iu	400 iu	See page 129 for instructions on sunning mushrooms.
For vitamin K$_2$ (RDA 80–300 mcg, higher if therapeutic)		
Goose liver pâté, 100 g	370 mcg	
Gouda cheese, 1 ounce	20 mcg	
Natto, 1 tablespoon	450 mcg	
Pastured eggs, 1	35–80 mcg	Amount varies depending on the chicken's diet and lifestyle.
Pastured butter and milk	20–40 mcg	Amount varies depending on the animal's diet and lifestyle.
Pasture-raised organ meats and dark meat chicken	60 mcg	
For phytoestrogens (RDA ≥50 mg)		
Red clover and other herbs, ½ cup	1,322 mg	Prepare in bone vinegar (page 231).
Soy, as milk, tofu, or fermented soy products, ½ cup	128 mg	Must be properly prepared (page 246).
Alfalfa, flaxseed, hops, lentils, mung beans, pomegranates, sesame seed	Lesser amounts	

something better comes along and use waxed paper instead of plastic wrap, even if the box says it's BPA-free. You don't know what else is in the plastic because there are no requirements, yet, to identify BPS as an ingredient in packaging.

Beans

Buy dry beans already sprouted or sprout your own following the "Sprouting Beans" instructions on page 48.

Favas are primeval beans with as many names as there are cultures that prize them. *Broad beans* is the most common alias for this member of the pea family.

Garbanzo beans are chickpeas and the basis for many friend-to-bone dishes including, famously, tahini (see the Tahini recipe on page 234).

White beans may be cannellini, great northern, or navy. The nutritional differences are marginal. All contain both soluble and insoluble fiber, which makes them an excellent source of prebiotics, and you may use them interchangeably in recipes.

Chocolate

For the pleasure of eating chocolate, choose organic dark chocolate. Dark chocolate is made with at least 70 percent cocoa solids. Do not eat chocolate that is laden with sugar and hydrogenated fat. Read the label. Whether it's cacao or cocoa, look for solids and butter. For cooking choose pure natural—not Dutched—cocoa powder. Dutching reduces the nutritional benefit by half or up to 90 percent depending on how much it is alkalized.

Bittersweet means cocoa solid and cocoa butter fat in about equal amounts with a bit of sugar (no more than one-third, but look for much less) added in.

Some chocolate purveyors proudly present products like nibs in raw, unfermented cacao form. These have high levels of phytic acid (see chapter 4 for an explanation of the adverse effect of phytic acid).

Cornstarch

Conventional cornstarch is almost always made with GMO corn, so it's important to use organic cornstarch.

Eggs

Ideally choose local eggs from pasture-raised chickens, or read labels carefully to find pastured eggs at the store. Cage-free is not the same thing as pastured; the term can be used to designate spaces so densely crowded the birds can barely move.

Flavorings

An essence, for example of vanilla, is a synthetic flavoring. An extract, which is created from the plant using ethyl alcohol and water, is natural.

Flour

Choose organic unbleached sprouted flour. Dozens of grains, seeds, and beans may be sprouted, dehydrated, and ground into flour. Sourdough calls for organic sprouted white flour; rye bread calls for sprouted rye flour. Flour prepared specifically for making bread is typically labeled *bread flour*.

Fruits, Citrus

Conventionally grown citrus fruit peels are routinely waxed and sad to say even sometimes tinted before sale. To guard against chemicals buy organic.

Fruits, Dried

Dried fruit is like fresh without the water, so ounce for ounce dried fruit contains much more sugar although also more fiber and concentrated nutrients. When buying dried fruit, even organic dried fruit, read the label. Bypass those with added sugar (typically cranberries) or coated with oil (typically cranberries and raisins) and do not buy sulfured fruit—fruit with sulfur dioxide as a preservative. (See "Molasses" on page 120.) Sulfur dioxide is a favorite for commercial apricots because it encourages retention of a bright Halloween-orange color. Instead choose Turkish apricots, which are all-natural, chewy, delicious, and nutritious. For the same reason choose organic prunes.

The amount of calcium in figs can vary from 2 percent up to 10 percent or more of RDA. Among those readily available dried, Black Mission and Turkish figs are the best sources of calcium and may contain up to 20 percent RDA in just two fruits.

Tiny chewy red goji berries and supersweet mulberries, which are harder to find and (when organic) very costly, are nutrient-packed medicinal staples and rich in calcium.

Buy organic whenever possible.

Garlic

Whenever possible buy organic garlic. In any case check that the cloves feel firm to the touch all around and that there are no green shoots popping through.

The most efficient garlic storage is a specialty garlic pot. Made of porous material, with a loose-fitting top and airholes, these containers are designed to prevent garlic from drying out or developing mold. For important information on how to prepare garlic for use in recipes, see the Chinese Broccoli with Oyster Sauce and Fried Garlic recipe on page 132.

Ghee

Known for centuries to offer bountiful health benefit, ghee is a pure butter oil obtained by culturing raw milk—which produces curd and buttermilk—and then removing water and milk solids from the curd. The remaining oil has the health benefits of cultured food and has a high smoke point so it is nutritious and useful.

Unfortunately the very properties attributed to ghee made it a prime candidate for marketing hype, and commercial so-called ghee is typically clarified butter. Best to make your own, as described in "How to Make Ghee" on page 243.

Herbs

Create your own herb collection by drying fresh stems, whether from your pesticide-free garden or from organically grown fresh market herbs.

Lentils

Lentils are high-protein seeds available in a variety of colors. Cooking times differ slightly among them. The nutritional differences are marginal though black caviar lentils (a.k.a. mungo beans) are distinguished by being high in anthocyanin, an intensely beneficial flavenoid, and having a very desirable omega-3 to omega-6 ratio. Black beans are similar to lentils in nutrition profile.

Milk Storage, Natural/Unpasteurized/Raw

To keep natural milk fresh for as long as possible, set the fridge temperature at 34°F (1°C). This temperature setting can cause fresh vegetables to freeze. To avoid this, place them in the crisper drawers, or at least keep them off the lowest shelf (cold air sinks).

Molasses

We specify unsulfured blackstrap molasses. Molasses is the byproduct of boiling sugarcane. The first boil produces the very sweet cane syrup. The second boil produces virtually no product because it isn't very sweet and it is bitter. The third boil produces blackstrap molasses. The sucrose is all but gone, leaving a treacle full with minerals, vitamins, and other beneficial nutrients along with a hint of sweetness.

Sulfur dioxide, a preservative, is toxic in high amounts. It has some antimicrobial properties and has the effect of sustaining color in fruits and vegetables. It is added to many products including dried fruits and molasses. Choose only unsulfured food products, including dried fruit and molasses.

Since molasses is the product of a boiling process, the amount of calcium remaining depends on the process. That's why there is a range of calcium RDA across different brands of molasses. We like Plantation brand because each tablespoon contains 20 percent of the US RDA for calcium.

Mushrooms, Sunned and Dried

Buy clean, fresh mushrooms, organic if possible. Mushrooms are 85 percent water and their flesh easily absorbs soil and air contaminants. In many supermarkets the difference in price between organic and conventionally grown is not as striking as it is with some other foods. Most mushrooms are quite lightweight, so you have a bounty in ½ pound. Wash just before using.

Keep fresh mushrooms in the fridge. Keep sunned dried mushrooms in the pantry in a glass storage container. Sunned mushrooms will retain their vitamin D for up to a year. For instructions on sunning and drying mushrooms, see the "Sunning Mushrooms" sidebar on page 129.

Many dried mushrooms are commercially available. Soak them before using them; you may find the liquor is bitter.

For instructions for growing your own shiitake mushrooms, see "Grow Your Own Shiitake Mushrooms" on page 247.

Nuts

You can sprout nuts yourself. Follow the "Sprouting Beans" instructions on page 48. You can also buy already sprouted nuts. Many Whole Foods Markets sell sprouted almonds. Blue Mountain Organics (see the resources section) has a wider selection.

Sometimes but not always raw nuts have been soaked and dried, which removes phytic acid. Roasting some nuts such as almonds may produce high levels of acrylamide, a chemical produced by cooking some foods at high heat that is currently of intense interest as a potential carcinogen. (See "AGE" on page 40.") Our best advice is to stick to sprouted raw nuts.

Oil

Choose coconut oil whenever possible for cooking. The bone health benefits are nothing short of spectacular. One study showed that the effects of virgin coconut oil on bone microarchitecture were much better than treatment with calcium.[2]

Beyond bone considerations, choose cold-pressed oil; that means oil extracted by mechanical means rather than something chemical.

Each type of oil has a different smoke point—the highest temperature it can withstand before nutrients break down or the oil releases toxic fumes. Olive oil has a relatively low smoke point; that of coconut and grape seed is higher; that of avocado oil is higher still. So within certain bounds you can mix and match oils—but respect the boundaries. Check the smoke point of both oils before you decide on a substitute.

Onions

Onions are members of the allium family of vegetables and have benefits similar to those of garlic. You may substitute any onion for any other in our recipes, though nutritional benefits differ slightly among red, yellow, and white onions.

No matter which you use, peel as little as possible after you remove any papery outer layer. In general about 75 percent of the beneficial compounds are in the outer layers.

Onions vary in sweetness and tear factor depending on the water and sulfur content. White onions are sweetest, lowest in sulfur, least likely to make you cry, and lowest in advantageous compounds—though this last is relative since all onions offer desirable nourishing compounds. Red onions have the added benefit of deep color, which means a relatively higher level of phytonutrients.

Pasta Sauce, Jarred

Always read the label when choosing a tomato or pasta sauce. Tomato should be the first ingredient listed. Choose a sauce that is organic and that does not include added sugar, hydrogenated vegetable oil, or thickeners such as carrageenan, which is produced from a red seaweed but has been linked to allergy, side effects, and illness.

Salt

Salts from the sea contain algae—which are not live yet are no less beneficial—and salts from different areas have different mineral compositions, so subtle taste differences exist and each chef must find the salt to which he or she is partial. See the "Salt" sidebar on page 39 for more about salt.

Seaweed

Edible seaweed including arame, wakame, nori, and kombu is rich in minerals and, harvested naturally, provides a host of health benefits. Arame and wakame are especially good sources of calcium. Wash raw seaweed just as you would earth plants—thoroughly—and for the same reason: Tiny organisms cling to plants and remain out of sight. Dry the seaweed in the sun and store in a glass jar or glass food storage container for up to two months in the pantry, up to four months in the fridge.

Seeds

The nutritious seeds we specify in our recipes include chia, hemp, pumpkin, sesame, and squash. Ideally you will sprout them, but that is a labor of love for someone with the time. Many recipes benefit from the taste of roasted or toasted seeds. Watch them carefully because they burn quickly.

Sesame seeds are calcium powerhouses. White sesame seeds are hulled; they are the sweeter of the two and make good food ingredients such as tahini. Black sesame seeds retain the hull, boast even more calcium than the white seeds, and make a lovely oil. Look for organic black sesame oil at specialty Asian food shops.

Sourdough Starter

Sourdough starter is dried wild yeast—yeast that lives in the air. Packaged baking yeast doesn't produce the same ferment or the same flavor.

If you know someone who keeps a viable starter, ask for a cup and feed it at home. Otherwise buy a commercial San Francisco Sourdough starter pack. Check consumer reviews before you buy.

Soymilk

You want soymilk made from fermented soybeans; otherwise you will be drinking anti-nutrients. Make your own (see "How to Make Soymilk" on page 246) or buy Eden brand soymilk.

Soy Sauce, Organic

Shoyu is the Japanese word for "soy sauce." Typically shoyu is made from soybeans plus koji, rice, or wheat and salt; the ingredients are fermented with *Aspergillus oryzae*. If you choose organic soy sauce you can be relatively confident that the sauce did not originate with genetically modified soybeans.

Soy sauce is available as dark or light. The difference is significant. Light soy sauce is made from soybeans fermented with wheat. It is thinner in consistency and much saltier than dark soy sauce. Dark soy sauce is made from soybeans without the addition of wheat, and the beans are fermented for up to a year. Dark soy sauce is thicker and less salty than light soy sauce. The designation *low sodium* does not suggest light or dark but typically means that after fermentation the sodium is removed.

Sprouts

You can buy organic seeds for sprouting at home. Sprouting at home is ideal because often those sprouts sold even in natural food and whole foods stores are not organic. We put mung bean sprouts at the top of the list. If you are looking for more phytoestrogen, substitute organic soy sprouts for mung. Be cautious when buying soybean sprouts, because conventionally grown soy sprouts are often a GMO product.

Stevia

Most commercially available stevia products, such as Truvia, are highly processed from the leaves of the stevia plant. They contain the sweetest glycoside, rebaudioside, and are processed using chemicals.

In Japan and South America the whole plant has been used for centuries in the form of whole ground green leaf powder. This whole leaf also contains another sweet glycoside, stevioside, which has a more bitter aftertaste.

If you are using sugar alternatives, use organic ground stevia leaf.

Sugar

Turbinado, demerara, and muscovado are minimally processed sugars and retain natural moisture and some natural molasses. Turbinado has the highest molasses and calcium contents. Commercial brown sugar is highly processed white sugar with molasses added back in. Animal byproducts and chemicals may be used to process sugar.

Tahini

Tahini is simply ground sesame seeds. Experiment to see whether you like the flavor of white, black, plain, or toasted seeds. To learn how to make your own tahini; see the Tahini recipe on page 234.

Tofu

Typically tofu is made via cooking and preparing soybeans, which yields soymilk and tofu curd. See "How to Make Tofu" on page 247.

If you buy commercial tofu, check that there is no added calcium carbonate or other calcium fortification and no preservatives. Whole Foods and some natural food stores sell artisanal locally made tofu packaged in filtered water. You should consume fresh commercially available tofu within a couple of days from purchase or divide it and freeze portions for later use.

Tomatoes, Sun-Dried

Although drying tomatoes leaves a higher concentration of carbohydrates, it also leaves the vegetable bursting with much higher concentrations of bone health goodness: Calcium, magnesium, niacin, and vitamin K feature among them.

Sun-dried tomatoes are a tasty snack and a fine addition to antipasto.

Vinegar

Raw organic apple cider vinegar contains mother of vinegar, which promotes mineral release. Do not buy pasteurized apple cider vinegar, even if it is organic. You can make your own from fresh apple cider, following the Apple Cider Vinegar recipe on page 244. We also recommend making your own bone vinegar (see the Bone-Building Calcium-Rich Vinegar recipe on page 231) because it is a self-contained bounty of minerals.

Other vinegars also promote mineral release though they are less powerful agents. Tasty vinegars such as balsamic vinegars and wine vinegars are made from grapes.

Water

When we use water in our recipes, we choose filtered water—water that has passed through a reverse osmosis filtration system—or mineral water from glass bottles.

Yogurt

The Greek yogurt style is the result of a filtering process that removes much of the whey—the liquid that's left when you add culture to milk and thereby create curds. It also removes a lot of the lactose, milk's natural sugar. So Greek yogurt is creamier and lower in carbohydrates. Unfortunately it is also one-third lower in calcium. Thus 6 ounces of regular-style yogurt provides 30 percent of the dietary requirement of calcium, while an equivalent amount of Greek-process yogurt provides only 20 percent. We still recommend choosing Greek yogurt, however, because of the lower sugar content; you can easily make up the calcium difference simply by eating an ounce of Gouda cheese.

Thus when it comes to Greek-style yogurt and all the others, it's a trade-off—but only if you start with both unsweetened. Added sugar nullifies the value of comparison. Choose full-fat yogurt unless your healthcare provider instructs you to limit cholesterol and/or animal fat or a recipe specifies something other than full-fat yogurt.

Of course ideally you would start your own with raw milk, but there are downsides. If the raw milk is not extremely fresh, then the bacterial content of the milk will battle with the yogurt culture. Then the taste may not be right. Also, yogurt made with raw milk can be very thin in consistency.

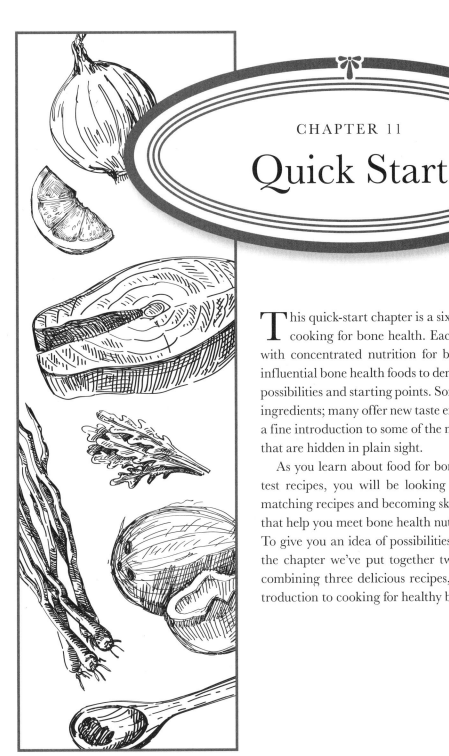

CHAPTER 11

Quick Start

This quick-start chapter is a six-recipe introduction to cooking for bone health. Each of the recipes is rich with concentrated nutrition for bone-health. Each uses influential bone health foods to demonstrate the variety of possibilities and starting points. Some call for mainstream ingredients; many offer new taste experiences and provide a fine introduction to some of the many bone health gems that are hidden in plain sight.

As you learn about food for bone health and begin to test recipes, you will be looking ahead to mixing and matching recipes and becoming skilled at planning meals that help you meet bone health nutrient daily allowances. To give you an idea of possibilities, in the second part of the chapter we've put together two sample meals, each combining three delicious recipes, to round out your introduction to cooking for healthy bones.

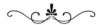

Nettle Infusion

MAKES 1 QUART

If you were going to do only two things to prevent and treat osteoporosis, use homemade bone vinegar (Bone-Building Calcium-Rich Vinegar recipe on page 231) on greens and drink this nettle tea. Both are herb infusions.

Nettle tea is a gift from traditional medicines. Think of it as a liquid vitamin and calcium pill with a very big difference: Nettle infusion not only gives you energy—consume a glass for a week and see—but it provides nearly everything you need to strengthen bones: calcium, magnesium, iron, vitamins B, C, A, D, and K, protein, trace minerals, potassium, zinc, copper, sulfur, and boron. Nettle is more nutritious than blue-green algae.

As do most whole nutritious foods, nettle supports general health, too. It nourishes the adrenal glands. It is an aid for many complaints from weak nails to allergies. In traditional medicine men take nettle as an antidote to frequent nighttime urination. In traditional cultures pregnant and lactating women take nettle tea as a tonic, as the tea's iron content can treat blood loss and/or anemia.

Nettle infusion provides energy and a rich source of calcium. And since the vitamins and minerals that calcium needs for absorption and transport are integral, nettle tea is safe, effective calcium supplementation. For bone strengthening, drink ½ cup/4 ounces every day.

1 oz. (28 g) dried nettle stalks and leaves
1 quart (1 L) boiling water

Using rubber gloves, fill a mason jar with the dried nettle, then fill the jar with the boiling water. Cover and brew overnight.

The next day strain out the plant material and, still using gloves, squeeze the herbs to get all the good stuff. Refrigerate. The tea will taste good for 2 days. If it goes sour, it makes a great food for plants.

Caution: Nettle (especially fresh) has tiny hairs that release the same irritating substance ants do when they bite, so when handling fresh or dried nettle stalks always wear rubber gloves and use tongs.

Nutrition Information: 1 cup nettle infusion tea: 125 mg calcium; 75 mg magnesium; 450 iu vitamin A; 4.1 g protein

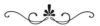

The Mix-Up Poke Bowl

SERVES 2

This is a fresh light meal for anytime. It leaves you feeling satisfied yet buoyant. It's sometimes served for breakfast in Laura's house.

Watermelon radishes are members of the famous brassica (cabbage) family of vegetables that contain powerful antioxidants. These magenta roots are gentle in taste and delicious with just about any food—but especially good with cheese, vegetables, herbs, and salad dressing.

If you want a more substantial meal, add rice. This is a flexible dish, so leave out or add from the options list. You can safely eat bok choy raw. Use snow peas raw or, for a softer flavor, lightly steam them.

The optional ingredients add variety and renew your interest in this wonderful dish. The suggested amounts are per serving. Experiment to increase or decrease according to taste.

Colorful dishes are lovely and offer the benefit of many different phytochemicals.

Sesame Shoyu Dressing (see page 162)

½ pound (230 g) marinated and/or seared and cubed wild-caught salmon or tuna or tofu

2 sunned marinated shiitake mushrooms, sliced (see "Sunning Mushrooms" on page 129 for instructions)

1 cup (70 g) raw bok choy

1 cup (145 g) raw or lightly steamed snow peas

2 green onions, chopped

¼ medium white onion, sliced

1 avocado, sliced

¼ cup (20 g) shredded toasted nori seaweed

3 watermelon radishes, sliced

1 Tbsp. fish eggs (roe)

2 Tbsp. sesame seeds (a mix of black and white)

OPTIONAL INGREDIENTS

¼ cup (46 g) adzuki beans (sprouted, lightly cooked, and cooled; or sprouted raw)

2 cherry tomatoes

¼ cup (38 g) Daikon Kimchi (see page 202)

1 Tbsp. shaved lotus root

3 macadamia nuts

¼ cup (41 g) chopped mango

¼ cup (26 g) mung beans (sprouted, lightly cooked, and cooled; or sprouted raw)

¼ cup (30 g) pea sprouts

¼ cup (26 g) shredded cucumber

1 tsp. shredded ginger, or to taste

Mix the shoyu dressing, and put ½ cup (120 ml) of it in a bowl with your tuna and salmon or tofu. Coat the fish gently with the shoyu and marinate for 2 hours or up to overnight in the fridge. Add 2 tablespoons of the dressing to the mushrooms and marinate in the fridge as for the fish or tofu. Refrigerate the remaining dressing.

When you are ready to eat, put the vegetables and fish eggs in a bowl. If you are adding optional ingredients, put them in at this point. Toss the ingredients well. Set the marinated fish or tofu on top and pour the rest of the dressing over all. Sprinkle with sesame seeds. Delicious.

> **Nutrition Information per Serving:** 34g protein; 250 mg calcium; 200 mg magnesium; 8,000 iu vitamin D; phytoestrogen

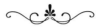

Helen's Hearty Hemp Seed Salad

SERVES 2

The keys to this rich anytime dish are fresh organic arugula still attached to the roots, a creamy avocado, and any Gouda, whether made with pasteurized or raw milk.

Either milk is fine because the bacteria used to produce Gouda cheese are the same bacteria that manufacture vitamin K_2 in your body and produce K_2 in the cheese irrespective of the milk medium. If you choose raw cheese, Beemster is so delicious it's worth trying to find.

We love to make this salad with fresh figs. The fructose in figs helps to promote calcium absorption.

2–4 cooked organic chicken thighs

1 bunch fresh arugula leaves, crisped in ice water

¼ small red onion

1 avocado at the peak of readiness

¼ cup hemp seeds

2 tsp. olive oil

4 fresh figs

4 tsp. virgin coconut oil

1 tsp. apple cider vinegar

1 oz. (28 g) grated goat milk Gouda

Molasses pecans, for garnish

Bake or broil the chicken thighs with or without the skin. Helen removes the skin before baking because she has familial high cholesterol. You may keep or remove the skin for serving.

Wash the arugula. Spread the leaves in an approximate single layer on a length of paper towel, roll up and give a gentle twist, then unroll the towel. If water remains, pat the leaves with another piece of paper towel until they're dry. If the stem ends are curled, clip them.

Slice up slivers of red onion to equal about 2 heaped tablespoons.

Tear the clean dry arugula leaves stem and all. Distribute half the leaves on each plate. Sprinkle leaves with the vinegar. Toss to coat evenly.

Scoop out the avocado, half for each plate, and pile onto the leaves.

Sprinkle 1 tablespoon hemp seeds on each plate. Distribute the red onion slivers. Drizzle with olive oil and vinegar. Slice and add the figs.

Add the chicken to the plate and tip the coconut oil over the avocado and the chicken. Top with Gouda and pecans.

Note: Thighs from pastured hens are best, but organic chicken thighs have less fat in the skin and provide much more healthy protein per ounce than battery hens.

Nutrition Information per Serving: 26 g protein; 80 mg calcium; 150 mg magnesium; 30 mcg zinc; 25 mcg K_2

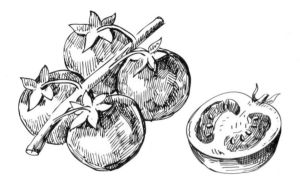

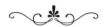

Swoon Breakfast
SERVES 1

You can tick a lot of bone health boxes if you have 10 minutes and one or two pastured eggs.

If you live in a state that sells raw cream, try making butter (see "Natural Milk Butter" on page 242) for this recipe. Unless you are on a restricted-sodium diet, add ½ teaspoon of salt to the poaching water. Salt helps the eggs to set. To help the white set completely, spoon some boiling water over the eggs once or twice during cooking. We recommend dill as a table seasoning because of its rich calcium content.

1 Tbsp. coconut oil
1 Tbsp. butter or ghee
1 portobello mushroom cap, chopped in big pieces
1 tomato, cut in half
8 collard leaves (you may substitute 10 lacinato kale leaves)
1 or 2 pastured eggs, as you wish
1 tsp. fish eggs (roe)
Pinch of salt
Salt, black pepper, finely ground chili pepper, dried dill, for seasoning at the table

Put the oil and butter in a frying pan. Turn the heat to medium. Once the pan is hot, add the mushrooms and the tomato halves, face-side down. Stir up the mushrooms to encourage cooking through. Add the greens. When the mushrooms begin to wilt, turn the tomato halves over, stir, and turn down the heat. Scoop the mushrooms and tomato into a heap at the center of the pan and put on the cover. Set to simmer.

Put about 4 inches (10 cm) of water in a small saucepan and add a pinch of salt. Put the water on to boil over medium heat.

When the water has reached a rolling boil, crack the eggs carefully against the side of the poaching pot and drop each egg into the water. Turn the heat down enough to keep the water from boiling over. If white foam comes to the top, ignore it. After 1 minute check to see whether the egg has come to the top. If not, help it along very gently with a spatula. Aim to keep the yolk intact.

When the white is cooked, use a slotted spoon to plate the mushrooms and tomatoes—leave the juices in the pan—and pop the eggs on top. Prick the yolks open with the tines of a fork. Pour the mushroom and tomato pan juices over all. Sprinkle on the fish eggs. They add a salty taste so you might not want to add salt. Add a little black pepper, a sprinkle of red pepper, and a generous dash of dried dill. Swoon.

Nutrition Information per Serving: 50 mcg vitamin K_2; 3,000 iu vitamin D; 60 mg calcium

---

⊰ Sunning Mushrooms ⊱

Set a mushroom in the sun and it makes vitamin D, just as we do. For best results, leave mushrooms gills-up through two days of sunshine, then store. The vitamin content will be robust for up to a year. You can sit the mushrooms gills-up on a sunny windowsill or in a conservatory to good effect. Sunned mushrooms produce D_2 and some D_3, which can supplement natural sources of vitamin D including D_3 from fish eggs, fish oil, fish, and the sun. Find more information about vitamin D on page 21.

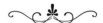

Charcoal-Fired Scallops with Arugula Microgreens and Roe Sauté
SERVES 2

Scallops are the ultimate last-minute gourmet dish. They cook quickly and need only greens as a backdrop. Serve as a starter or make them a main dish.

Sea scallops—barrel-shaped and about an inch high—are perfect on the grill. Oil before seasoning. Bay scallops are tiny. In a sauté they're done before you turn your back to the pan. Buy dry scallops from a trusted fishmonger. The plump wet ones are usually soaked in phosphate solution to make them plumper, which compromises the texture. Some grocery stores display fish for up to a week.

12 large scallops
Arugula microgreens (or arugula, watercress, lamb's lettuce, or a mixture to taste)
1 avocado
1 lime wedge per person
1 or 2 spring onions roasted on the fire and served whole (optional)
1–2 Tbsp. avocado oil (optional)
Garlic powder
Black pepper
3 or 4 chunks jicama or Jerusalem artichoke per person

ROE SAUTÉ

2 Tbsp. coconut oil
1 small clove garlic, minced
12 scallop roe
Sea or Himalayan pink salt in a grinder

Wash the scallops and dry them on paper towels. Light the grill and set at high, or get the charcoal going till it's red-hot.

Wash, then thoroughly dry, the microgreens. Slice the avocado, put into a bowl with the pit, cover, and refrigerate. Prepare luncheon- or dinner-sized plates with a helping of microgreens, a lime wedge, and a selection from the recipe note.

Rub oil on the spring onions. Lightly sprinkle garlic powder over the scallops. Use a stronger hand to sprinkle on the black pepper. Turn the scallops carefully and repeat the garlic and pepper.

Place onions and scallops on the grill. Move swiftly so they'll all be done at just about the same time. Cook the scallops for 2 minutes on each side.

Remove the onions and scallops to the serving plates atop the microgreens. Add sliced avocado and jicama or Jerusalem artichoke chunks to the plates.

For a richer dish, finish with Fig Balsamic Glaze (see page 162).

Roe Sauté: Heat the oil to medium high. Add the garlic, immediately turn the heat down to medium, and add the roe. Sauté, turning gently with a wooden spoon, until they are done through—about 2 minutes. Turn one twist of the salt over the roe and serve with the scallops.

Cook roe separately from the scallops because they cook—if anything—more quickly. The roe can be grilled rather than cooked in a pan, but it takes a very deft hand and a tightly woven grate. If there are two of you, one can sauté the roe and one grill the scallops. Otherwise, prepare the roe just before grilling the scallops.

Note: You can add a tiny, delightful touch of color to this dish with one small cherry tomato cut in half, a slice of roasted red or purple beet, a stick of red bell pepper, or a tiny sprinkle of wild blueberries. Or, for a vibrant color presentation, serve these scallops with roasted asparagus and black rice.

Nutrition Information per Serving: 32 g protein; 200 mg calcium; 120 mg magnesium; 800 iu vitamin D; 400 mg phosphorus

Bone Shrub

In the 17th century shrubs were all the rage. They started life as medicinal cordials that arrived in England from Italy, where they were first produced during the Renaissance. According to an anonymous text of the time, shrubs served to "renew the natural heat, recreate and revive the spirits, and free the whole body from the malignity of diseases." A shrub is a concoction of fruit, vinegar, and sparkling water, sometimes combined with alcohol. There is an old adage that taking a teaspoon of apple cider vinegar in the morning cures many ills; likewise drinking shrub.

Some shrub cordials were a bright-yellow hue and contained flecks of gold leaf, and so took their name from the "cordial vertues" of the rays of the sun, which some alchemists thought the medicines contained. And in a way the alchemists were right—the plants use the sun's rays to produce the enormous and varied benefits they provide to us as foods.

By the 19th century, typical American recipes for shrubs used vinegar poured over fruit—traditionally berries—and left to infuse anywhere from overnight up to several days. Then the fruit would be strained out and the remaining liquid would be mixed with a sweetener such as sugar or honey and reduced to create a syrup. The sweet-and-sour syrup could be mixed with either water or soda water and served as a soft drink, or it could be used as a mixer in cocktails. With the advent of home refrigeration, shrubs fell from favor.

Making a shrub is an ideal way to take your bone-building vinegar. Contemplate the difference between popping an industrially made supplement and sitting in the sun absorbing your vitamin D while you sip this tart fruity gift from nature. The herbs in the bone-building vinegar, one ingredient in every shrub, contains all the vitamins and trace minerals you need for bone health. Nettle alone contains over 400 mg of calcium in a cup. Your tasty, fruity shrub will provide you with all the base nutrition you need to foster healthy bones.

How to Make Shrub

Making shrub is not a precise process. The basic idea is to take whatever fruit rinds and fruit scraps you have on hand, put them in any jar with a clean, tight-fitting cover, and pour bone-building vinegar over them. See the Bone-Building Calcium-Rich Vinegar recipe on page 231.

Add a teaspoonful of your Ginger Bug (see page 222)—the ginger goes well with the herbs in the bone vinegar. Let the brew sit, covered, at room temperature for a few days.

Strain the liquid through a sieve, mashing the fruit pulp to get the fruit flavor. Add 2 Tbsp. of honey or sugar.

The resulting syrup can be enjoyed by adding it to some sparkling water and an ice cube.

Use a tablespoon of the fruity sweet vinegar, mixed with sparkling water or something sweeter if you like.

We encourage you to adapt and explore, and make this as simple or as complex as you like.

Serving it with Sweet Hibiscus Tea (see page 224), an ice cube, and some fizzy water is lovely. You can also put it in our homemade sodas—see "Homemade Sodas" on page 221. Our bone vinegar has a lovely spice to it, which goes really well with the ginger beer.

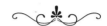

Bone-Friendly Meal One

SERVES 4

Super-Easy Seared Wagyu Beef with Mushroom Shoyu Sauce

Wagyu is a breed of cow originally reared in Japan, now also raised by some farmers in the United States. The meat is fine, marbled and high in unsaturated fat. This is the one meat you don't want to marinate—it's so tasty as is. We love this dish as a small plate with a large salad or soup. It's also perfect as a main dish for two.

Wagyu beef is costly, and often the animals have been fed a grain-dominated diet. Check with your supplier to see how the animals were raised. Alternatively, choose some other type of pasture-raised or organic steak, or the best you can afford. It will pay off in taste.

1 16-oz. (455 g) Wagyu steak, or any fine aged, well-marbled steak
¼ cup (65 g) Mushroom Shoyu Sauce (see page 162)
1 Tbsp. roasted sesame seeds

Put the steak in the freezer for 30 minutes. Then remove it and cut it into very thin strips while you heat a cast-iron pan or griddle at medium heat for 5 minutes. Sear the strips for 20 seconds on each side; plate in a pile. Drizzle on mushroom shoyu sauce and sprinkle on the sesame seeds. Serve right away with Chinese broccoli and freshly boiled and peeled sweet potato, or with rice. This meat is simply delicious.

Nutrition Information per Serving: 25 g protein; B vitamins; 2.5 mg iron; trace minerals

Chinese Broccoli with Oyster Sauce and Fried Garlic

1¼ cups (300 ml) peanut oil
Whole head of garlic, smashed and chopped
Salt
1 tsp. sesame oil
1 Tbsp. Oyster Sauce (see page 163)
3 bunches Chinese broccoli

Cook the garlic in the peanut oil until golden brown. Remove and place on paper towels to drain off excess oil.

In a small bowl combine 1 teaspoon of the garlic-infused oil with the sesame oil and oyster sauce. Mix well until combined and then add 1 tablespoon hot water. Stir and set aside. Reserve the remaining garlic oil for another use.

Boil 2 quarts of water, add a pinch of salt, turn the heat down and simmer the Chinese broccoli until just tender, about 4 minutes. Drain well on paper towels or in a salad spinner and place on a serving platter. Drizzle the mixed oyster sauce on top and sprinkle with the fried garlic.

> **Nutrition Information per Serving:** 200 mg calcium; 28 mg vitamin C; 1,400 iu vitamin A; 75 mg magnesium

Kabocha Squash with Maple Syrup, Shoyu, and Ghee

Kabocha, with delicate, nutritious edible green or red skin, is a cross between pumpkin and butternut squash and sweeter than either one. One serving of kabocha squash is a tasty nutrient bounty: It has all the vitamin E, vitamin C, and potassium for a day along with lots of vitamin A, many of the B vitamins, folate, and a host of minerals including 45 mg of calcium, 35 mg of magnesium, and most of the copper you need per day.

Shoyu is a soy sauce typically made from soybeans and koji, rice, or wheat fermented with *Aspergillus oryzae*.

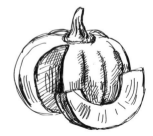

1 kabocha squash
2 Tbsp. shoyu
2 Tbsp. maple syrup
1 Tbsp. ghee (see page 243)

Preheat the oven to 350°F (177°C).

Slice the kabocha squash in half, then into 1- to 2-inch-wide (2.5 to 5 cm) pieces. Save the seeds for roasting (see the Spiced Pepitas recipe on page 229). Line a cookie sheet with foil and place the squash pieces on their sides. Roast for 25 to 30 minutes, turning them after 15 minutes. While the squash is cooking, in a small saucepan mix the shoyu, maple syrup, and ghee. Heat gently until warm. When the squash is done cut the pieces in half and put in a bowl. Pour on the sauce and coat the squash pieces.

> **Nutrition Information per Serving:** 3,500 iu vitamin A; 150 mg vitamin C; omega-3 fats; 15 mcg vitamin K$_2$

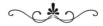

Bone-Friendly Meal Two
SERVES 2

Pescaditos and Habas Secas Granadinas con Aioli La Pilareta

Another title for this meal could be the Natural Spanish Bone Health Supplement Option.

La Pilareta, formerly Bar Pilar, is an institution in El Carmen, Valencia's old town neighborhood.

Helen was thrilled to find that two of their signature dishes, both among her favorites, are ideal for bone health: Boquerones Aceite Olive—little fish fried in olive oil—and Habas Secas Granadinas, broad beans (a.k.a. fava beans), popular in the southern Spanish style of cooking—in this case a recipe typical of Granada.

These two are so good for bones in so many ways we think of them as our go-to bone health supplement. Wonder why?

One reason is that people eat these little fish skin, bones, and all. Plus they contain the healthy fats of fish in the greater herring family. And fava beans contain calcium, phosphorus, potassium, and a relative gold mine of magnesium. Add in the aioli—raw garlic probiotic plus vitamin K_2 from the aioli's egg yolk—and you're sitting bone pretty.

Boquerones Aceite Olive

In Spain tiny fry—very young fish—make popular tapas dishes. Typically the chef chooses boquerones, a white anchovy with soft bones and an aromatic fishy flavor. Of course little soft-boned fish make their way into many national cuisines—think sprat in Scotland, sild in Norway, whitebait in the UK. Baked, grilled, or fried, you can eat any fry skin, bones, and all for a solid calcium infusion.

Make bread crumbs from sourdough bread you've allowed to dry and put into a blender or crushed between sheets of waxed paper with a meat tenderizer or a rolling pin.

Two dozen small fry
Flour
Bread crumbs, finely ground to a powder
Olive oil, for frying

Wash the fish, dry in paper towels, and then air-dry until the skins are perfectly dry. Rub the fish with a hint of olive oil.

Make a coating mix by mixing equal parts flour and pulverized bread crumbs. Shake the fish around in the coating mix.

Add oil to a fry basket or frying pan and heat it to barely bubbling. Add the coated fish and fry until the coating is slightly browned—about 4 minutes.

Nutrition Information per Serving: 23 g protein; 180 mg calcium; omega-3

Habas Secas Granadinas

Yerba buena is also known as *hierbabuena*, which translates as "good herb" and refers to wild-growing plants of the mint family—most often spearmint. We use ¹/₂ cup (75 g) dried beans per serving, but you can adjust as you like depending on what part—appetizer, side dish, main course—the beans will play in your meal. If you don't have a pressure cooker, you can use an electric slow cooker or put the ingredients in a saucepan, cover tightly with foil, and cover the pan with a tightly fitting lid. Double the cooking tim but check the beans often.

2 cups (300 g) dried fava beans
A few sprigs of yerba buena
1 *guindilla* (whole red cayenne pepper)

Soak the dried beans for 24 hours (see "Soaking Beans" on page 47). Put the beans in a pressure cooker for 10 to 15 minutes with salt, yerba buena, and the whole cayenne pepper (remove the seeds first if you want a milder flavor). Remove the beans from the cooking water with a slotted spoon, allowing the water to run off them, and serve hot or cold drizzled with olive oil and accompanied by a fish or seafood tapa. Serve with a side of aioli, which is basically garlic mayonnaise.

Nutrition Information per Serving: 45 mg calcium; 10 g protein; 45 mg magnesium; phytoestrogen

Aioli

Aioli is so good in so many ways, it's worth a bit of experimentation: You can vary the garlic and lemon tastes to suit yourself, for instance. Use a food processor or a mortar and pestle to make this garlic mayonnaise but not a blender; in the end you'll have more on the sides and in the bottom than in your serving dish.

2–4 cloves garlic
1 tsp. or a bit more fresh lemon juice
Pinch finely ground sea salt
1 egg plus 1 yolk
¾ cup (180 ml) olive oil

Process the garlic, lemon juice, and salt in a food processor or by hand with a mortar and pestle. Add the egg and the yolk, blending until they're thoroughly incorporated. With the machine running—or your pestle whipping around (but you'll need a helping hand for this)—stream in ½ cup (120 ml) of the olive oil. Keep mixing till it looks like mayonnaise. Add additional olive oil until the mixture reaches the consistency you want.

Nutrition Information per Serving: 40 iu vitamin D; 50 mcg vitamin K_2

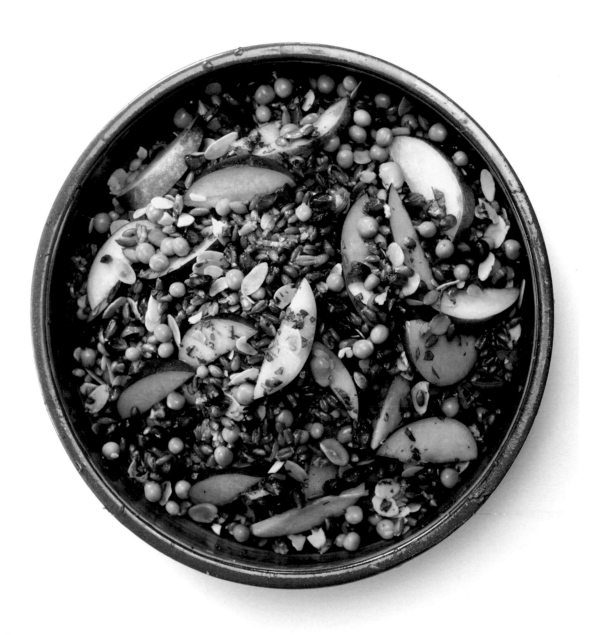

Figure 14. Nectarine, Pea, Broad Bean, and Spelt Salad, page 155. *Photograph courtesy of Reynolds*

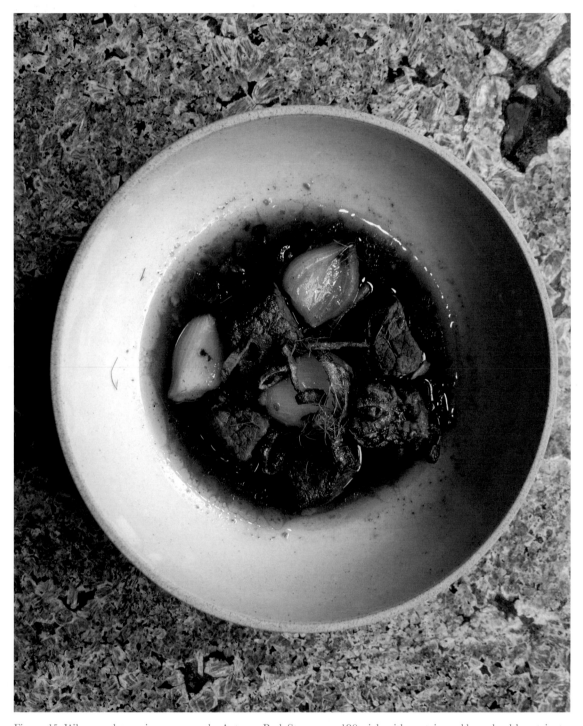

Figure 15. When apples are in season, make Autumn Pork Stew, page 180, rich with protein and bone health nutrients.

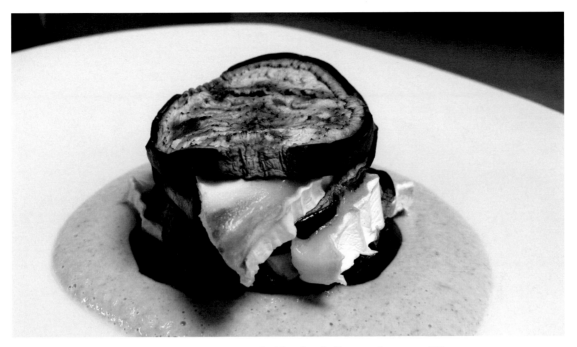

Figure 16. Berenjena Torre, an eggplant tower served with yellow bell pepper jam, page 172.

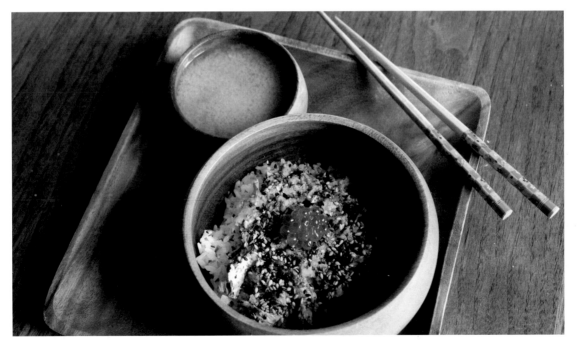

Figure 17. Japanese Bowl Set, page 184.

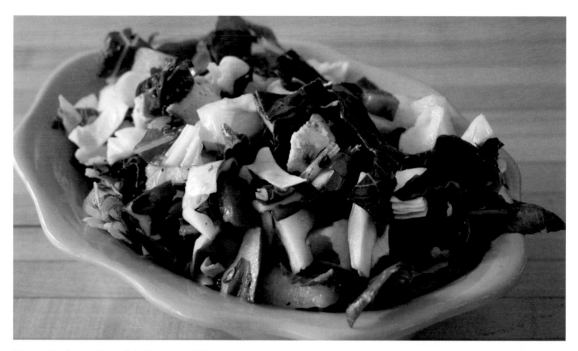

Figure 18. Super-Basic Stir-Fry, page 193.

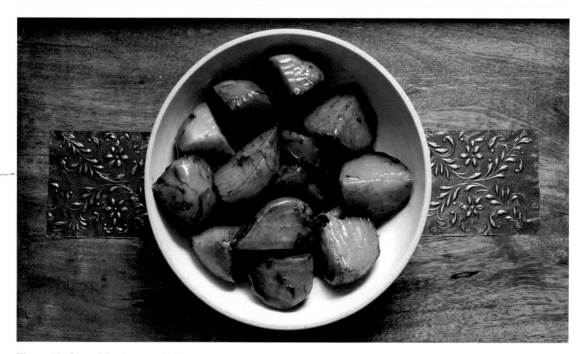

Figure 19. Glazed Beets, page 202.

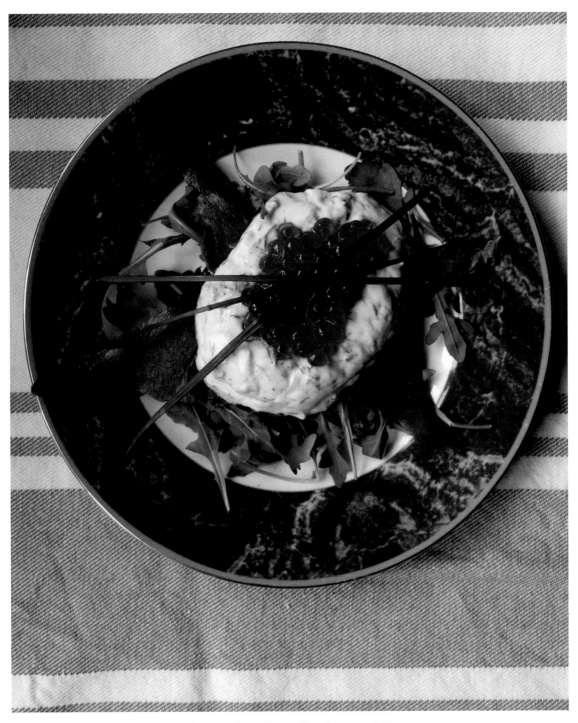

Figure 20. Smoked Salmon with Fish Roe and Zesty Yogurt Dressing, page 207.

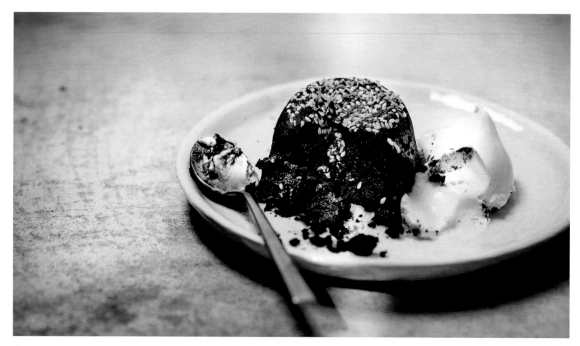

Figure 21. Tahini Chocolate Cake, page 216. *Photograph by Jenny Zarins.*

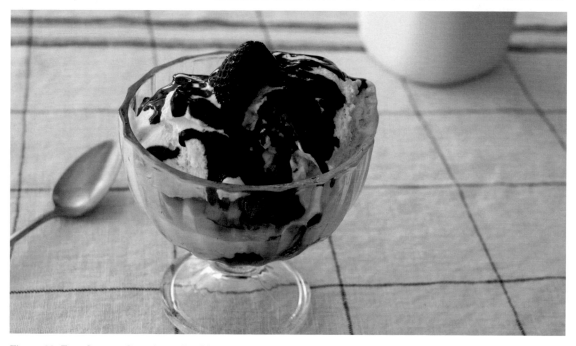

Figure 22. Four Seasons Strawberry Parfait, page 212.

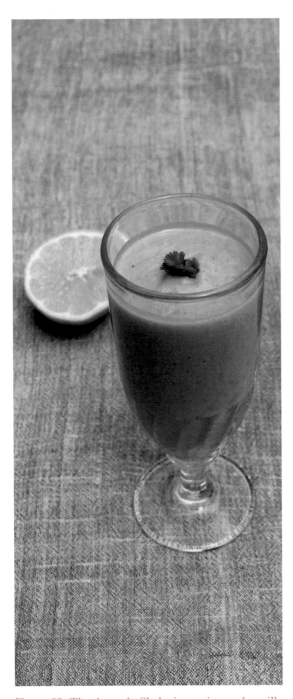

Figure 23. The Avocado Shake is a twist on the milk-shake tradition, see page 220.

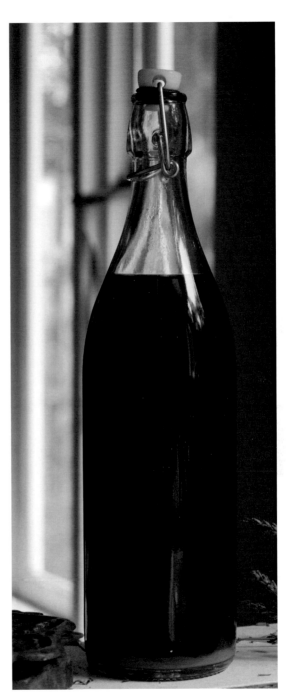

Figure 24. Bone-Building Calcium-Rich Vinegar (page 231) is a mainstay of bone health and a powerful ally in preventing and treating bone loss.

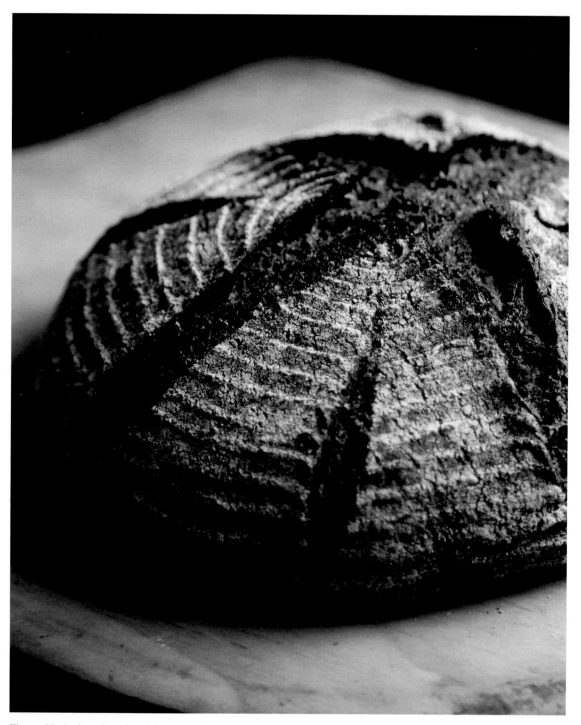

Figure 25. Artisan Sourdough Rye Bread, page 240. *Photograph courtesy of Eric Rusch*

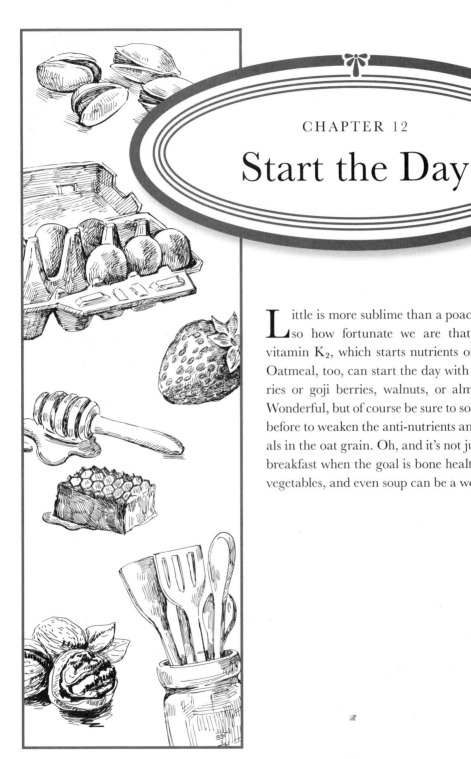

CHAPTER 12

Start the Day

Little is more sublime than a poached pastured egg—so how fortunate we are that the yolk contains vitamin K_2, which starts nutrients on the road to bone. Oatmeal, too, can start the day with the likes of mulberries or goji berries, walnuts, or almonds for breakfast. Wonderful, but of course be sure to soak the oats the night before to weaken the anti-nutrients and release the minerals in the oat grain. Oh, and it's not just eggs or cereal for breakfast when the goal is bone health; salads with fruit, vegetables, and even soup can be a welcome change.

Marinated Charentais Melon with Greek Yogurt, Pumpkin Seeds, and Honey

SERVES 4–6

A lovely light breakfast on the sweeter side, with delicate yet strong flavors and bone health ingredients to start strengthening your bones from the get-go. This recipe is from Reynolds, a UK purveyor of fine food.

2 Tbsp. coconut sugar

1 cup (240 ml) water

1 orange

1 thumb-sized piece of fresh ginger

4–5 whole star anise

2 Charentais melons

24 oz. (680 g) Greek yogurt (homemade or store-bought)

5 Tbsp. honey

5 Tbsp. pumpkin seeds

Place the sugar and water into a large saucepan and bring to a boil, making sure that all the sugar has dissolved. While the syrup is boiling, use a peeler to take ½-inch (1.25 cm) pieces of rind from the orange and set aside. Cut the orange in half and squeeze out the juice into a small bowl. Peel the ginger and cut into matchstick-sized pieces. Add the orange skin and juice, ginger, and whole star anise to the stock syrup. Return to a boil.

Cut each melon in half, and then remove the seeds and the skin. Cut into approximately ¼-inch (.6 cm) cubes. When the stock syrup has returned to a boil, remove it from the heat and add the melon. Allow this to cool at room temperature (about an hour), then pour it into a mason jar and store in the fridge. It is recommended that you leave the mixture in the fridge overnight to allow all the flavors to infuse prior to use.

Serving Suggestion: Put about 1 cup (300 g) of Greek yogurt into a bowl for each portion; add honey to each serving. Using a slotted spoon, take the melon out of the liquid and place on top of the yogurt. Garnish off with a handful of pumpkin seeds.

Nutrition Information per Serving: 110 mg calcium; 100 mg magnesium; 200 mg vitamin C; 100 mg phosphorus

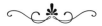

Chickpea Breakfast Soup

SERVES 4

The traditional bessara, an Egyptian bean soup, is made with fava beans and eaten for breakfast (see Sprouted Fava Bean Soup, page 146). Here's an even more bone-friendly version made from chickpeas. Chickpeas, also called garbanzos, have a beautiful balance of nutrients: protein, calcium, and magnesium in harmony along with phosphorus and vitamins. That's everything bone-friendly in one place. We add a soft-boiled egg to make a complete, delicious bone health breakfast.

2 cups (305 g) spouted chickpeas (see "Sprouting Beans" on page 48)

2 cloves garlic, smashed and finely chopped 10 minutes before using

4 cups (1 L) chicken bone broth, vegetable broth, or water

2 Tbsp. olive oil

1 tsp. ground cumin

½ tsp. salt

¼ tsp. red pepper flakes

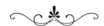

OPTIONAL CONDIMENTS

Cilantro

Olive oil

Paprika

Cumin

Minced garlic

Chopped chilies or chili flakes

Yogurt

Soft-boiled eggs, left in the shell

Put the beans, garlic, and broth (or water) in a pot, bring to a boil, and simmer for about an hour until the beans mash easily. Pour the beans and liquid into a large bowl and add the olive oil, cumin, salt, and pepper flakes. Puree with a hand blender. You can thin the soup with more water if you want.

Set out any condiments you are offering with the meal; encourage people to add to suit to their taste.

> **Nutrition Information per Serving:** 230 mg calcium; 230 mg magnesium; approximately 50 mcg vitamin K$_2$ (with egg); 45 g protein; 67 iu vitamin A; 350 mg phosphorus

❧ Hot Breakfast Tips ❧

- Soak rolled oats overnight in water and yogurt, buttermilk, or vinegar. Rinse and cook as usual for breakfast.
- Soak whole wheat flour overnight in water and unpasteurized buttermilk before using it in, say, pancakes or waffles.
- Substitute sprouted grain flour for your typical whole grain flour. If you have a grain grinder, you can sprout the grain yourself, dry it, and grind it into fresh flour.

Bone-Friendly Oatmeal with Goji Berries, Walnuts, and Almonds

SERVES 2–3

Thanks to the energizing complex carbohydrates in oats and the healthy fats in goji berries and nuts, this is perfect post-workout or pre-busy-day. Oats are one of the best dietary sources of silicon. Some vitamins in oats are fat-soluble; serve oats with butter or cream and those vitamins will be absorbed. Buy sprouted nuts or plan ahead to soak nuts for 8 hours before serving to remove phytic acid (see "Soaking and Fermenting Grains," page 50, to learn about phytic acid).

2 cups (162 g) uncooked steel-cut or rolled oats

2 Tbsp. raw buttermilk or 1 tsp apple cider vinegar

Water

Pinch of salt

1 Tbsp. butter or cream

Handful of goji berries (or your favorite dried fruit)

Handful of walnuts and almonds
  (or your favorite nuts)

Powdered cinnamon and/or raw honey to taste

In the evening, place the oats and buttermilk or vinegar in a bowl. Stir them together. Add water just to cover the oats. Cover the bowl with a clean towel or cloth. Leave on the counter overnight.

In the morning, drain the liquid (reserving it), rinse the oats, and drain in a colander. Bring the reserved liquid and salt to a boil. Stir in the rinsed oats, cover, reduce the heat to a simmer, and cook the oats for 5 minutes. Add the butter or cream, goji berries, walnuts and/or almonds, and cinnamon and/or raw honey.

> **Nutrition Information per Serving:** 130 mg calcium; 100 mg magnesium; 10 g protein; 2 mg iron

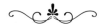

Upside-Down Savoyarde Eggs

SERVES 2

Savoyarde, formerly Savoie, is a historical region that once embraced parts of France, Switzerland, and Italy. Cuisine in this area is rich and delicious.

In this recipe, the pastured eggs and Gouda will give you enough K_2 for the day (but it's fine to have even lots more K_2 later in the day), and the maitake will get your vitamin D off to a galloping start. The Gouda provides about 300 mg of calcium. Oregano is very high in phytoestrogen. Fresh oregano dries nicely on the windowsill and keeps well stored in a jar.

½ tsp. ghee
1½ cups (100 g) maitake mushrooms, or sunned
    shiitake, sliced (see "Sunning Mushrooms" on
    page 129)
10 sprigs dried oregano
Truffle salt or sea salt
¼–½ cup (about 2 oz. [55 g]) shredded raw or
    pasteurized Gouda
¼–½ of a chopped onion
2 pasture-raised eggs

Heat half the ghee in a pan, put in the sliced mushrooms, rub the dried oregano off the sprigs and add to the pan. Sprinkle with salt. Cook for 7 minutes, turning the mushrooms. After the mushrooms have cooked for about 4 minutes, start cooking the cheese and eggs.

In a small egg pan, heat the rest of the ghee on high heat. Toss in the cheese, spreading around evenly. This will create a lattice of cheese. Reduce the heat to medium-low. Cook the cheese lattice for 3 minutes. Slide it out of the pan.

Toss in the onion. Cook on medium heat for 2 minutes. Mix the eggs in a small bowl with a fork or a whisk. Pour the eggs into the pan with the onion. Move the mix around with a wooden spatula. It's best to fold rather than stir. Cook about another minute until the eggs are set.

Put the eggs on a plate and the mushrooms on top. Place the cheese lattice over the top. See the image on page 6 of the color insert.

> **Nutrition Information per Serving:** 200 mg calcium; 800 iu vitamin D; 70 mcg vitamin K_2

The Osteoporosis Enemy Breakfast

SERVES 1

Helen's first food remedy was The Breakfast. It was a labor of love each morning that paid off within 15 months. The ingredients list is long, and some advance preparation is required. We've included lots of tips for making things convenient. If you have osteopenia or osteoporosis, it's worth the time; for prevention, include it every so often.

To treat bone loss, organic ingredients are optimal. Choose black Mission and Turkish figs, which provide 20 percent of your calcium daily requirement. Macadamia nuts have outstanding ratios of

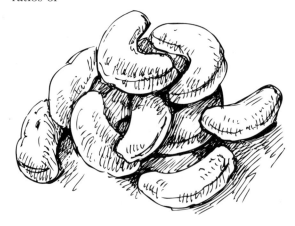

omega fatty acids. Look for sprouted seeds, or try sprouting your own.

1 Tbsp. ground seeds, such as chia, hemp, golden flax, white sesame, black sesame, poppy
1 tsp. pumpkin seeds (sprouted is optimal)
1 tsp. sunflower seeds (sprouted is optimal)
1 or 2 black Mission or Turkish figs, or 2 fresh figs
1 dried apricot half, unsulfured
1 Brazil nut
Any 8 nuts from this collection: macadamias, almonds, cashews, filberts, pecans, pistachios, and/or walnuts
1–2 Tbsp. unsulfured blackstrap molasses
½–¾ cup (120–180 ml) raw milk
¼ cup (37 g) blueberries, or ¼ cup (40 g) sliced strawberries, or ⅓ cup (40 g) raspberries, or ½ banana

OPTIONAL ADDITIONS

Goji berries
Mulberries
Goldenberries
Oil-free raisins

Using a seed grinder, coffee bean grinder, or mortar and pestle, grind the seeds. Put in a breakfast bowl. Cut the fig or figs and the apricot into bite-sized pieces and add to the seeds. Add the optional dried berries and fruit, if you're using. Add 1 Brazil nut and 2 each of four or more nuts. (Vary your choice of nuts daily.) Add 1 or 2 rounded tablespoons of unsulfured blackstrap molasses.

Shake the milk well; pour ½ to ¾ cup (120 to 180 ml) of it over the mixture. Stir gently until the molasses is mixed in. Top with fresh fruit. Enjoy. Your bones are saying thank you.

◄ Making Things Easy ►

Premixing your seeds and nuts will simplify assembling this breakfast. Buy several types of bagged seeds and mix them all together in a big bowl. Then refill the original bags with the mix or store in glass jars or BPA-free ziplock freezer bags. Label each jar or bag as MIXED SEEDS. Keep one bag or container out and store the rest in the freezer or fridge.

To do the same with nuts, combine ¼ pound (115 g) Brazils, ½ pound (225 g) macadamias, and ½ pound (225 g) each of the roasted nuts—filberts, pecans, almonds, cashews, pistachios, walnuts. Use sprouted nuts when possible. Shell the pistachios. Place them into the big bowl. Add the other nuts. Mix well and package in jars or bags. Freeze until you need them.

Variation: To add vitamin K_2, expand your breakfast to include 2 pastured organic eggs. You can substitute raw goat's milk or properly prepared soymilk (see page 246 for cow's milk). Substitute kiwi fruit, melon, mango, papaya, persimmon, or apple for the berries or banana.

Nutrition Information per Serving: 747 mg calcium; 300 mg magnesium; 15 mg protein; 75 mg vitamin C; 125 mcg vitamin A; 3.2 mg iron; 90 mg phosphorus

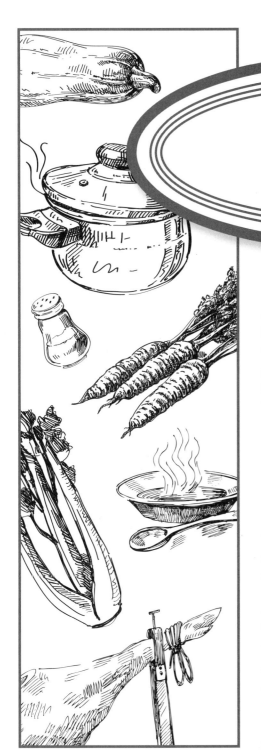

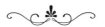

CHAPTER 13

Soups

Soup is a great food. It whets the appetite and allows the cook a lot of leeway. On the practical side, people who start a meal with soup eat less of the rest—which is good news unless the main course is your signature dish. Soups are great for seasonal cooking and some, like bone broth, are bone health VIPs.

Bone Broth

MAKES 1 GALLON (3.8 L)

The simplest, most effective way to create collagen is to make bone broth. Bone broth affords elements that are the ideal ratio of amino acids to build this structural protein.

About Bone Broth

This preparation is rich in minerals that are found in bones and marrow, including calcium, magnesium, iron, silicon, phosphorus, sulfur, and other trace minerals. The other substances are marrow, cartilage, gelatin, glycine, and proline. Cartilage, marrow, and gelatin are forms of collagen; proline and glycine are amino acids that are foundational components of collagen.

Traditionally prepared bone broth has been the mainstay of many ancient and some modern cultures where building and preserving bone is an integral part of long life in health. In traditional cultures, including in Chinese medicine, bone broth is used as a base for feeding infants who cannot breast-feed or are otherwise milk-intolerant. To those ends, dried medicinal herbs were often, and in some cultures always, added to the cooking pot. Many people do still use medicinal herbs when making bone broth, and although a comprehensive text on the compendium of herbs useful for this purpose is beyond the scope of this book, some examples are ginger, Da Zao (jujube dates), and Gou Qi Zi (wolfberry). You can find out more about Chinese herbs by consulting a licensed Chinese medical practitioner.

Adding the vinegar when you are starting the soup helps pull minerals from the bones. Apple cider vinegar provides the most thorough pull. Adding parsley near the end creates an additional pull on the minerals and preserves the parsley's essential oil flavor.

Bone broth needs a long boil. For fish bones, simmer the bones covered for at least 2 hours; for poultry, at least 8 hours; for beef, at least 12. The optimum for beef is 24 hours.

Good Bones for Broth

You can use any bones including non-oily fish and any bones from poultry, lamb, and beef. If you are using beef bones, for added flavor you can roast them before adding them to the broth water. If you are using chicken bones, include chicken feet if possible. Animal feet are particularly rich in gelatin. That may help explain why even today traditional Chinese chefs present beautifully cooked chicken feet to guests, including at breakfast. Helen learned this firsthand when she and her husband were guests of a Guangdong province business association. Officers told her that at one time feet were the only parts of a chicken considered edible so except for the male organ, which is a ceremonial symbol of good luck, the rest was discarded.

Pig trotters are widely available. To find chicken feet, ask at a traditional butcher shop or supermarket meat counter. Some online suppliers ship organic pastured chicken feet. Keep a freezer stash of bones from roasted chicken or beef. You don't get quite the same collagen harvest as you do using raw bones but you do get some, so it's a good way to add collagen for you and additional value to the life of the animal.

Whenever possible, choose organically raised animal parts for making broth.

2–3 pounds (900–1400 g) bones
1 chicken, calf's, or pig's foot
2 Tbsp. apple cider vinegar
4 quarts (4 L) cold filtered water
1 bunch parsley, curly- or flat-leaf, about 10 stalks

OPTIONAL INGREDIENTS FOR ADDED GELATIN

4–6 meaty oxtail bones
Additional 2–3 chicken feet
1 additional sliced calf's foot
1 additional pig's trotter

OPTIONAL FLAVORINGS

1–3 onions
2–3 carrots
2–3 celery stalks

3 cloves fresh garlic, peeled and rough-chopped
Freshly ground sea salt, preferably
    pink Himalayan

Put the bones, feet, vinegar, water, and any medicinal herbs and optional flavorings (whole or roughly chopped) in a stainless-steel pot or slow cooker. Let stand for 30 minutes to 1 hour. Turn on the heat and bring to a boil. Skim any scum off the surface of the water. Reduce the heat, cover, and simmer as directed previously in the "About Bone Broth" section. During the last hour of simmer, add the parsley. Continue cooking for 1 further hour. Strain while hot so the fat does not clot the colander; let the broth cool.

You may remove congealed fat that rises to the top but be careful to retain the marrow. Marrow contains omega-3 fatty acids, minerals, vitamin A, and stem cells, precursors to red and white blood cells and platelets. Consuming animal bone marrow helps with rebuilding after marrow suppression, typically following chemotherapy and radiation treatments. Marrow can also help to redress iron deficiency anemia.

Examine the beef bones for retained marrow, scrape it out with a slender knife, and leave it in the soup. Refrigerate the cooled broth until it is cold.

Cold broth will be gelatinous. It should shimmer, much as chicken soup does when refrigerated. If the soup is thin, increase the bones-to-water ratio next time.

Refrigerate what you will use within 7 days. Immediately freeze the rest.

Nutrition Information per Serving: collagen; calcium; magnesium; trace minerals; silicon; iron; phosphorus; sulfur

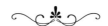

Bone Broth Fish Soup

SERVES 2

This is Helen's mixed-up fish soup. Mostly the base is plain bone broth—the bones, a bit of vinegar at the start, and parsley in the last hour. That is the start of soups like this one rich with olive oil and garlic, tempting with al dente vegetables, and interesting with a lovely piece of fish. Helen uses haddock or cod because it becomes so juicy and scrumptious once in the soup. Chris prefers monkfish. Halibut is successful, though expensive.

3 oz. (85 g) haddock, cod, halibut, or monkfish
2 cups (480 ml) bone broth
3–4 Tbsp. olive oil, divided
2 cloves garlic, sliced
1 tsp. red pepper flakes or 1 dried red chili
    pepper, crushed
1 small carrot, cut in ¼-inch (.6 cm) slices
6–8 small cubes organic natural tofu
1–2 spring onions or scallions, sliced into rounds
3–4 medium shiitake mushrooms, stems and
    caps sliced
1 small vine-ripened tomato (optional)

Wash the fish and dry it with paper towels. If you are using monkfish, cut it into large chunks. Set the fish aside.

Set the bone broth in a small saucepan. You'll need a lid.

In a small frying pan, add 1½ to 2 tablespoons of the olive oil and 1 slice of garlic; turn the heat to medium. When the garlic just begins to sizzle, reduce the heat slightly and add remainder of the garlic, carrot, tofu, scallion(s), chopped mushrooms, and tomato, if using.

Heat the broth to simmering. As soon as it reaches a simmer, cover to prevent reduction.

Sauté the vegetables quietly, adjusting the heat as needed, until the garlic is brown, the mushrooms are cooked through, and the carrot is al dente. Pour the sauté into a large soup bowl, but do not scrape. Cover the soup bowl with a plate to retain the heat.

In the frying pan, add the remaining olive oil, heat to medium, and sauté your fish until it is no longer translucent. Cook about 7 minutes or until the fish flakes when you insert a fork.

Pour the piping-hot spicy bone broth into the bowl and add the fish. Enjoy.

> **Nutrition Information per Serving:** collagen; calcium; magnesium; trace minerals; silicon; iron; phosphorus; sulfur

Bone Broth Sausage Soup

SERVES 2

A hearty full-meal soup for cold nights, or any time to feel restored. And here's a tip: When you make this recipe, make sure you prepare a few extra tofu chunks to eat while you cook—they are irresistible.

½–1 chicken-and-garlic sausage per serving, prepared ahead of time (see below)

1 tsp. olive oil

1 scant tsp. white miso paste

4 cups (960 ml) meat or poultry bone broth (see Bone Broth, page 141), divided

¼ sweet Vidalia onion

1 clove garlic, sliced very thin

8–10 ½-inch (1.25 cm) tofu chunks

¼ zucchini, any size, cut into small chunks

2 tomatoes, cut in half

2–4 Tbsp. toasted or untoasted sesame oil (optional)

A few ribbons of lacinato kale, torn into small pieces (optional)

Split the sausage or the sausages lengthwise. Add a teaspoon of olive oil to a small cast-iron griddle or fry pan. Heat the pan until the oil skitters a bit and turn the heat to medium. Place the sausage cut-side down on the griddle. Fry for at least 5 minutes on each side and then until done to your pleasure.

Mix the miso paste in ¼ cup (60 ml) of the cold bone broth. Set aside.

Using the sausage pan, sauté the onion and garlic until the aroma rises and the onion is heading toward translucent. Add the tofu and sauté until the chunks are browned and look crunchy. Add the zucchini chunks and tomato halves. Sauté until the two are just softened. Turn off the heat. You may set this all aside for a while or keep it covered in the refrigerator along with the cooked sausage for a few hours or overnight.

Heat the remaining bone broth till bubbles form around the edge, indicating the soup is near a boil. Add the chopped sausage. Add the contents of the sauté pan. (You may wish to include the sesame oil sometimes for flavor variation.)

Add the miso mixture to the soup pot and stir. If you are including lacinato kale, now is the time to add the chopped ribbons to the soup.

Dip the ladle deep into the soup, stir up the vegetables and sausage, and scoop up a ladleful for each soup dish. Repeat until you have as much as you like in each bowl. Top up with a little extra broth.

> **Nutrition Information per Serving:** calcium; magnesium; trace minerals; silicon; iron; phosphorus; sulfur

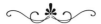

Truffled Jerusalem Artichoke Soup

SERVES 2

This is a luscious anytime soup—rich, filling, with perfectly balanced flavors. The Jerusalem artichoke is a vegetable with many names, including sunroot, sunchoke, and topinambour. It is actually a species of sunflower. These grow easily and you can store them; they have little starch and a high ratio of inulin; they make a great prebiotic for your gut bugs. Black truffles can be very costly; you can substitute porcini mushrooms. Thanks to Reynolds for this recipe.

1½ lb. (680 g) Jerusalem artichoke
½ lemon
2 Tbsp. unsalted butter, divided
1 clove garlic
2 cups (480 ml) vegetable stock
¾ cup (180 ml) raw double cream
Salt and pepper
1 oz. (28 g) black truffle, thinly shaved on a
   mandoline
4 tsp. black truffle oil

Peel and dice the Jerusalem artichokes and place them into water with the lemon. Use the half lemon as is; do not squeeze the juice into the water.

Place a medium-sized pan over medium heat and add half of the butter. Once the butter has melted, add the Jerusalem artichoke and the garlic clove and sweat for 5 minutes, taking care they don't become too brown. Add the vegetable stock and the double cream and simmer for 30 minutes.

Season to taste. Blend the soup in a food processor with the remaining butter then pass it through a chinois—a sieve with a very fine cone-shaped mesh. When you are ready to serve, pour into shot glasses and top with a black truffle shaving and a drizzle of the truffle oil.

Nutrition Information per Serving: 75 mg calcium; vitamin C; excellent prebiotic; great source of trace minerals; 4 mg iron (about 30 percent of bone RDA)

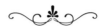

Butternut Squash and Natto Powder Soup

SERVES 2–3

Now that research confirms the benefits to bone and general health of vitamin K_2—and that natto is nothing short of a K_2 factory—some specialty food manufacturers have sought to develop a palatable form of natto for Western consumers—and succeeded. It's a powder, and we use it because we prefer it to the consistency and smell of natto.

Here is an excellent soup recipe that includes natto powder. One tablespoon of natto powder per bowl supplies 450 mcg (100 percent RDA) of MK7, the long-lasting form of vitamin K_2.

1 medium-large butternut squash
2 Tbsp. ghee
1 yellow onion, chopped
Sea salt and ground black pepper to taste
½ cup (120 ml) warm chicken bone broth or water
2–3 Tbsp. natto powder

Cut the butternut squash in half lengthwise. Scoop out the seeds and save them for roasting. Cut the squash into chunks and bake at 350°F (175°C) for 20 minutes or until soft. Cool and remove the skin.

In a saucepan, heat the ghee, then add the onion, salt, and pepper. Cook until the onion softens, then add the squash chunks and mix. Remove from the heat and use an immersion blender to make a thick soup. Add the warm bone broth or water to thin to your desired consistency.

Ladle the soup into individual serving bowls and stir 1 Tbsp. of natto power into each bowl. The natto adds a pleasant, slightly malty flavor.

> **Nutrition Information per Serving:** 75 mg calcium; 50 mg magnesium; 450 mcg vitamin K$_2$; 50 mg vitamin C; 14,000 iu vitamin A

Sprouted Fava Bean Soup

SERVES 4

Ancient Egyptians were suspicious of beans and gave them a long soak. Today Egypt's popular soup called bessara is served with stems of fresh arugula, pickles, and bread. Talk about the wisdom of the body. Favas—also called broad beans—are high in L-dopa, and are being studied for their ability to help with symptoms of Parkinson's disease.

This bessara variation is a popular breakfast in Morocco. Soak the beans for between 3 and 4 days. They are ready to use at the first sign of a sprout. Hull before cooking.

2 cups (250 g) sprouted hulled fava beans (see "Sprouting Beans" on page 48)
2 large cloves garlic
4 cups (960 ml) filtered water
2 Tbsp. extra-virgin olive oil
1 tsp. ground cumin
½ tsp. salt

OPTIONAL CONDIMENTS

Cilantro
Olive oil
Paprika
Cumin
Minced garlic
Chopped chilies
Chili flakes
Yogurt

Put the sprouted beans, garlic cloves, and water in a pot, bring to a boil, and simmer for 45 minutes to an hour, until the beans are mashable. Drain the beans and garlic, put them in a large bowl, and toss with the olive oil, cumin and salt. Puree with a hand blender (also called an immersion blender). Taste and thin the soup with additional water if you wish. Serve with an array of condiments, varying them each time you serve this soup.

> **Nutrition Information per Serving:** 60 mg calcium; 50 mg magnesium; 14 g protein; phytoestrogen; trace minerals including almost 100 percent of daily copper needs

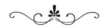

Mexican Fava Bean Soup

SERVES 2–4

This is the version from Mexico. Within this recipe is a version of an ancient Mayan spice mix called *recado*. It is often used as a marinade for meat. Here it complements the hearty fava bean beautifully.

2 cups (250 g) fava beans, sprouted and hulled
4 cups (960 ml) water
1 chopped heirloom tomato or equivalent heirloom cherry tomatoes
1 clove garlic, smashed then chopped
1 small yellow onion, chopped

½–1 tsp. salt

1 tsp. black pepper

1 Tbsp. olive oil

½–1 tsp. ground cumin

2 tsp. crushed saffron threads

OPTIONAL GARNISHES

Cilantro leaves, finely chopped

Saffron threads

Olive oil

Ground cumin

Chopped raw garlic

After sprouting and hulling the fava beans, bring them to a boil in the water. Simmer, loosely covered, for 45 minutes.

While the beans cook, prepare the *recado*. Mix the tomato, garlic, onion, salt, pepper in a blender. In a large saucepan, heat the oil on medium-high. Brown the cumin for about 2 minutes, stirring constantly, then add the tomato mix; stir so it doesn't stick, about 5 minutes.

Mix the fava beans and saffron into the *recado*, stirring to keep the mixture from sticking. Cook for about 10 minutes more.

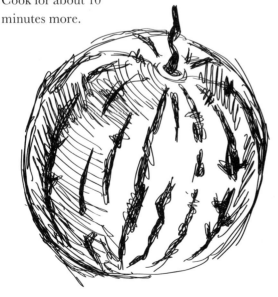

Serve chunky or blend further with a hand-held immersion blender or hand mixer. Top with garnishes if desired.

> **Nutrition Information per Serving:** 60 mg calcium; 50 mg magnesium; 14 g protein; phytoestrogen; trace minerals; 800 mcg copper

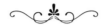

Watermelon Gazpacho with Basil Oil
SERVES 2–4

The ingredients for this soup seem an odd combination, we know. However, on the theory of equal and opposite reaction, the taste is amazing. It's light and refreshing and if there are kids around, you'll be glad when they ask for seconds, as it is full of goodness.

1 large heirloom tomato or equivalent heirloom cherry tomatoes

2 cups (305 g) watermelon with seeds

1½ tsp. red wine vinegar

¼ cup (60 ml) olive oil

1 tsp. virgin coconut oil

2 Tbsp. chopped red onion

½ cucumber, minced

2½ Tbsp. minced fresh dill

2 small cloves garlic

½–1 serrano chili

1 cup (150 g) raw feta cheese

Salt and pepper

BASIL OIL

1 cup fresh basil leaves

¼ cup olive oil

¼ tsp. salt

Put all the ingredients into a blender. Puree until the color and consistency are even. Put the mixture into a bowl and top with a drizzle of Basil Oil and a fresh basil leaf.

Basil Oil: Put the basil oil ingredients in a blender and puree until smooth.

> **Nutrition Information per Serving:** 200 mg calcium; 30 mg vitamin C; 1,600 iu vitamin A

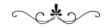

Mushroom Soup

SERVES 6

Basic mushroom mix—mushrooms, garlic, onions, and butter—makes the base for so many delicious dishes. Here we use it as the starter for a luxurious soup.

To create intense flavor, use at least four but hopefully more varieties of mushrooms: maitake, shiitake, cremini, oyster, trumpet, portobello, porcini, enoki, straw, or any of the others you may seek out or come upon in your grocery store or at a local produce stand.

6 cups (1.5 L) mushrooms, four or more varieties
6 cups (325 g) Bone Broth (page 141)
¾ cup (1½ sticks [170 g]) unsalted butter, divided
2 Tbsp. extra-virgin olive oil
1 large double shallot or two small double
    shallots, chopped
4 cloves garlic, minced
2 Tbsp. unbleached sprouted white flour
1½–2 cups (360–480 ml) heavy cream, divided
1 Tbsp. fresh or dried thyme
Nutmeg (optional)
Sea salt and freshly ground black pepper
Truffle oil

Chopped chives (optional)
Chopped flat-leaf parsley (optional)

Wash the mushrooms, drain in a wire strainer, and dry on paper towels. Trim off the lower ends of the stems and chop the rest—stems and all.

In a stockpot, bring the bone broth to a simmer. Turn off the heat.

Melt ½ cup (115 g) of the butter in a large frying pan and add the olive oil. Sauté the shallot and garlic for 2 minutes or until a garlic aroma rises. Turn up the heat, add the mushrooms, fold in the butter-oil mix, cover the pan, reduce the heat, and cook until the mushrooms are limp. They should give a goodly amount of juice.

In a small frying pan, make a roux by melting the remaining butter and whisking in the flour. Cook on the lowest heat for 3 minutes. Watch to make sure the flour doesn't brown.

In a stream add ½ cup (120 ml) of the hot bone broth; whisk until the broth is incorporated and starts to thicken. Add ½ cup (120 ml) of the cream. Whisk and stir over low heat until the mixture thickens. Add the mixture to the rest of the bone broth.

Add the mushrooms and thyme, and nutmeg if desired. Season with salt and black pepper as needed. Stir over low heat until the soup is hot and bubbles form. Add the remaining cream and nutmeg. Heat on low until just heated through. Whiz with an immersion blender for a few seconds to thicken the soup while retaining the textures. For a thicker soup, add additional cream while cooking.

To each serving add a few drops of truffle oil. Top with chives or parsley if you like.

> **Nutrition Information per Serving:** 100 mg calcium; 800 iu vitamin D; trace minerals; collagen

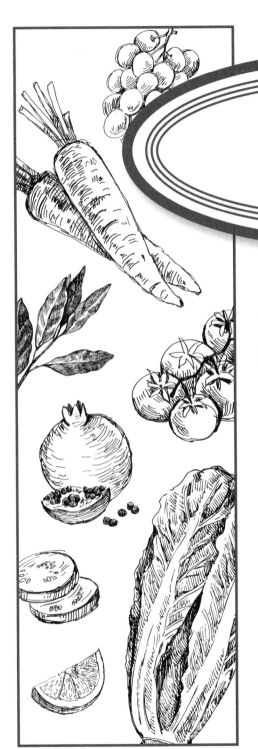

Salads

The compounds that give fruits and vegetables their rich color palette are phytochemicals—*phyto* meaning "plant." Phytochemicals are non-nutrients; that is, they provide no standard nutrients. Yet as antioxidants and as cell-signaling molecules, they are vital to health. Each color represents its own group of phytochemicals, and they all fall under the heading of flavonoids.

Carotenoids make pumpkin, squash, and carrots orange. There are numerous forms of carotenoids, precursors to vitamin A. Another carotenoid, lycopene, makes tomatoes and watermelons red. Lycopene is a strong antioxidant; it appears to protect against prostate cancer and cardiovascular disease.

Anthocyanins provide color to red-purple grapes and berries, which are also intensely antioxidant. Scientists hypothesize that the anthocyanins in blueberries are highly protective against Alzheimer's disease.

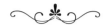

Seaweed Salad with Yuzu Dressing

SERVES 2

Chefs and beauty care specialists alike use yuzu, a leathery-peel Chinese citrus fruit prized for its high vitamin C content and ability to rejuvenate skin. It is said that a hot yuzu bath on winter solstice wards off winter colds and flu. Fresh yuzu are seasonally available in some food markets. Juice from fresh is preferable to bottled yuzu juice, which is widely available on the Internet.

Wakame nears the top of the list in vegetarian sources of omega-3 fatty acids. Of late Westerners have embraced this subtle, sweet seaweed. Compounds in seaweed help burn fatty tissue.

3 Tbsp. wakame seaweed
½ cucumber, chopped
1 head butter lettuce
1 tsp. toasted sesame seeds

DRESSING

1 Tbsp. sugar
1 Tbsp. hot water
3 Tbsp. miso paste
1 tsp. sake
1 tsp. mirin
1 Tbsp. yuzu juice

Soak the seaweed in cool water for 30 minutes. Drain it and mix it with the cucumber and lettuce in a large bowl. Dress the salad with Yuzu Dressing and sprinkle the sesame seeds on top.

Dressing: Mix the sugar into the hot water in a small bowl. Add the remaining dressing ingredients and mix well.

Nutrition Information per Serving: 150 mg calcium; 100 mg magnesium; 50 mg vitamin C; phytoestrogen

The 7-Eleven Salad

SERVES 1

Late one night at the airport in Copenhagen, Laura was hungry and the only source of food was a 7-Eleven—where people buy packaged food, donuts, and late-night corn dogs, right? Nope, not here. There were fresh-grilled vegetable sandwiches and crisp appetizing salads. Do customers in Denmark shun processed fat, sugar, and carbs?

Our salad is in homage to the 7-Eleven stores in Denmark, and a reminder that market forces can bring us high-quality nutrition. In this bean and grain dish, phytic acid is a distant memory.

½ cup (10 g) raw arugula
1 cup (70 g) chopped raw bok choy
¼ cup (38 g) sprouted garbanzo beans, cooked and cooled (see "Sprouting Beans," page 48)
¼ cup (46 g) sprouted raw adzuki beans (see "Sprouting Beans," page 48)
½–1 cup (90–185 g) quinoa, cooked
½ can (about 4 oz. [115 g]) wild-caught salmon with bones, or 4 oz. (115 g) fresh sashimi-grade salmon
½ cup (145 g) Zesty Yogurt Dressing (page 207)
Salt and pepper

Sprouting the beans takes a few days, and quinoa preparation takes about half a day, so preplan these ingredients for the most effective bone health results. Once these are available, however, this salad is simple and straightforward to prepare. Simply mix all the ingredients in a bowl. Enjoy, and think of the joys of travel.

Nutrition Information per Serving: 200 mg calcium; 140 mg magnesium; 30 g protein; phytoestrogen; probiotics

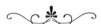

Colorful Arugula Salad with Fresh Lemon Dressing

SERVES 2

Yellow vegetables are among the antioxidant leading lights. This is a simple salad you can dress up with red beets or expand the yellow theme by adding Cape gooseberries—also called ground cherries—sold in American grocery stores as physalis. They have a characteristic papery skin.

Yellow-green comes from zeaxanthin and lutein, both xanthophylls in the carotenoid family. Think avocado, or melon. In particular these two compounds accumulate in the retina and are specifically protective against ophthalmic diseases and overall, against aging.

4 boiled golden beets
2 cups (40 g) fresh arugula, washed, stems removed
2 purple or red tomatoes, cut into wedges
Goat cheese (optional)
A few physalis, halved, or whole blueberries (optional)

DRESSING

½ cup (120 ml) olive or pistachio oil (or a mix)
1 Tbsp. red wine vinegar
1 tsp. bone vinegar
2 Tbsp. fresh lemon juice
⅓ cup (38 g) chopped Vidalia or other sweet onion
Salt and pepper to taste

Boil the beets in their skins until a cake tester slips right through easily, about 20 minutes. Allow the beets to cool, then peel them and cut them into wedges. As the beets are cooling, swish the arugula leaves in a bowl of very cold water, then drain dry and tear the leaves.

Combine all the vegetables and optional ingredients in a bowl and toss, or set out the arugula on a platter and arrange the remaining optional vegetables and cheese into a pattern that pleases you.

Dressing: Mix all the ingredients in a bowl and blend with hand blender. Pass the dressing with the salad.

Nutrition Information per Serving: 150 mg calcium; high in the phytonutrient betalain and in trace minerals

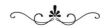

About Arugula

You may know arugula as rúcula or rocket. It is richly nutritious—a member of the celebrated Brassica family that includes broccoli, bok choy, and cauliflower—and is your bones' star green. The young, bright-green leaves are subtle in flavor, and the darker leaves can be piquant and peppery. And it's a gardener's dream: It's easy to grow and maintain even in cool climates; the leaves regenerate for months; and, the entire plant—flowers, seeds, and leaves—is edible.

But with a bone health hat on, we love arugula because it is relatively low in oxalic acid—and it includes in its extensive nutritional armory higher-than-average-for-greens calcium, potassium, and vitamin K.

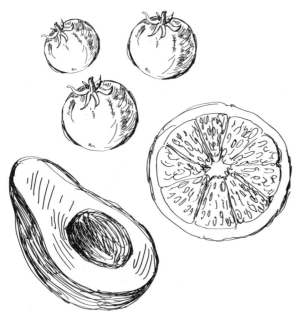

Breakfast Salad

SERVES 1

Though a morning staple in many countries, salad may not have breakfast appeal in the West. But take a look: No lettuce leaves and vinaigrette for this one. Instead tropical fruits and a creamy dressing smooth with avocado and sweet with the natural sugar of oranges and honey.

Fresh and light and full of nutrients to start off your morning, this is a dish to enjoy for breakfast or serve for brunch. Choose it as a great alternative to a smoothie or include it as a complement to a more substantial egg or breakfast rice dish.

1 cup (16 g) chopped kale
5 heirloom cherry tomatoes, halved
½ mango, diced
½ avocado, diced
5 sprouted roasted almonds
¼ cup (25 g) sunflower sprouts
¼ cup (25 g) radish sprouts (optional)
¼ cup (25 g) soybean sprouts (optional—if you need a phytoestrogen boost)
2 slices cooked unpreserved bacon, in pieces (omit for vegan)
½ tsp. poppy seeds
2 tsp. Spiced Pepitas (page 229)
Pinch of salt
Pinch of cayenne pepper

DRESSING

½ avocado
Juice of ¼ lime
Juice of ½ small orange
1 clove garlic, whole
Pinch of salt
2 Tbsp. olive oil

Pinch of black pepper

1 tsp. honey

Prepare the kale, tomatoes, and mango. Cut an avocado in half and gently slide the two halves apart. Leave the pit in one half and set it aside for the dressing. Dice the other half. Combine the vegetables and fruit with the rest of the ingredients in a bowl and toss, then dress and toss the salad again. The optional radish sprouts would add a strong spicy flavor, and the soybean sprouts offer a phytoestrogen boost.

Dressing: Put all the ingredients into a blender and puree. Toss over the salad.

Variation: Substitute ¼ cup (70 g) Zesty Yogurt Dressing, page 207, for the orange juice and honey. Enjoy the bacon on the side.

Nutrition Information per Serving: 110 mg calcium; 150 mg magnesium; 13 g protein; phytoestrogen; probiotics

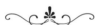

Caesar Salad

SERVES 2

Caesar Cardini first made this storied salad at the restaurant in Tijuana he ran during Prohibition days so people could eat *and* drink. Or so the story goes. This is scrumptious and quickly prepared with a bowl, a whisk, and six ingredients. And your bones love this treat, too. The yolk is rich in K_2; anchovies have bones; and vitamin K, vitamin A, and folate top the list of romaine's bounty. Rinse the eggshells before cracking; salmonella bacteria live on the shell, not inside the egg. This is much less a worry if the eggs are from pastured hens.

1 large clove garlic

2 pastured egg yolks

1 head or 2 hearts of fresh romaine lettuce

4–6 anchovies in olive oil

½ cup (120 ml) olive oil

Big squeeze of fresh lemon juice

Dash of Worcestershire sauce

Dab of Dijon mustard

About 1½ oz. (42 g) shaved raw milk
   Parmigiano-Reggiano, crumbled into bits

Shake of cracked black pepper

Fifteen minutes before making the salad, put the garlic through a garlic press and set aside.

Rinse the shells of two eggs in cold water. Wash the lettuce leaves whole; dry thoroughly in paper towels. Separate the egg yolks from the egg whites. If you plan to use the whites, you can refrigerate them for up to 4 days or freeze for up to 6 months in a freezer compartment.

Put the yolks into a small deep bowl. Whisk in the minced garlic. Whisk in the anchovies until they are chopped into tiny pieces but not yet melted away. Pour in the oil in a steady stream slowly but continuously to incorporate it, whisking all the time, until the mixture has thickened into a lovely creamy Caesar vinaigrette. Whisk in the lemon, Worcestershire, and mustard. Fold in the Parmesan and black pepper.

Tear the lettuce leaves into a bowl or leave whole, and dress the salad.

Note: Notice there's no salt in the ingredients list. The anchovies provide that along with their bones. Using anchovies packed in olive oil makes the anchovies easier to mash. And no croutons, please, unless they're made from your own sourdough bread.

Nutrition Information per Serving: 375 mg calcium; 60 mg magnesium; 50 iu vitamin D; 40 mcg vitamin K_2; 18 g protein

> ### ❧ Coring Lettuce ❧
>
> You can core a head of iceberg lettuce the same way you core a head of romaine. Push a bit of wet paper towel into the space where the core was and store the lettuce in a BPA/BPS-free plastic bag or lettuce keeper. Even organic and untreated it will keep crisp and fresh in the fridge for days.

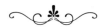

French Salad

SERVES 2

Lamb's lettuce, also called cornsalad and mâche, is a smooth-leaf salad green that is lovely on the tongue especially when dressed in the very lightest of vinaigrettes. Lamb's lettuce is one of the richest vegetable sources of vitamin A, and higher than any other in vitamin C. If you cannot find lamb's lettuce for this salad, use watercress with a slightly more robust dressing of richer olive oil—or use romaine lettuce, which is richer in minerals than most other lettuces, and balsamic vinegar. Lore has it that Roman soldiers ate a lot of this lettuce as part of keeping fighting fit; thus the name. Well, that's the story and we're sticking to it.

2 medium vine-ripened Beefsteak tomatoes, washed and dried in paper towels
2 medium red beets, boiled and then peeled
1 small red onion, peeled
2 cups (70 g) lamb's lettuce, washed and spun dry or dried very gently in paper towels

Slice the tomatoes quite thick so they look meaty and substantial. Slice the beets in medium slices.

Slice the onion thinly and separate into rings. Place the onion, tomatoes, and beets into a shallow bowl and marinate in Lightly Lightly Vinaigrette dressing (page 163) for 15 minutes or up to an hour.

Distribute the lamb's lettuce into a shallow bowl. We like to use a large, flat pasta bowl. Dress with the vinaigrette to taste. Distribute the vegetables over the lettuce. Toss and serve.

Note: Roasted beets are delicious, but boiling reduces anti-nutrients. If you have the time and inclination, skin the tomatoes before slicing them.

Nutrition Information per Serving: 40 mg calcium; 50 mg magnesium; trace minerals; 0.8 mcg boron

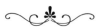

Italian Salad

SERVES 2

This salad also uses either lamb's lettuce or romaine, but introduces richer flavors of goat cheese and citrus.

2 cups (70 g) lamb's lettuce
2–4 oz. (57–115 g) medium-aged goat cheese
1 orange, cut into thin slices, each slice peeled and quartered
1 Tbsp. dried cranberries
2–3 Tbsp. sprouted pumpkin seeds

Wash the lamb's lettuce in cold water, dry in paper towels, and dress to taste. Cut the goat cheese into small chunks. Add the orange pieces and goat cheese to the salad and toss. Sprinkle with dried cranberries and sprouted pumpkin seeds.

Variation: Substitute roasted red and gold beets for the oranges.

Nutrition Information per Serving: *Using Lamb's Lettuce:* 80 mg calcium; 60 mg magnesium; 38 mg vitamin C; 330 mcg vitamin A; 53 mg phosphorus; *Using Romaine Lettuce:* 90 mg calcium; 60 mg magnesium; 1.2 g protein; 210 mcg vitamin A; 24 mg phosphorus

lemon zest and season well. Mix all the ingredients (except the almonds and pumpkin seeds) together with the dressing. Let stand for 1 hour for flavors to develop. Sprinkle with almonds and seeds.

Nutrition Information per Serving: 300 mg magnesium; 30 g protein; prebiotics; 50 percent of daily iron requirement

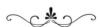

Nectarine, Pea, Broad Bean, and Spelt Salad

SERVES 4

Broad beans are fava beans by another name. This recipe, shared with us by the Reynolds company, results in a salad that is sweet and tender, and surprisingly filling. It's a lovely spring dish, and looks beautiful on the table. Peas are actually a fruit, and have been around since the dawn of agriculture. This salad is best served at room temperature.

1 lb. (500 g) fresh peas in shell
1 lb. (500 g) fresh fava beans in shell
6½ Tbsp. (100 ml) smoked olive oil
Juice and zest of 2 lemons
2 ripe nectarines, stoned and sliced
1 lb. (500 g) cooked spelt
½ cup (20 g) flat-leaf parsley, picked
¼ cup (10 g) mint leaves,
  roughly chopped
Seeds from ½ pomegranate
1 bunch spring onions, chopped
Salt and pepper
½ cup (50 g) flaked almonds, toasted
2 Tbsp. (20 g) pumpkin seeds

Pod, blanch, and refresh the fresh peas. Pod, blanch, refresh, and peel the broad beans. Whisk together the smoked olive oil, lemon juice, and

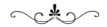

Fresh Mint Salad

SERVES 2–3

This spicy salad with its light lemon dressing is a fine complement to heavier dishes like Fava Bean and Pork Falafel (page 183).

A quarter cup (15 g) parsley offers 250 percent of a day's vitamin K_1 and 25 percent of vitamin C. It contains luteolin, a powerful antioxidant. Mint can alleviate stomachache.

Za'atar, an herb mixture dating from biblical times, today simply refers to a blend of Middle Eastern flavors and is a favorite of chefs who specialize in Middle Eastern food because each can make a signature mix. With this za'atar we offer ours.

2 cloves garlic
1 head romaine, chopped
2 tomatoes, chopped
½ medium cucumber, chopped
¼ cup (15 g) chopped fresh parsley,
  flat-leaf or curly-leaf
¼ cup (25 g) chopped fresh mint
1 lemon, juiced
4 tsp. olive oil
2 Tbsp. za'atar

ZA'ATAR

1 Tbsp. ground oregano, fresh or dried

1 Tbsp. sumac (optional, hard to find in supermarkets)

1 Tbsp. thyme

1 Tbsp. cumin

1 tsp. salt

1 tsp. ground black pepper

1 tsp. ground turmeric

1 Tbsp. sesame seeds

Smash garlic cloves whole and in the skin. We use the flat side of a meat tenderizing hammer. Celebrity chefs like the flat side of a knife, but we avoid that technique. If you have a heavy plastic glass, smash the garlic with the bottom of the glass. Remove the garlic skins—they will come off easily. Use a paring knife to lop off the stem end and chop the rest into small pieces. Mix all the ingredients in a medium-sized bowl. Toss it well.

Za'atar: Using a mortar and pestle, grind the oregano with the sumac (if you have it), thyme, and cumin. Add the salt, pepper, and ground turmeric and stir. Tip the mix into a clean jar, add the sesame seeds, and shake to mix. It keeps well on a pantry shelf.

Note: Poison sumac and sumac are different species.

Nutrition Information per Serving: 135 mg calcium; 70 mg magnesium; 7 g protein; phytoestrogens

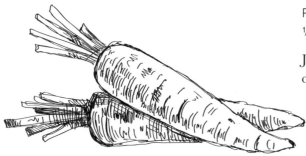

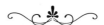

Jicama Red Summer Salad

SERVES 2–3

Here's another refreshing salad. Red cabbage contains abundant calcium, vitamin C, vitamin A, and 50 percent of a day's requisite vitamin B_6. In the Netherlands Cohort Study on Diet and Cancer, it was found that eating any cabbage once a week dropped the risk of colon cancer by more than 60 percent. Also, the anthocyanins stimulate digestion.

Jicama is a potent prebiotic—but you must peel it before eating it. Use homegrown sprouts (for instructions, see page 48) or buy fresh organic.

1 jicama root, peeled

1 large carrot

½ head red cabbage

¼ cup (25 g) sunflower sprouts

¼ cup (25 g) radish sprouts

¼ cup (25 g) soy sprouts

½ cup (120 ml) Dressing

DRESSING

1 fresh lime

1 tsp. minced chili or chili flakes

1 Tbsp. chopped shallot

1 Tbsp. apple cider vinegar

1½ tsp. red sherry vinegar

Pinch of sugar

Pinch of salt

⅓ cup (80 ml) olive oil

Julienne the jicama and the carrot. Shred the cabbage. Put the vegetables into a bowl along with the rest of the ingredients. Mix well.

Variation: To make this salad a complete meal, add ½ cup (95 g) sprouted cooked and cooled chickpeas or pinto beans (canned beans cannot be sprouted, so either buy already sprouted beans or start with dry and see "Sprouting Beans" on page 48); ¼ cup (46 g) cooked sprouted quinoa; and ¼ avocado. Mix everything in a big bowl and toss with Red Summer Dressing.

Dressing: Cut the lime into quarters and squeeze into a small jar. Mince a dried whole chili with the back of a teaspoon. Add the minced chili or already prepared pepper flakes to the jar along with the remaining ingredients. Shake until the oil and seasonings are well mixed.

> Nutrition Information per Serving: 200 mg calcium; 125 mg magnesium; 13 mg protein; phytoestrogen; prebiotics

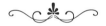

Long Life Salad

SERVES 4

Laura made this one summer when it was so hot, eating anything seemed a bridge too far. This salad was so pleasing to eat and so nutritious, it became a summer staple.

It does take a bit of advance planning, yet it is so nutritious we think you'll agree that it's worth the effort, especially since we can safely say that adding this to your diet improves the chances you'll live longer. Sounds like snake oil but it's sound nutritional science.

1 cup (150 g) chopped green beans
3 stalks celery, chopped
1½ cups (380 g) homemade teriyaki tofu cut into bite-sized chunks (see "How to Make Tofu" on page 247 and Marvelous Marinade on page 165)

½ cup (50 g) fresh raw sprouted mung beans (not dried, see "Sprouting Beans" on page 48)
1 avocado cut into bite-sized chunks
½ cup (120 g) sprouted, cooked, and cooled garbanzo beans
¼ cup (25 g) radish sprouts and/or alfalfa sprouts
¼ cup (46 g) fresh raw sprouted adzuki beans
2 peeled chopped raw carrots
4 chopped marinated shiitake mushrooms
½ cup (17 g) chopped watercress

DRESSING · Makes ½ cup (120 ml)

Pinch of salt and freshly ground black pepper, or more to taste
3 Tbsp. apple cider vinegar
3 Tbsp. olive oil
1 Tbsp. coconut oil, at room temperature

Prepare a bowl of ice water. Drop the green beans into a pan of boiling water and boil for 3 minutes. Drain the beans and plunge them into the ice water. Leave the beans to cool.

If the celery isn't fresh and crisp, using a separate bowl, pop it into some ice water. It should crisp by the time the beans have cooled. Then drain and dry it thoroughly on paper towels before chopping.

Combine all the ingredients in a large bowl. Dress with Long Life Dressing.

Dressing: Put the ingredients in a bowl and mix well, or put them into a jar with a tight-fitting lid and shake to mix.

> Nutrition Information per Serving: 185 mg calcium; 350 mg magnesium; 800 iu vitamin D; 20 g protein; phytoestrogens; prebiotics; probiotics

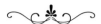

Persimmon Jicama Pomegranate Salad

SERVES 4–6

This lovely salad created by Molly Watson, Local Foods Expert at About.com, is one of the most bone-friendly salads we've come across. Prepare this for a scrumptious lunch or robust side salad.

Don't shy away from persimmons. Fuyus have neither seeds nor tannins, so they are sweet and easy to enjoy, and their modifications arose safely through hybridization. When they're paired with romaine, jicama, and pomegranate in this delicious dressing, there's no pucker—just pure nutrition.

Pepitas—the word is Spanish for "little squash seeds"—are shelled pumpkin seeds.

1 head romaine lettuce
1–2 fuyu persimmons
½ small jicama
1 pomegranate
½ cup (65 g) roasted pepitas
 (candied optional)

DRESSING

1 small clove garlic (optional)
3 Tbsp. olive oil or virgin coconut oil
1 Tbsp. lime juice
½ tsp. agave syrup or raw honey
½ tsp. sea salt
¼ tsp. freshly ground black pepper
⅛–¼ tsp. ground cumin

Tear or cut the romaine lettuce into bite-sized pieces, rinse, dry, and keep cool in the fridge.

Hull the persimmons by using a sharp knife to cut around the top and pull off the hull along with whatever is attached. Cut the persimmons in half, set the halves cut-side down, and cut half-moon slices. Peel the jicama and cut into thin slices or matchsticks.

To remove the seeds from the pomegranate, press down while rolling the fruit. Then cut it into quarters. Submerge the quarters in a bowl of cool water and gently squeeze the seeds loose. The pith will float up while the seeds sink. Pick off the pith and pour the water through a strainer, saving the pomegranate seeds.

Put the lettuce in the salad bowl and toss gently but thoroughly with the dressing to coat the leaves evenly. Lay the persimmon slices and jicama sticks on top. Drizzle with the reserved dressing. Sprinkle with pomegranate seeds and pepitas to taste. Serve right away.

Dressing: Combine all the ingredients in a large salad bowl. Whisk vigorously to incorporate the seasonings into the oil. Remove 2 teaspoons of the dressing and set aside in a small cup or bowl.

Nutrition Information per Serving: 100 mg calcium; 140 mg magnesium; 100 mg vitamin C; 2,000 iu vitamin A; phytoestrogen; prebiotics

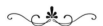

Napa Cabbage Salad

SERVES 4–6

Napa cabbage belongs to the Brassica family, a cousin of brussels sprouts and kale. As such it is much more nutritious than it might seem likely for such a light leaf. Apart from the antioxidant phytonutrients, there's half your daily dose of vitamin C and vitamin K_1, along with a large dose of folate, for almost no calories. Add in the edamame, the seeds, and the seaweed and suddenly you have a nutritional powerhouse hidden in a light tasty salad.

1 whole napa cabbage, washed and sliced into shreds

1 cup (240 g) non-GMO edamame, shelled, soaked, and boiled for 5 minutes

¼ cup (10 g) arame, soaked for 20 minutes and drained, and/or 1 sheet of nori, chopped

⅓ cup (42 g) toasted sunflower seeds, sprouted

2 Tbsp. black sesame seeds, sprouted

DRESSING

⅓ cup (80 ml) olive oil

¼ cup (60 ml) brown rice malt syrup

¼ cup (60 ml) brown rice vinegar

1 Tbsp. tamari

1 Tbsp. sesame oil

1 small or medium onion, grated

1–2 cloves raw garlic, minced

Place the cabbage in a large salad bowl with the edamame and the seaweed. Toss in the seeds and mix. Then in a smaller bowl, combine all the ingredients for the dressing and mix well. Pour it over the salad and toss well to coat.

Nutrition Information per Serving: 180 mg calcium; 150 mg magnesium; 8 g protein; phytoestrogen; high in trace minerals

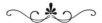

Sprouted Lentil Salad with Honey Almond Dressing

SERVES 4–6

Any plant-based diet requires the consumption of high-protein plant-based foods. Along with beans, legumes such as lentils are an excellent way to fill that need! Lentils are delicious, easy to store and prepare, and a very inexpensive plant-based protein source.

Lentils have been eaten for generations all over the world as a side dish as well as main courses and soups. They do, however, contain anti-nutrients like phytic acid and enzyme inhibitors, which can make them hard to digest. Still, that's easily avoided: Sprouting them can neutralize these naturally occurring properties and make them a safe part of your diet.

¼ cup (60 ml) olive oil

4 Tbsp. toasted slivered almonds, divided

2–4 Tbsp. apple cider vinegar

1 Tbsp. raw honey or vegan sweetener

1 tsp. whole-grain mustard

Salt and pepper to taste

1 bunch red kale, washed, deveined, and chopped

2 cups (155 g) sprouted lentils

1 small bunch green (spring) onions, chopped

Make your dressing by combining the olive oil, 3 tablespoons of toasted almonds, the apple cider vinegar, sweetener, mustard, salt, and pepper in a blender until smooth. Combine your kale and sprouted lentils in a bowl and pour the dressing over. Toss to coat all ingredients with the dressing. Sprinkle onions and remaining almond slivers on top and serve.

Store any leftovers in the fridge. The kale won't wilt, so it makes a great second meal.

Nutrition Information per Serving: 240 mg calcium; 130 mg magnesium; 24 g protein; phytoestrogen; prebiotics

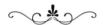

Niçoise Salade

SERVES 4

Alice Waters, founder of Chez Panisse Restaurant and Café in Berkeley, California, created Niçoise Salade as a simple, delicious luncheon entrée. This recipe is from her book *The Art of Simple Food*,[1] and we are delighted that Alice has given us permission to include it here.

This compound salad is based on a recipe from Provence. The summer vegetables are set off by piquant anchovies and rich hard-cooked eggs.

SALADE

3 salt-packed anchovies

¾ lb. (340 g) ripe tomatoes

¼ lb. (115 g) green beans, trimmed

1 sweet red pepper, cut in half, stem, seeds, and veins removed

2 medium or 1 large cucumber

2 eggs

VINAIGRETTE

1½ Tbsp. red wine vinegar

Salt

Fresh-ground black pepper

1 garlic clove, peeled and crushed

4 Tbsp. extra-virgin olive oil

5 basil leaves, chopped

Soak for 15 minutes and fillet the anchovies. Cut the anchovy fillets lengthwise into strips and coat them with a bit of olive oil. Wash and core the tomatoes. Cut into small wedges and season with salt. Blanch green beans in salted boiling water until tender. Drain and lay out to cool. Cut red pepper in half. Remove stem, seeds and veins. Cut into thin strips. Peel and cut the cucumber into bite-sized wedges, large pieces, or slices. Place the eggs in a saucepan of water and bring to a boil. Cook at a gentle boil for 5 minutes, then cool in cold water. Peel the eggs.

Make the Vinaigrette: Mix red wine vinegar, salt, black pepper, and garlic in a small bowl. Stir to dissolve the salt and then let sit a few minutes to macerate. Whisk in olive oil and basil leaves. Taste for salt and acid and adjust as necessary.

Prepare Ingredients for the Salade: Cut cooled eggs into quarters. Season the cucumbers, peppers, and green beans with salt and then toss with three-quarters of the vinaigrette.

Assemble the Salade: Arrange on a plate. Dress the tomatoes, tossing gently, and arrange around the vegetables. Garnish the salad with the eggs and the strips of anchovy fillet.

Variations: For a more substantial salad, grill or pan-sear ¾ pound (340 g) fresh tuna, such as skipjack, leaving it quite rare. Break the tuna into pieces, dress with a bit of the vinaigrette, and arrange on the plate with the vegetables.

Serve the salad on a bed of lettuce or arugula.

Roast the peppers, then peel and seed them, and cut into strips.

Nutrition Information per Serving with Skipjack Tuna: 300 iu vitamin D; 18 g protein; prebiotics; high in selenium and trace minerals

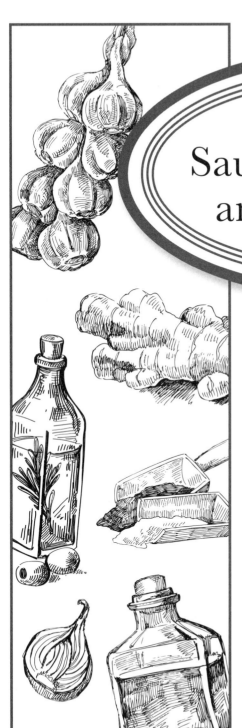

CHAPTER 15

Sauces, Dressings, and Marinades

For years Helen didn't make her own sauces, marinades, or salad dressings, imagining there were some culinary tricks she didn't know. Fortunately that reluctance is a distant memory. Making dressing is as simple as mixing oil and vinegar or a vinegar alternative and seasoning it. And what could be easier than enlisting a sweet vinegar to free minerals from nutritious food? Your homemade dressing will stay good in the fridge for weeks—if it lasts that long. Ditto marinades. Sauces are sometimes more involved and always satisfying to make.

In our homes there are no store-bought sauces, dressings, or marinades, because we don't like the manufacturing practices used in making them or the additives they contain. This chapter includes several of our favorite sauces. And at the end of this chapter we've listed other sauce and dressing recipes from throughout the book, along with page numbers for ready reference.

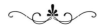

Fig Balsamic Glaze

MAKES 1 CUP (240 ML)

This is beautiful over scallops (see Charcoal-Fired Scallops with Arugula Microgreens and Roe Sauté, page 129), chicken, steak, even grilled fruit. The recipe calls for some sugar, and we advise you to be cautious in adding it. Taste it as you go because the balsamic vinegar has some innate sweetness. You may find you prefer the glaze with very little added sugar.

2 Tbsp. ghee or coconut oil
2 Tbsp. minced shallot
¼ cup (60 ml) balsamic vinegar
¼ cup (60 ml) water
8 fresh ripe figs, mashed into a paste
1–2 tsp. coconut or turbinado sugar
Pinch of salt

Heat the oil in a skillet. Add the shallot and cook for 2 minutes. Add the vinegar and the water for another minute. Add the fig paste, sugar, and salt. Reduce for about 10 minutes. The sauce should be the consistency of a rich glaze.

Nutrition Information per Serving: 180 mg calcium; 30 mg magnesium; 4 g protein

by adding *Aspergillus oryzae*, a probiotic fungus, and later brine to a mix of soybeans and cracked wheat. The mixture will sit for about a year.

Mirin is a Japanese sweet wine made from a rice culture, koji, and shochu, a sweet wine whose alcohol content can be between 1 and 35 percent. Mirin itself is typically 14 percent alcohol. If you are advised to avoid alcohol in your diet, check the label for alcohol content.

2 cloves garlic, halved and smashed
¼ cup mirin
1 Tbsp. rice vinegar
4 tsp. shoyu (all-purpose soy sauce)
¼ cup toasted white sesame seeds
¼ cup olive or avocado oil
¼ cup peanut oil
2 tsp. toasted sesame oil

Mix everything in a small bowl. Cover and let the mixture sit in the fridge for a few hours, or overnight, or until you will use it. It will be fresh for 3 days.

When you are ready to serve the dressing, remove the garlic.

Nutrition Information per Serving: 200 mg calcium; 70 mg magnesium; 5 g protein; phytoestrogen; probiotics

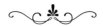

Sesame Shoyu Dressing

MAKES 1 GENEROUS CUP (240 ML)

Soy sauce is fermented soybeans. If you choose organic soy sauce, you can be relatively confident that the sauce did not originate with genetically modified soybeans. Shoyu soy sauce is a fermentation of soybeans and cracked wheat. You can make shoyu

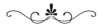

Mushroom Shoyu Sauce

MAKES 1 GENEROUS CUP (240 ML)

3 Tbsp. unsalted butter
2 Tbsp. minced shallots
1 cup (7 g) sliced sunned shiitake mushrooms
1 clove garlic, smashed

Splash of mirin

3 Tbsp. shoyu

Combine all the ingredients in a saucepan, cover the pan, and simmer for 10 minutes. Remove garlic clove. This sauce is delicious for drizzling over Wagyu beef (see Super-Easy Seared Wagyu Beef with Mushroom Shoyu Sauce, page 131) or any meat.

> **Nutrition Information per Serving:** 100 mg calcium; 50 mg magnesium; 400 iu vitamin D; 28 g protein

Lightly Lightly Vinaigrette Dressing

MAKES 1 SCANT CUP (240 ML)

We love the light texture and refreshing flavor of this dressing. If you want a richer dressing, add an anchovy.

⅓–½ cup (80–120 ml) avocado oil,
    depending on taste

1 Tbsp. apple cider vinegar

1 Tbsp. red wine vinegar

1 tsp. stone-ground mustard

1 small clove garlic, finely chopped

1 shallot, finely chopped

Pinch of salt, pinch of pepper

1 anchovy (optional)

Mix all the ingredients in a small bowl, or in a small jar with a lid to shake. If you're using an anchovy, fork-mash it into the mixture and stir until it dissolves.

> **Nutrition Information per Serving:** phytoestrogen; probiotics; omegas

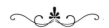

Oyster Sauce

MAKES 2 CUPS (480 ML)

This oyster sauce is the traditional sauce used over Asian vegetable dishes. It is the real thing, which sadly most commercial oyster sauces are not; and worse yet, the commercial products are not suitable for bone health. Start with fresh oysters, of course, because oysters are terrific for bones: calcium, protein, and a huge boost of omega-3, not to mention zinc and vitamin C.

1 cup (240 ml) water

16 oz. (455 g) fresh oysters

¼ cup (½ stick) butter

½ small onion, minced

1 clove garlic, smashed and minced

1 Tbsp. minced fresh ginger

1 tsp. thyme

1 tsp. oregano

1 tsp. fresh basil

2 Tbsp. flour

½ cup (120 ml) chicken bone broth

½ cup (120 ml) cream

¼ cup (60 ml) dark soy sauce

Cornstarch (optional)

Black pepper to taste (optional)

Heat the water in a pan, add the oysters, cover, and steam until the oysters open. Save the broth (cooking water) in a bowl. Finely chop the oysters.

Melt the butter and sauté the onion, garlic, and gingerroot over medium heat until the onion is soft. Add the minced oysters, thyme, oregano, and basil. Sift in the flour, mixing constantly, until the flour is cooked into the mixture. Whisk in 1 cup (240 ml) of the oyster broth and the chicken broth, cream, and soy sauce.

Pour the sauce through a sieve, removing any solids. Return the remaining liquid sauce to the pan. Mixing constantly, cook the sauce over medium heat until thickened. If it isn't thickening properly, add a small amount of cornstarch and water and cook until it's thick enough. If desired, add ground black pepper to taste.

> **Nutrition Information per Serving:** 80 mg calcium; 15 g protein; 50 mg zinc; phytoestrogen

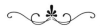

Fresh Cherry Sauce

MAKES 2 GENEROUS CUPS (480 ML)

Laura likes to make this with sour cherries. Sour cherries make this sauce perfect for desserts yet also for savory meats and cheeses.

3 cups (415 g) pitted cherries (sweet or sour, whichever you prefer)
¼ tsp. ground cinnamon
¾ cup (150 g) sugar
2 Tbsp. water, divided
1 tsp. cornstarch

Put the cherries, cinnamon, sugar, and 1 tablespoon of the water into a saucepan on medium heat. Simmer for 10 minutes. Mix the cornstarch and the other tablespoon of water in a small bowl until the cornstarch is fully mixed. Stir into the cooking cherries and cook 4 more minutes or until the sauce begins to thicken.

> **Nutrition Information per Serving:** 20 mg vitamin C

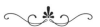

Spice Shake

MAKES 3 CUPS (720 ML)

This is a super-versatile shake-on seasoning that brings out the best in vegetables, beans, grains, tofu, salads . . . and it is bone-friendly. In Japan the name is furikake. You'll may find it on shelves in the Asian food section; Eden foods makes one we like. You can buy it premixed, but we like to make our own. It's simple.

The optional ingredients allow you to make your own version that is spicier or sweeter than the basic mix, as you prefer.

2 cups (290 g) toasted white sesame seeds
2 cups (290 g) toasted black sesame seeds
1 cup (110 g) ground toasted nori seaweed
¼ cup (12 g) shiso leaf powder

OPTIONAL INGREDIENTS

1–2 Tbsp. chili flakes
1 tsp. ginger powder
1 tsp. ground orange peel
1 tsp. ground lemon peel
  1 Tbsp. bonito or salted shrimp
    ½ tsp. turbinado sugar

Put all the ingredients into a clean jar. (If you started with toasted nori sheets, you can break up the sheets by hand and pulverize the bits in a spice grinder.) Turn the jar a couple of times to mix the ingredients, and close the jar tightly.

Store the spice shake with your spices. It will keep for 6 months.

Notes: Shiso leaf powder is available at grocery stores; it's a pickled, salty powder, so when you use it in a dish, there's no need to add salt. Eden sells shiso leaf powder in a small bag.

Bonito and salted shrimp can be purchased dried in stores or online. Bonito is flakes of dried tuna. If you use bonito or salted shrimp, shelf life of the furikake is 2 months.

Nutrition Information per Serving: 100 mg calcium; 40 mg magnesium; 2 g protein; phytoestrogen

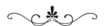

Delectable Marinades

These two are among our favorite marinade recipes. The first is delicious with salmon, tuna, tofu, shiitake mushrooms, or lotus root. The second is perfect for mushrooms.

Marvelous Marinade
MAKES 1 CUP (240 ML)

3 Tbsp. peeled finely grated fresh ginger
¼ cup (60 ml) soy sauce
1 Tbsp. rice vinegar
1–2 tsp. sugar, depending on taste
1 Tbsp. mirin (Japanese rice wine)
1 Tbsp. coconut oil
1 Tbsp. peanut oil
1 tsp. sesame oil

Mix the marinade ingredients in a bowl and add whatever you wish to marinate. Put the bowl in the fridge and allow the contents to marinate for a minimum of 4 hours and up to 12. Turn the contents occasionally.

Nutrition Information per Serving: 200 mg calcium; 70 mg magnesium; 5 g protein; phytoestrogen; probiotics

Marinade for Mushrooms
MAKES ¼ CUP (60 ML)

2 Tbsp. balsamic vinegar
1 Tbsp. olive oil
½ tsp. dried basil
½ tsp. dried oregano
2 cloves garlic,
    smashed
    and minced
Pinch of salt
    and pepper

Using a wire whisk, blend all the marinade ingredients in a medium-sized bowl. Add the mushrooms and marinate for 2 to 8 hours in the fridge. Stir occasionally.

Nutrition Information per Serving: 200 mg calcium; 70 mg magnesium; 5 g protein; phytoestrogen; probiotics

⇥ About Herbs ⇤

Use fresh basil leaves or organic dried basil. Chop or tear fresh basil leaves before adding to the pot in order to release oils.

Dry oregano leaves at home. Fresh oregano will dry in about 4 days on a windowsill; or you can hang the stems using a string and paper clips or clothespins anywhere the air is fresh.

When you add dried herbs, pour them into your palm and rub your palms together over the pot to release the oils and raise the flavor.

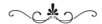

Grandma Doris's Homemade Spaghetti Sauce

SERVES 4–6

Helen's mother-in-law, Doris Kelly, was famous in the family for her spaghetti sauce. She used sliced Polish sausage and a heap of cremini and portobello mushrooms. Of course she never would tell us how much of anything, including mushrooms, so we've replicated her recipe by trial and error (but only after gaining the permission of her daughters). Helen keeps the very important portobellos because when stir-fried they give juice—an essential ingredient in this sauce—but expands the repertoire to include trumpet, shiitake, maitake, or enoki mushrooms and only pure meat sausages—no fillers or colors added.

For a meatless meal, omit the sausages. This sauce is delicious either way and keeps perfectly well for several months in the freezer.

1 large yellow onion

12 cloves garlic, smashed and chopped small

6 Tbsp. olive oil (plus a bit for drizzling once the sauce is done)

6 cups (325 g) chopped mushrooms, including at least 2 cups (110 g) of chopped portobello caps

2 large cans whole plum tomatoes in tomato puree—about 6 cups (1.4 kg) of tomatoes

½–1 Tbsp. dried basil or 2–4 basil leaves

3 Tbsp. dried oregano or leaves from about 6 sprigs of home-dried oregano

Salt and pepper to taste

½ tsp. dried chili

4 pure meat sausages, optional

Chop the onion and garlic and let them sit for about 10 minutes.

❧ About Tomatoes ❧

Tomatoes can make or break your sauce. Whether they're canned whole, crushed, or fresh, the tomatoes must be organic and should be a variety of plum tomato. Flavored canned tomatoes— say, with garlic or basil—are acceptable. Don't use canned tomatoes in juice— they make the sauce watery—but we always keep a small can on hand in case we don't get the chili out in time.

Fresh tomatoes change a sauce recipe substantially. Use about 15 fresh plum tomatoes for one large can along with half a can of tomato concasse to make up for the puree. Concasse is pure tomato paste—no oil, no salt. Purists say peel the tomatoes but we say use as they are if you wish; we don't mind the skins.

Tomatoes and chili are perfect partners. To control the heat, omit the dried chili flakes and instead put chunks of fresh hot chili pepper into the sauce before you start the simmer; remove these with a slotted spoon when the sauce is hot enough for you. Lots of tasting goes on here. Helen isn't complaining. If the sauce gets too hot, add 6 to 8 fresh tomatoes or a few whole canned tomatoes.

In a large saucepan, heat the olive oil until a snippet of garlic begins to bubble. Add the chopped garlic and onion and sauté on low heat until the onion is translucent and the garlic is only browning around the edges, if at all. Turn up the heat a bit, add the mushrooms, and stir. When the mushrooms have wilted, cover the pot and cook, continuing to check and stir the mixture until the mushrooms give juice. Remove the pot cover.

Add the plum tomatoes and the puree. Snip the tomatoes with a small scissors to release the juice. Cook for 15 minutes. Then, using a potato masher, crush the tomatoes until they are just integrated with the sauce but still slightly chunky.

Rub in the dried herbs; add salt, pepper, and dried chili. Turn the heat to the lowest setting—if you have lower than simmer, that's good—and barely simmer for 2 hours. If simmer is your lowest setting, scoop the bottom every 20 minutes or so to be sure nothing sticks.

Add optional sausage, whole or sliced. You can add sautéed eggplant and zucchini chunks instead of sausage to provide texture and additional flavors.

> **Nutrition Information per Serving:** 25 mg calcium; 400 iu vitamin D; 18 mg protein; 200 mg vitamin C; 1,200 iu vitamin A; prebiotics

More Sauces, Dressings, and Marinades

SAUCES

Aioli (page 134)

Mexican Mole (page 194)

Plum Sauce (page 192)

Tomato Sauce for Raw (Vegan) Lasagna (page 177)

DRESSINGS

Avocado Dressing for Breakfast Salad (page 152)

Dressing for Lauren Rae's Napa Cabbage Salad (page 159)

Honey Almond Dressing for Sprouted Lentil Salad (page 159)

Dressing for Plum All Around Dinner Salad (page 192)

Two Ways with Black Beans Dressing (page 181)

Yuzu Dressing for Seaweed Salad (page 150)

Zesty Yogurt Dressing for Smoked Salmon with Fish Roe (page 207)

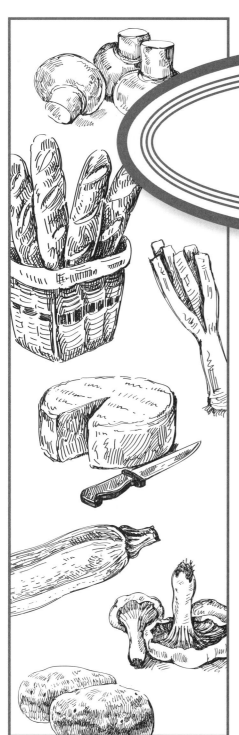

CHAPTER 16

Small Plates

I t seems that upon small plates there always sits something exotic, delicate, beautifully prepared. As the hostess or waiter sets the plate in front of you, you relax, enjoy the sight, and take your time picking up the fork, savoring the first bite.

This is the French way of dining, at home, at a dinner party, or in a restaurant. No matter the stresses of the day, when it's time to eat the mind rests, the body unwinds, and the five senses open to the experience. Mindful of the deleterious effect of stress on our bones, we make every effort to re-create the small-plates experience in our own homes, and hope you will discover this pleasure in yours.

Small plates might include *amuse-bouches*, tiny tasters that stimulate an appetite, followed by perfectly dressed salads, pâté, creamy baked Brie en croûte, a small fish, some shrimp or squid cooked just until done—and flavored with melted garlic butter or made spicy with chopped garlic and chopped fresh red chili, atop fresh arugula or watercress.

To bake Brie en croûte, wrap a small whole Brie or a large wedge in homemade or ready-made pastry, place in a Brie baker or any small covered casserole, and bake in the oven at 350°F (177°C) until the crust is golden and crisp, about 20 minutes. Cool for 10 minutes and serve. If you prefer to skip the pastry, bake the Brie and serve with small rounds of sourdough, crisp crudités, or a bit of fig jam.

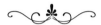

Chris's Thai Fish Cakes

MAKES 12–15 FISH CAKES; SERVES 3–4

A few years ago, Helen and Chris were on vacation in Koh Samui, Thailand. What had once been a quiet hidden gem was now a robust tourist town, so they went in search of authentic Thai cooking in the alleyways behind town where locals went to eat after work. There they found Rainbow, a restaurant run by just one enterprising and very talented young woman operating in a lock-up garage. She fed Helen and Chris for several nights right along with her family, and the dream of local food came true. Chris especially remembers the fish cakes. The owner of Rainbow made them using a fresh-caught local fish that tasted like salmon, so Chris has recreated the recipe using salmon.

1 lb. (455 g) salmon fillet, boned and skin removed
2 Tbsp. Thai red curry paste
½–1 tsp. red chili pepper flakes
2 Tbsp. chopped cilantro
5 small scallions, finely sliced
1 Tbsp. light brown sugar
1 tsp. nam pla (fish sauce)
1 Tbsp. freshly squeezed lime juice
2 oz. (55 g) young green beans, finely chopped
1 Tbsp. coconut oil

Cut the salmon fillet into 1-inch (2.5 cm) chunks and place these into the processor. Add all the other ingredients except the green beans and coconut oil. You will add these later. Process the fish-herb-spice mix until it's just approaching minced. You do not want a fish paste, so take care not to overprocess.

Empty the mince into a medium-sized bowl, add the green beans, and stir them into the mix.

Divide the mix and flatten into patties. You will have enough mix to make 12 to 15 patties. Cover the bowl and place in the fridge for 1 hour to help the patties set. If you want them uniform, dip into flour just before frying.

Heat the oil in the frying pan; when it's hot, fry the fish cakes about 2 minutes on each side until golden brown. Serve with roasted asparagus, broccolini, or your favorite dipping sauce.

> **Nutrition Information per Serving:** 50 mg magnesium; 28 g protein; 1,000 iu vitamin D; prebiotics

Pâté de Foie de Poulet (Traditional Chicken Liver Pâté)

SERVES 2; SERVES 4 FOR HORS D'OEUVRES

We are pleased to present this recipe from Paleo Leap. Their approach and recipes are a boon to people with epilepsy who must be on a very high-protein/low-carbohydrate diet and who also want to take care of their bones.

In some cultures, Paleo Leap tells us, hunters would feed muscle meat to the dogs and keep the organs for themselves. That's no surprise given the bountiful nutritional gift from gizzards. Of course some people shy away from those, but that's just habituation. The great Julia Child tore down that wall when she presented her boned turkey with chopped gizzard gravy.

Enjoy this pâté as a snack on celery sticks, on lettuce leaves, or on cucumber rounds. Enjoy it the French way on toast triangles; add a bit of fig jam or a few baby arugula leaves.

½ lb. (225 g) chicken livers
3 thin slices bacon, chopped into cubes

1 large onion, diced

1 clove garlic, minced

¾ cup (1½ sticks [170 g]) butter

¼ cup chopped parsley

3 Tbsp. sherry (you can use 1 Tbsp. apple cider vinegar instead)

Salt and pepper to taste

Fresh nutmeg

Prepare the livers by cutting out the white stringy part.

Heat a large pan over medium-high heat and cook the bacon for about 3 minutes. Add the onion, garlic, and ¼ cup (55 g) of the butter and soften for another 3 or 4 minutes. Add the livers to the pot and cook for about 7 to 10 minutes with a little more of the butter. Once cooked through, add the parsley, sherry, and salt, pepper, and fresh nutmeg to taste. Remove from the heat and pour the mixture into a blender or food processor; blend until smooth. Pour the smooth mixture in a serving dish.

Melt the remaining butter and pour over the pâté evenly. Cover and put in the refrigerator to cool until the fat hardens.

Nutrition Information per Serving: 30 mg vitamin C; 53,000 iu vitamin A; all trace minerals; B vitamins

Fritto Misto

SERVES 4–6

This is simple to make and simply delicious. Eating the beans right out of the bowl may be problematic because you may already have eaten them right out of the pan! White beans are a nice alternative to garbanzo beans in this recipe, and

we use navy or cannellini (white kidney) beans. If you have never enjoyed fennel—at all or just this way—you will be surprised and delighted. Slice the fennel in ½-inch (1.25 cm) julienne strips. The fiber in some types of beans is valuable for maintaining gut health, and they're a rich source of nutrients for bone health, too.

6 cloves garlic, rough chopped

¼ cup (60 ml) olive oil

1 can or carton sprouted garbanzo beans (14–16 oz. [400–455 g]), rinsed thoroughly and dried in paper towels

2 fennel bulbs, stem end and ferns removed, bulb rinsed and dried thoroughly

¼ tsp. salt

½ tsp. cardamom powder

Fry the garlic in the olive oil over medium heat until the garlic begins to turn golden. Add the beans to the garlic immediately. Move the beans around occasionally until they are well browned. Remove with a slotted spoon to a shallow bowl. Drain on paper towels.

Repeat the frying and draining for the slices of fennel. Toss the vegetables with salt, plate them, and sprinkle with the cardamom powder. Eat immediately. You may not be able to stop.

As an alternative, leave the fennel raw—the raw fennel with the fried beans is a delicious alternative, with fewer calories, and the enzymes from the raw vegetable help with digestion and absorption.

Note: You can substitute 1¾ cups (350 g) dried garbanzo beans for the canned beans. Soak them overnight, then dry them in paper towels.

Nutrition Information per Serving: 200 mg calcium; 230 mg magnesium; 39 g protein; prebiotics

❧ Health Benefits ❧ of Fennel

Fennel has unique phytonutrients that are very potent antioxidants. The most intriguing phytonutrient compound in fennel is anethole. In animal studies, the anethole in fennel has repeatedly reduced inflammation and helped prevent cancer. It is believed that this works by shutting down an intercellular signaling system. In this way, the anethole prevents activation of a potentially strong gene-altering and inflammation-triggering molecule.

Fennel is high in vitamin C and contains some folate, calcium, magnesium, vitamin B₉, and phosphorus.

Salt

Pepper

Fresh-squeezed lemon juice

Freshly chopped flat-leaf parsley

Sweet cherry tomatoes (optional)

Use a sharp vegetable slicer to create very thin zucchini strips.

Season the goat cheese with salt and pepper and a sprinkle of fresh-squeezed lemon juice. Mix until the seasoning is absorbed. Place a heaping teaspoon of cheese mixture at one end of a zucchini slice. Roll up and put in a pasta bowl, end-side down. Continue to roll up the rest of the slices and add them to the bowl. When you have rolled all the stuffed slices, grate the goat cheese coarsely over the top and sprinkle the parsley.

If fresh cherry tomatoes are available, use them to dot the edge of the bowl. Serve with freshly baked sourdough rolls.

> **Nutrition Information per Serving:** 60 mg calcium; 5 g protein; 35 mg vitamin C

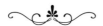

Calabacín Carpaccio Raw Vegetarian

SERVES 4

When we began assembling recipes for this book, Helen remembered two delicious vegetable dishes she had enjoyed at La Forcola—a favorite Italian restaurant in Valencia, Spain. Each dish featured a small amount of fine, aged goat cheese. *Calabacín* is zucchini (courgette); *berenjena* is eggplant. We have made this many times now and can confirm that you do want aged cheese for these dishes.

2 medium zucchini

Aged goat cheese

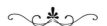

Berenjena Torre

SERVES 4

This is an eggplant tower that is served with yellow bell pepper jam and sun-dried tomatoes. Andrea told us proudly that he'd sun-dried the tomatoes himself just that week, and we were grateful that he had because the flavor was heady. In this recipe, we use brandy to deglaze the pan, which lends flavor to the mix.

3 oz. (85 g) fresh goat cheese, divided

Salt

Pepper

1 or 2 Tbsp. finely chopped fresh coriander
6 champignons (ordinary white mushrooms)
Extra-virgin olive oil
1 large clove garlic, minced
½ cup (120 ml) brandy
2 eggplants
4 sunned portobello mushroom caps

YELLOW PEPPER MARMALADE

1 lb. (455 g) yellow bell peppers
½ cup (100 g) cane sugar
Juice and zest of 1 unwaxed lemon

Mash the goat cheese with salt and pepper and a pinch of chopped coriander until it will hold its shape in a mound. (If you wish, do this in advance and refrigerate until needed.)

To make the sauce, first wash the white mushrooms and slice them.

Put a tablespoon of olive oil in a pan and fry the garlic lightly. Do not allow the garlic to brown. Leave the garlic in the pan but push it to one side. Season the mushrooms with a pinch of salt and pepper and stir-fry until they are soft. Remove the mushrooms and garlic to a medium-sized bowl. Deglaze the pan with the brandy on medium heat and return mushrooms to the pan. Stir until the mushrooms are coated with the glaze. Return the mushrooms to the bowl and use an immersion blender to blend until the mushrooms form a thick sauce. Add 1 or 2 tablespoons of the goat cheese mixture to thicken the mixture further. Set aside or refrigerate if you will be assembling the dish at a later time.

Wash and slice the eggplants into 1-inch (2.5 cm) slices. Salt the slices and put weight on them for at least 1 hour. Rinse and dry thoroughly in paper towels.

Slice the portobello mushrooms into thin slices across the whole of the mushroom rather than into vertical slices. You will have about eight thin, flat slices.

Heat a toaster oven or oven to 350°F (177°C).

Lightly grease a griddle pan with a few drops of olive oil that you rub around with a small piece of waxed paper or your finger. Fry the mushroom slices until they are glazed and limp. Remove to a small casserole, cover, and keep warm in a 150°F (66°C) oven or toaster oven.

Add more olive oil. Fry the eggplant slices on low/medium heat, turning frequently until each piece is cooked through but still firm. Drain on paper towels.

To build a tower of three eggplant slices, mushrooms, and goat cheese: Place the first eggplant slice on a plate; add mushroom slices and 1 teaspoon of seasoned goat cheese. Place the second eggplant slice on top of the mushrooms and cheese and repeat with the same filling. Place a third slice of eggplant on top of the mushroom and cheese. Press very gently on the tower to firm it. Put a tablespoon of olive oil into a 2-quart (1.9 L) baking dish, swirl to coat the bottom of the dish, and set the tower into the casserole. Make more towers and add them to the dish.

Heat in a 350°F (177°C) oven until the tops are just slightly browned and the whole is heated through.

Put two dollops of mushroom sauce strategically on a flat plate and put one eggplant tower on top of each. Present with a tablespoon of Yellow Pepper Marmalade and decorate with sun-dried tomatoes, blueberries, or tiny peppers. Sprinkle each plate with chopped coriander.

Yellow Pepper Marmalade: Cut the peppers in half. Scrape out the pith and seeds. Slice the halves into thin slices and put into a bowl with the remaining ingredients. Leave, covered, for 1 hour. Pour the peppers and liquid into a small pan. Heat on low until the mixture begins to thicken. Turn up the heat slightly, stirring constantly, and let the mixture thicken to the jam consistency you like.

Nutrition Information per Serving: 100 g calcium; 24,000 iu vitamin D; 100 g phosphorus

Mushroom Artichoke Napoléon

SERVES 4

When it comes to dishes created in layers, usually of contrasting and complementary textures, the napoléon was originally Neapolitan, meaning from Naples.

Layering food *à la napoléon* is popular in many cultures, and the sweet versions are household words. A popular French pastry is the mille-feuille—millefoglie in Italian—which is a pastry of "a thousand leaves" typically filled with custard or pastry cream. Greek baklava is a similar pastry infused with honey and filled with chopped nuts.

Mushrooms are the start of the many treasured savory napoléons. Ours includes Yukon Gold potatoes, which have double the vitamin C content of most other potatoes. Vitamin C is an antioxidant and also contributes to the manufacture of collagen—the substance that makes up most of bone matrix.

4 Tbsp. extra-virgin olive oil
6 artichoke hearts—from fresh artichokes or commercially available hearts, not marinated
6 large sunned portobello mushroom caps
1 pound (455 g) Yukon Gold potatoes
Juice of ½ fresh lemon
3 Tbsp. grated Gouda cheese
6 oz. (190 g) soft fresh goat cheese (or burratta cheese)

4 medium-sized cloves garlic, minced
½ tsp. fresh thyme
½ tsp. fresh sage
Salt and pepper to taste
3 Tbsp. freshly grated raw milk Parmesan cheese
¼ cup extra-virgin olive oil
1 cup chicken broth, chicken bone broth, or vegetable broth (see chapter 13 for recipes)

Slice the artichoke hearts into ½-inch (1.25 cm) rounds. Remove the mushroom stems. Thinly slice the mushrooms as follows: Cut in half vertically. Turn the cut side to the right. Slice along each half. Cut the bottom off the mushroom stem. Slice in rounds. Peel and thinly slice the potatoes (if you do this in advance, coat lightly with olive oil or place in a bowl of water and a teaspoon or so of lemon juice).

Preheat the oven to 425°F (218°C). Butter an 8 × 10-inch baking dish or six individual baking dishes. Arrange the potato slices in the bottom of the dishes, then top with artichoke hearts and mushroom slices. Squeeze on a bit of lemon juice. Coarsely crumble half of the gouda and goat cheeses over. Sprinkle with half of the garlic, thyme, sage, salt, and pepper, then 1 tablespoon of the Parmesan. Drizzle with 1 tablespoon of the oil. Repeat the same process to make a second layer. Pour the broth over the mixture, then top with the remaining potatoes and cheeses. Cover with foil. Bake 30 minutes.

Reduce the oven temperature to 400°F (204°C). Uncover the pan and sprinkle the top with the remaining 1 tablespoon Parmesan. Bake uncovered until the potatoes are tender and the top is brown, about 15 minutes.

Nutrition Information per Serving: 300 mg calcium; 800 mg magnesium; 800 iu vitamin D; 40 mcg vitamin K$_2$; prebiotics

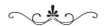

Mushroom Bruschetta

SERVES 4

Mushrooms, yogurt, goat cheese, and sourdough star in this recipe provided by Chobani. The yogurt and cheese are not cooked or even hot so the probiotics and milk enzymes remain intact.

2 Tbsp. first-cold-press virgin olive oil
8 oz. (225 g) sliced sunned mushrooms (maitake, shiitake, porcini, cremini, chanterelle)
1 garlic clove, finely minced
1 Tbsp. finely chopped fresh thyme
Salt and pepper
18 ½-inch-thick slices sourdough baguette or 18 ½-inch-thick diagonally cut baguette slices, toasted
4 oz. (115 g) fresh goat's-milk cheese, raw/ unpasteurized
½ cup (120 ml) full-fat Greek yogurt

TO SERVE COLD

Put the oil into a medium-sized skillet. Add the mushrooms and sauté over medium heat until golden, about 6 minutes. Reduce the skillet heat to medium. Stir in the garlic, thyme, salt, and pepper. Cook for 1 minute. Do not let the garlic brown. Put into a bowl and set aside until cool.

Toast the bread slices lightly on both sides.

Whisk goat cheese and yogurt until mostly smooth. An electric mixer makes things easy, but you can do this by hand with a strong wire whip.

Spread the yogurt-cheese mixture on the toast and top with the mushroom mixture.

TO SERVE HOT

Prepare the yogurt/cheese spread before cooking the mushrooms. Toast the bread while the mushrooms are cooking. Spread the sauce onto the bread and top with hot mushroom mix.

Nutrition Information per Serving: 300 mg calcium; 22 mg magnesium; 15 g protein; probiotics

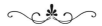

Nick's Kale and Collard Greens

SERVES 4

This is a basic recipe for many greens including Swiss chard, any kind of kale, or any other dark leafy green you like. Laura likes to add nettle leaves.

"It is a staple in our house," Laura's husband Nick says, "when the Southern California nights get chilly." You can do any of the greens separately or mixed, depending on what you have on hand and as you enjoy eating.

2 bunches collard greens, or kale, or a mix
½ cup (120 ml) shoyu
2 Tbsp. ghee
1 cup (240 ml) water

Chop or rip up the collard greens. Put everything in a pot with a lid. Bring the water to a boil then cook on low for 15 to 20 minutes. Check after 10 minutes to make sure the water hasn't all been absorbed; if it has, add more.

Serve over rice, or prepared quinoa (see "Preparing Quinoa," page 151). For a triple magnesium boost, serve

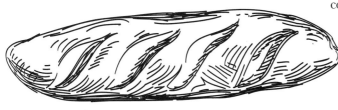

❧ Start the Day with Kale ❧

While Helen was making coffee one morning, her nephew's eight-year old came bounding in. His eyes panned the counters—but Helen wasn't ready for pancake brigade yet, so she offered orange juice. "I could get that myself, Aunt Helen," he said, "but I don't want that. Where's your juicer? Can't you make my kale juice?"

Clearly his parents already knew what Helen had yet to learn: that compounds in naturally grown kale enrich you from the cells out and may influence beneficial genetic expression. Kale seems to reduce inflammation and the risk of five different cancers while also lowering LDL cholesterol. Kale has nearly four dozen flavonoids—pigments that scavenge free radicals.

And on the *life's not perfect but this is better than most* side, kale's calcium remains more bioavailable than that in pasteurized milk thanks to its relatively low levels of anti-nutrients. Likewise for kale's magnesium.

with sprouted beans (see "Sprouting Beans," page 48) or with steamed fish (see Steamed Whole Fish, page 196) or sliced seared beef (see Super-Easy Seared Wagyu Beef with Mushroom Shoyu Sauce, page 131).

Nutrition Information per Serving: 300 mg calcium; 200 mg magnesium; 8 g protein

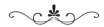

Parmigiano Pannacotta
SERVES 4–6

Pannacotta is a glass custard, so called because it is made with milk and cream or sometimes buttermilk but rarely with egg yolk, so it looks clear. That's one of the reasons we love this one: The custard is perfect, and there are the yolks to provide that K_2 we treasure from pastured eggs.

1 cup (200 ml) double cream
1 cup (200 ml) milk
8.8 oz (250 g) Parmigiano-Reggiano
3 pastured egg yolks
4 gelatin leaves, soaked in cold water

Bring the cream and milk to a boil in a saucepan. Remove from the heat and mix in the grated Parmigiano, stirring well until completely melted; leave to cool slightly.

Whisk the egg yolks in a bowl and pour over the warm cream mixture. Squeeze off the excess water from the gelatin leaves and add to the cream mixture. Stir well until the gelatin has dissolved, then pass through a fine sieve.

Pour into greased dariole molds and place into the fridge to set.

Nutrition Information per Serving: 300 mg calcium; 50 mcg vitamin K_2

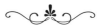

Parmesan and Basil Crisps
SERVES 2–6

Try serving the crisps together on a plate with the Parmigiano Pannacotta, and dress it up with micro red basil leaves. This is another tasty recipe from Reynolds that looks as good as it tastes.

100 grams (3.5 oz.) Parmigiano-Reggiano, finely grated

Fresh basil leaves

Micro red basil leaves

Preheat the oven to 200°C (392°F) and the fryer to 190°C (374°F).

Line a baking tray with a silpat baking sheet and spread the grated Parmigiano evenly across it. Place in the oven for 10 minutes or until all the cheese has melted together and is golden brown.

While the cheese is still warm, transfer it to a chopping board and cut out desired shapes for garnish; this will have to be done promptly as the cheese will turn brittle quickly.

Select some nice-sized basil leaves and place them in deep fryer until they are crisp but still retain their green color. Transfer to a tray lined with paper towels to soak up excess oil. Sprinkle with fresh red basil leaves.

Nutrition Information per Serving: 250 mg calcium; 8 g protein

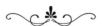

Raw (Vegan) Lasagna

SERVES 4–6

Eating a raw meal once in a while is a pleasure. It is light on your digestive system and full of fresh, available nutrients and live enzymes. This lasagna from Carlota Cassou is like a raw vegetable napoléon, and makes a great side or main dish. The filling is our stand-in cheese sauce.

Carlota's recipes reflect our aligned view that food is the best first port of call for prevention, treatment, and longer life in health, that interlinking forces influence health, and also that we humans can be gently proactive in harnessing those forces for our own and the planet's good.

Note that you'll need to set up the sweet potatoes to marinate the night before you want to serve this dish.

MARINATED SWEET POTATOES

1 Tbsp. olive oil

2 tsp. sesame oil

1 Tbsp. rice vinegar

1 Tbsp. soy sauce

1 tsp. Herbes de Provence

1 sweet potato, very thinly sliced

FILLING

½ cup (65 g) macadamia nuts

½ cup (70 g) cashews

1 Tbsp. nutritional yeast

1 Tbsp. olive oil

½ cup water

Pinch of salt

PESTO SAUCE

1 Tbsp. filling

½ avocado

1 cup (30 g) spinach leaves

Big handful of fresh basil leaves

2 Tbsp. olive oil

Pinch of salt

TOMATO SAUCE

4 dried tomatoes

2 small tomatoes

1 tsp. chili pepper flakes

1 Medjool date

1 Tbsp. olive oil

Pinch of salt

1 tsp. Herbes de Provence or oregano

OTHER INGREDIENTS

1 zucchini, cut lengthwise into strips

Parsley for garnish

Whisk all ingredients for the sweet potato marinade in a bowl or a large glass storage container. Add the sweet potato slices, stir to coat, cover, and put in the fridge to marinate overnight.

The following day, when you are ready to cook, make the filling by putting macadamias, cashews, and nutritional yeast in a blender. Once this mixture is well crushed, split off about 2 Tbsp. of powder to serve as the "Parmesan." Then add the oil, water, and salt, and blend until it resembles a cheese sauce.

To make the pesto sauce, put all the pesto ingredients in a blender and process. Wash out the blender.

Then make the tomato sauce by blending all of the tomato sauce ingredients in the blender.

To assemble the lasagna, use an 8-inch-square serving dish or an 8 × 12 or 8 × 13 rectangular serving dish—in any case, a dish with high sides. At the base place 3 or 4 zucchini strips, then a thin layer of tomato sauce, another layer of strips of zucchini, a thin layer of filling, a layer of marinated sweet potatoes, a layer of pesto, and finally a thin layer of zucchini. Dust the surface with "Parmesan."

To serve, cut the lasagna into rough portions with a sharp knife and enjoy.

> **Nutrition Information per Serving:** 100 g calcium; 200 g magnesium; 10,000 iu vitamin A

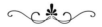

Tuna Sandwich/Salad

SERVES 1

Fish sandwiches are a favorite and there are so many variations—but here is an especially delicious one without mayo and with another opportunity to include vitamin K₂ as well as calcium. Fresh wild-caught tuna cooked to just done makes the juiciest sandwich. If you're using commercially prepared tuna, choose chunks from a jar or thoroughly drained from a can. Skipjack is the best tuna source of calcium.

3 oz. (85 g) tuna
1 pastured egg, hard-boiled (5 minutes)
1–2 Tbsp. finely chopped scallion/spring onion, shallot, or mild sweet Spanish onion
Pinch of rubbed dill, or more to taste (optional)
Ground black or white pepper
1 heaping Tbsp. hummus
Fresh arugula, washed and spun or paper-towel-dried
Tomato, sliced for a sandwich, scooped out for filling with tuna in a salad (optional)
Salt (optional)
2 pieces sliced sourdough or rye bread (page 240)

Fork-mash the tuna and egg. We like to leave it a bit chunky. Add the onion, optional dill, optional salt, and ground pepper. Add the hummus and turn through the mixture until it's thoroughly incorporated.

For a Salad: Tear the arugula, line a plate with it, then heap the tuna on top; or heap inside the tomato. Try serving this with carrot sticks and black olives.

For a Sandwich: Gently warm the bread in the toaster. Put the tuna on the bread and top with arugula—and, if you wish, very thinly sliced tomato.

> **Nutrition Information per Serving:** 175 mg calcium; 115 mg magnesium; 50–75 mg vitamin K₂; 40 g protein; phytoestrogen; prebiotics

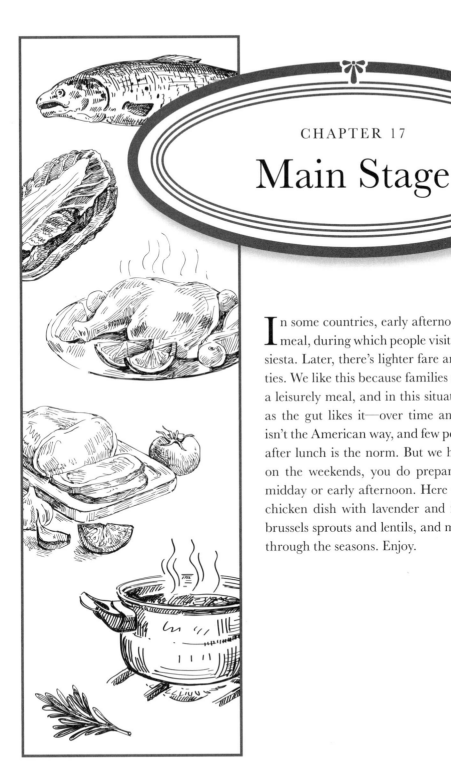

CHAPTER 17
Main Stage

In some countries, early afternoon is time for the main meal, during which people visit and after which people siesta. Later, there's lighter fare and the evening's activities. We like this because families share a table and enjoy a leisurely meal, and in this situation digestion proceeds as the gut likes it—over time and restfully. Okay, that isn't the American way, and few people work where a nap after lunch is the norm. But we highly recommend that on the weekends, you do prepare your main meal for midday or early afternoon. Here we offer a pork stew, a chicken dish with lavender and figs, wild salmon with brussels sprouts and lentils, and more—main dish meals through the seasons. Enjoy.

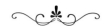

Autumn Pork Stew

SERVES 2

This dish is sweet. That doesn't mean sugared; it means the ingredients lend a lovely richness that practically demands chunks of cold crunchy apples. What better time to make this than when the air turns deliciously crisp and local apple crops abound? We like organic Fuji best but gala and pink lady, for instance, will also be bliss. Or, use your own favorite locally grown varieties.

Pork is one of the animal protein sources of the MK4 subtype of vitamin K_2 (see "Vitamin K_2: The Dark Horse Star" on page 22).

Sesame oil needs low heat. Notice that we sweat the garlic and onion in this recipe instead of frying them.

2 Tbsp. sesame oil

2 Tbsp. olive oil

10 cloves garlic, rough-chopped and left to sit for 10 minutes

6 shallots, prepared as for garlic

1 lb. (455 g) pork shoulder braising steak

⅓ cup (80 ml) sake

Pinch of salt

Pinch of black pepper

½–1 small punnet (basket) of heirloom cherry tomatoes

Leaves from a few sprigs of flat-leaf parsley, finely chopped

2 Fuji apples

Heat the oils to just hot in a 2-quart cast-iron or other heavy pot. Put one chunk of garlic or shallot into the oil. When it begins to sizzle, add the rest of the garlic and shallots and sweat the vegetables. Sit the shoulder steak on top of the vegetables. Pour in the sake. Season with salt and black pepper. Cover and simmer on the lowest heat your stove can sustain for 6 hours. Add the tomatoes, cover, and simmer for a further 30 to 40 minutes until the tomatoes fall in upon themselves. Use a fork to mash the tomatoes down. Heat the stew to piping hot and serve in bowls. Garnish with a sprinkle of the parsley.

Cut the apples into wedges or chunks. Eat the wedges with bites of the stew, or strew the chunks of apple on top and dig in.

> Nutrition Information per Serving: 60 mg calcium; 50 mg magnesium; 20 mcg vitamin K_2; 25 g protein; prebiotics

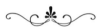

Two Ways with Black Beans

SERVES 2–4

Carlota Cassou describes this as a versatile lunch or lighter dinner main dish, and we agree. This wrap is equally delicious made with lettuce or a warmed tortilla.

Once more persimmons. Choose them very ripe or allow them to ripen before you eat them. Use one succulently soft hachiya and two very ripe fuyu.

Celery helps lower blood pressure, and coriander leaves supplement the calcium in your beans. This dish is equally good wrapped in lettuce or a healthy tortilla, where healthy means no hydrogenated or trans fats.

1½ cups (265 g) black beans, measured after they have been sprouted and cooked

1 ear of corn

2 fuyu persimmons

4 lacinato kale leaves

1 carrot

2–3 sticks of celery, leaves off

2 tomatoes

1 avocado

2 leaves butter lettuce for each serving or
   1–2 tortillas for each serving

Fresh coriander leaves, chopped, for garnish

DRESSING

1 hachiya persimmon (or ½ ripe mango)

Juice of 1 lemon

3 Tbsp. olive oil

¼ cup water

1 tsp. peeled freshly grated ginger

½ tsp. sea salt

Sprout and cook the black beans in advance.

Blend the ingredients for the dressing.

Boil the corn for 3 minutes, then let it cool enough to handle and shave off the kernels. Core and peel the persimmons and discard the seeds. Tear the kale leaves off the stems and chop. Chop the carrot, celery, tomatoes, persimmons, and kale and mix them in a bowl with the black beans. Cut up the avocado and fold in. Pour the dressing over the vegetables.

For a lettuce base, place 2 lettuce leaves on each plate. Mound a spoonful of bean and corn mixture on each leaf. Eat open-faced as a salad or roll into wraps. Garnish with fresh coriander.

For tortillas, warm them in a 350°F (177°C) oven for 2 minutes. Mound the salad and wrap.

If you want a chilled salad, pop the bean salad into the fridge for 20 minutes before dressing it.

Nutrition Information per Serving: 210 mg calcium; 180 mg magnesium; 18 g protein; phytoestrogen; prebiotics

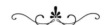

Chicken Stuffed with Lavender and Figs

SERVES 2

Early Romans and Greeks served whipped sugar and lavender as a condiment for meat, and Queen Elizabeth I drank lavender tea for migraines. Adams County, Pennsylvania, Master Gardener Madeline Wajda tells us that the best lavender varieties are Munstead and Hidcote, as other varieties are overly redolent of camphor. She advises shopping for culinary lavender.

Fresh and dried are fine for cooking. Dried flowers are herby; fresh flowers are sweeter and stronger. To substitute fresh flowers for dried, use one-half the amount specified for dried and infuse for a shorter time.

We prize this recipe for the MK4 and calcium.

4 pasture-raised chicken thighs with bones and skin

4 fresh figs, cut into small pieces

1 4-oz. (115 g) package plain goat cheese

3–4 whole lavender flowers, snipped into
   small pieces

2 strips preservative-free bacon, cut in half

Butterfly the chicken thighs: Lay each thigh flat, hold one hand on top of it, and with a very sharp, small knife cut through from side to side right through to the bone. Remove the bone but don't cut the thigh in half. Lay the thigh flat with the skin side down.

Remove the stems from the figs. Blend the goat cheese and lavender flowers in a small bowl. Add the figs and blend.

Stuff the thighs with this mixture, then pin them closed with long toothpicks. Wrap bacon over the top. Place into a small heavy casserole dish so they are pushed up against each other.

Bake uncovered at 350°F (177°C) for 45 minutes to 1 hour 15 minutes, depending on size. Remove the bacon strips for the last 10 minutes to brown the skin. Replace the bacon and serve. For extra deliciousness, top with Fig Balsamic Glaze (page 162).

Note: You may find goat cheese already blended with lavender at a farmers market or food store, and it will serve well in this recipe, too.

Variation: For those who like savory instead of sweet, make the stuffing using ½ cup (75 g) raw feta cheese and 1 marinated portobello mushroom or three shiitake mushrooms instead of the figs and goat cheese. To marinate the mushrooms, slice them, put them into Marinade for Mushrooms (page 165), and leave them in the fridge for up to 4 hours. Half a cup of feta contains about 350 mg of calcium.

> **Nutrition Information per Serving:** 80 mg calcium; 35 mg magnesium; 20 mcg vitamin K_2; 22 g protein; phytoestrogen; probiotics

⤙ About Lentils ⤚

We love lentils for bone health. They offer abundant vitamin B_9/folate; lots of manganese and molybdenum; and a generous provision when it comes to magnesium, phosphorus, and potassium. But, being seeds, they are high in phytates, so it would be good to soak your lentils or buy them already sprouted. Puy lentils take the longest of any lentil to cook and they also hold their shape better than any of the others, so give them a full 20 minutes or more.

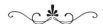

Wild Pacific Salmon with Lentils and Brussels Sprouts

SERVES 1

All three wild Pacific salmon are delicate, delicious, and rich in omega-3, vitamin D, and vitamin B_{12}. Wild Alaskan sockeye is the firmest and strongest-tasting of the three, and the easiest to overcook, but it has the highest vitamin D content of any fish and reputedly of any food. Wild Pacific king is the fattiest and most velvety—it's our choice when we can find it. And wild Alaskan silver is between the two in richness and the mildest in flavor. Choose a thick-cut piece of the fish and cook it until just done.

¼ cup (50 g) sprouted Puy lentils

2 cups (480 ml) water, filtered if possible

Sea salt

2 spring onions/scallions

2 cloves garlic

4 oz. (115 g) baby brussels sprouts or mature cooked sprouts cut in quarters

1 Tbsp. fresh raw butter

1 Tbsp. cold-pressed virgin olive oil, plus more for drizzling

1 slice thick-cut, lean, preservative-free bacon, chopped into tiny chunks—about the size of the spring onion rounds—and sautéed with onion and garlic (optional)

4–6 oz. (115–170 g) wild salmon

4 sprigs fresh parsley

Freshly ground black pepper

Freshly grated raw-milk Parmesan, for garnish (optional)

Parsley, for garnish (optional)

Rinse the lentils, check for impurities, and drain. Bring 2 cups (480 ml) water to a boil. Add the

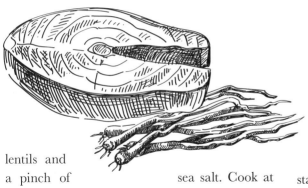

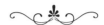

Fava Bean and Pork Falafel

SERVES 2–3

One cup of fava beans contains nearly half our daily RDA for folate. Favas are high in iron, magnesium, and manganese. They, like the spices we use here, are rich sources of plant isoflavones/phytoestrogens. Turmeric is a standout anti-inflammatory. Pork is high in complete protein and vitamin B_6, which helps to ensure that calcium doesn't sit in soft tissue. Pork also contains the MK4 subtype of vitamin K_2, another key on the key ring to keep your calcium in your bones. Omit the pork and substitute chickpeas for a vegan version; chickpeas also appear in the pescatarian version. Both are just as delicious.

If you are pregnant, use lemongrass with caution or ask your doctor.

½ lb. (225 g) ground pork
1 turmeric root, chopped fine
1 tsp. turmeric powder
2 Tbsp. minced lemongrass
2 Tbsp. smashed and minced garlic
½ cup (80 g) shallots, minced
2 Tbsp. minced ginger
1 tsp. salt
2 cups (250 g) sprouted cooked fava beans, hulled
¼ cup (23 g) sprouted chickpea flour
½ tsp. cayenne or chili powder
¼ cup (60 g) chopped tomato
1 Tbsp. peanut oil
Whole coriander leaves, for garnish
Lemon, for garnish
Freshly ground pepper

Mix the pork, turmeric root, and turmeric powder in a bowl, cover with a towel, and set aside. Pound the lemongrass, garlic, shallots, ginger, and salt in a large mortar or food processor until

lentils and a pinch of sea salt. Cook at a simmer, uncovered, for 20 to 30 minutes. They are done if they don't crack when you bite into them. Drain very well and cover.

While the lentils are cooking, chop the spring onions in rounds about ¼ inch (.6 cm) thick. You want them to retain their shape in the sauté. Rough-chop the garlic. Don't put it through a garlic press—you don't want it to melt down.

Add the brussels sprouts to boiling water. Cook baby sprouts for 2 minutes, mature ones for 4. Drain—and chop if you are using the large ones.

Melt the butter and olive oil in a high-sided nonstick frying pan. Add the spring onion, garlic, and bacon (if you're using it). Sauté for 2 minutes or until the garlic is golden and the onions wilt. Add the lentils to the pan and sauté, covered, for 5 minutes, until the lentil mixture is just heated through. Stir until the vegetables are well mixed. Sit the salmon on top of the lentil mix, then add a pinch of salt and black pepper to taste, a few drops of water, and a drizzle of additional olive oil. Cover. Cook on low until the salmon is steamed through and hot but still moist and velvety—about 7 minutes. Serve with a few sprigs of parsley and optional freshly ground Parmesan.

Nutrition Information per Serving: 400 mg calcium; 300 mg magnesium; 1,800 iu vitamin D; 45 g protein; trace minerals; selenium; 1,000 mg phosphorus it becomes a coarse paste. In a small bowl, mash the cooked fava beans.

Blend the paste, the fava beans, chickpea flour, chili, and tomato into the meat. Form into patties that are 1 to 2 inches (2.5–5 cm) round.

Heat the peanut oil to medium high. Cook the patties for about 3 minutes on each side or until nicely browned. Top with ripped coriander leaves and a generous squeeze of lemon and black pepper.

Note: This dish makes an excellent pairing with Fresh Mint Salad (page 155).

PESCATARIAN FALAFEL VARIATION

½ lb. (225 g) white flaky fish, chopped, such as tilapia, branzino, or bussa (swai)
2 cups (330 g) sprouted cooked chickpeas
1½ Tbsp. sprouted chickpea flour

Prepare this dish as for the pork and bean falafel, but substitute the fish for the pork, and chickpeas plus chickpea flour for the fava beans.

> **Nutrition Information per Serving:** 145 mg calcium; 160 mg magnesium; 10 mcg vitamin K₂; 35 g protein; phytoestrogen

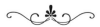

Japanese Bowl Set

Japanese cuisine is lovely to look at and designed to provide ultimate nutrition in a calorically economical way. This Japanese Bowl Set meal provides abundant nutrition for healthy bones. Although it contains no dairy products, this dish is high in calcium, vitamin K_2, vitamin D, folate, protein, potassium, isoflavones, and other vitamins and minerals. One pastured egg contains over half the daily requirement of vitamin K_2. Sesame seeds are high in calcium.

This dish is also high in iodine, which is essential for thyroid health. (A healthy thyroid ensures proper hormone production, which in turn helps overall health as well as healthy bones.)

The main bowl is a fish bowl, accompanied by a bowl of vegetable miso soup and a small dish of pickles.

Vegan Miso Soup
SERVES 1–2

2 cups (480 ml) water
3 strips kombu
3–4 Tbsp. white miso paste
1 cup (104 g) sprouted mung beans

Place the water and the kombu in a pot. Let sit for a minimum of 30 minutes (overnight is fine, too).

Put the pot on the heat and just before the water starts boiling, remove the kombu (if you like a stronger taste you can boil the kombu, but we prefer the subtler taste for a vegetable miso). Turn off the heat. Whisk in the white miso paste to taste. Do not boil the miso, which would kill the beneficial bacteria. Toss in the sprouted mung beans.

> **Nutrition Information per Serving:** 150 mg calcium; 150 mg magnesium; phytoestrogen; trace minerals

❧ About Miso ❧

Miso paste is filled with beneficial bacteria that taste great and, according to the National Cancer Institute, can with daily consumption influence about a 50 percent reduction in breast cancer. The isoflavones in the miso are an invaluable asset in strengthening bones. For clarity on the soy debate, see "Consuming Soy," page 78.

Fish Bowl
SERVES 1

1 pastured egg that has been boiled for 5
minutes, peeled, and soaked in ¼ cup (60 ml)
tamari for 20 minutes

½ cup (125 g) amaranth, cooked, or white rice

1 cup (150 g) wild-caught sardines in olive oil,
drained (oil reserved)

2 Tbsp. furikake (see Spice Shake on page 164),
divided

½ tsp. bone vinegar (page 231)

Prepare the egg, and the rice or amaranth. Place the cooked grain a bowl. Add the fish.

In a separate bowl mix a teaspoon of the olive oil from the fish, 1 tablespoon of the furikake, and the vinegar. Slice the soft-boiled egg and place it in the bowl. Pour the oil mixture over the bowl. Sprinkle with the remaining furikake.

Note: Amaranth is gluten-free, a complete protein, and great source of iron. Of all the grains it is the highest in calcium, with about 60 mg per ½ cup (120 g).

Nutrition Information per Serving: 380 mg calcium; 225 mg magnesium; 175 iu vitamin D; 50 mcg vitamin K_2

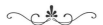

Chicken with Mushrooms and Marc
SERVES 4

Start the meal with the traditional Italian taster course of bruschetta or tomato/basil/buffalo mozzarella over arugula served with sourdough rolls. Add some fruity olive oil for dipping and a small plate of chili-, garlic-, or anchovy-stuffed olives—all for the table. Serve the main dish with a green of your choice. With its cream and brandy, it makes a fine dinner.

The mushroom mix is also delicious as a gravy for London broil, flank steak, or any braised meat.

4 large portobello mushroom caps and stems,
sliced thinly on the diagonal

½ lb. (225 g) organic mushrooms, stems included

Mix of 12 boneless chicken drumsticks and
chicken thighs

¼ cup olive oil

6 cloves garlic, crushed

1 large yellow onion, sliced thinly in rings

1 heaping Tbsp. oregano, fresh-dried at home
if possible

Salt and freshly ground black pepper

2½ Tbsp. butter

3 Tbsp. all-purpose flour

1 cup (240 ml) natural cream

2 Tbsp. cognac

Snip off and discard the ground-end stems of all the mushrooms. Wash them, drain in a wire-mesh colander, and dry well in paper towels. Wash the chicken and dry it well in paper towels.

Heat the olive oil in a large, high-sided frying pan. Brown the chicken quickly and remove with a slotted spoon, allowing the oil to drip and leaving any bits in the pan. Add the garlic and onions to the pan and sauté just until the garlic aroma rises. Add the mushroom slices. Cover and cook until the mushrooms give their juice and are tender. Return the chicken to the pan, sprinkle in the oregano, salt, and pepper, and cook for a further 15 to 20 minutes depending on the size of the thighs.

While the chicken and mushrooms are cooking make a roux of the butter and flour: Melt the butter until it begins to foam. Whisk in the flour a bit at a time until it's all incorporated. Add the cream in a thin stream, whisking all the while, until the cream is incorporated.

When the chicken is nearly done, pour in the cream mix, cover the pan, and allow the dish to thicken on simmer, stirring occasionally to make sure nothing sits too long on the bottom. Pour the cognac over all and let it rest.

Note: If you want a completely alcohol-free dish, add the cognac to the pan with the mushroom slices just after sautéing the garlic and onions.

> **Nutrition Information per Serving:** 100 mg calcium; 500 iu vitamin D; 10 mcg vitamin K$_2$; 28 g protein

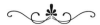

Lentils, Gizzards, and Duck or Chicken Livers with Penne (Rigate)

SERVES 4

In Lombardy and other northern regions of Italy, duck hunting is popular and earthy, rustic pasta dishes are common. This preparation can also be made with chicken gizzards and livers, which are easier to procure. We make duck often in summer—it's a barbecue natural—and by winter, with a little help from a local supermarket and the freezer, we have enough duck livers to achieve the melt-in-your-mouth taste of this fine winter dish.

This recipe is slightly adapted from one that appeared in the award-winning cookbook *A Mediterranean Feast*, by Clifford Wright. The most important thing to know about this preparation, Wright says, is that the gizzards and liver must be cooked separately and the livers are not cooked for more than 2 minutes.

Preparation time is 40 minutes.

3 Tbsp. extra-virgin olive oil, divided
¼ cup (19 g) brown lentils
1 small clove garlic, finely chopped
1 medium zucchini, diced

4 duck gizzards and hearts, thinly sliced while still partially frozen
4 duck livers, thinly sliced while still partially frozen
Salt and freshly ground black pepper to taste
¾ pound (340 g) whole wheat penne rigate
2 Tbsp. chopped fresh basil
Water as needed

Fill a pot with 6 quarts of water, salt abundantly, and add 1 tablespoon of the olive oil. Set on the stove.

Put the lentils in a saucepan and cover with water. Turn the heat to high and cook until tender, 20 to 25 minutes. Drain and set aside.

Set a skillet on medium-high heat. Add the remaining olive oil and garlic; heat until sizzling. Then add the zucchini and gizzards, season with salt and pepper, and cook, stirring, about 8 minutes, until the zucchini is soft and the gizzards are tender.

While the mix is sizzling, bring the salted water to a rolling boil over high heat. Add the pasta in handfuls. Cook over high heat, stirring occasionally so the pasta doesn't stick, until al dente. Drain well. Do not rinse the pasta.

Add the livers and basil to the skillet. Cook for 1 to 2 minutes until the liver loses any pinkness. Deglaze the skillet with 3 tablespoons water while stirring.

Toss the pasta with the liver mixture and serve immediately. Pass a grater and raw Parmigiano-Reggiano or conventional Romano.

Serve with watercress, rocket, or lamb's lettuce salad.

Our Adaptation: For extra calcium, cut a low-fat mozzarella cheese into tiny cubes and toss with the pasta and duck liver mix.

> **Nutrition Information per Serving:** 40 mg calcium; 70 mg magnesium; 60 mcg vitamin K$_2$; 25 g protein; trace minerals

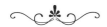

Mamma Lasagna

SERVES 4

Ricotta cheese that is handmade from the milk of pastured cows is as different from commercial ricotta as freshly ground French Roast coffee is from powdered instant. But for lasagna, handmade ricotta cheese has one drawback: Liquid may collect in the bottom of the pan. To avoid this, try adding ½ cup of commercial Parmesan to the ricotta—typically it has an anticaking agent that will thicken the ricotta—or an extra egg. We simply pour off the liquid before baking and save it for making tomato soup. Just be sure to dry the lasagna sheets before setting them in the pan.

You can make this for meat-eaters or vegetarians—or vegans if you leave out the cheese.

8 oz. (225 g) mozzarella or scamorza cheese, ideally of raw milk from pastured cows
1 large eggplant
2 portobello mushrooms, including stalks
6–8 large cloves garlic, peeled
Yellow onion, peeled (optional)
10–16 oz. (285–455 g) ricotta cheese, ideally of raw milk from pastured cows
1 pastured egg
2 Tbsp. freshly crushed dried oregano leaves
Sea salt
Freshly ground pepper

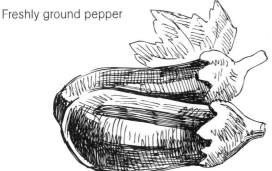

Olive oil
5 homemade lasagna sheets or equivalent commercial lasagna strips
1 jar commercial or homemade spaghetti sauce (see Grandma Doris's Homemade Spaghetti Sauce, page 166)
½ lb. ground grass-fed beef, browned
4 cooked pure sausage (no fillers)

Preheat the oven to 350°F (177°C). Line a 13 × 9 × 2-inch baking pan with aluminum foil.

Shred the mozzarella into strings or small pieces. Remove the stem end of the eggplant. Rinse it and wipe thoroughly dry with clean paper towels. Remove the earth end of each mushroom stalk. Separate mushrooms and stalks. Slice the garlic cloves, eggplant (skin on), and mushrooms—and onion, if you're using it—into lengthwise thin slices. For the eggplant, that means stem end to bottom end, not in round slices across the middle. Mix the ricotta cheese with the egg, oregano, salt, and pepper. Brush the eggplant slices on both sides with olive oil; salt one side lightly. Wipe any excess brush oil onto the aluminum foil. If you prefer, you can mist the eggplant slices and foil with an oil mist pump. Lay the eggplant slices in one layer.

Roast for 15 minutes. Then fold up the aluminum foil to cover the slices and allow them to steam. Heat olive oil in a frying pan on medium heat. Reduce the heat to low, add the garlic and mushrooms, and heat until the vegetables are just soft. The garlic should not be allowed to brown. Use the slotted spoon to remove the vegetables to a small bowl.

Boil a big pot of water. Add a teaspoon of salt and a tablespoon of olive oil. Add the lasagna sheets, stir gently, and boil for 2 to 3 minutes, until they're softened but not done enough to eat.

Tilt the pan to spill the sheets slowly into a strainer. Rinse the sheets in cool water and place each one absolutely flat on one section of paper toweling. Handle with care so the sheets don't tear.

Put 2 or 3 tablespoons of sauce on the bottom of the baking pan. Lay 1 lasagna sheet on top of the sauce. Layer the ricotta cheese mixture to about ¼ inch (.6 cm) thick. Sprinkle on some mozzarella or scamorza. Layer eggplant slices over the cheese. Cover with a thin layer of sauce.

Lay another lasagna sheet over the sauce. Repeat with the cheese, this time covering the cheese with slices of mushroom and garlic. Don't skimp. Cover the mushroom/garlic layer sauce.

Lay another lasagna sheet over the sauce. Cover with a thin layer of sauce. Set out the remaining eggplant and mushrooms, add a bit more sauce, and sprinkle on the mozzarella.

Bake at 350°F (177°C) for 45 minutes. Remove from the oven and cover tightly with aluminum foil. Allow to sit for 7 to 10 minutes before cutting into portions.

Serve with freshly-grated raw milk Parmigiano-Reggiano.

Notes: You may prepare and cook the vegetables a day ahead but not the lasagna sheets except in a pinch.

Scamorza is similar to mozzarella, easier to shred but harder to find. Cheesemakers tie and dry scamorza and sometimes smoke it before selling. If you use scamorza, choose unsmoked.

MEAT-EATER'S OPTION

Reduce the vegetables slightly and sprinkle on meat with each layer.

Nutrition Information per Serving: 283 mg calcium; 43 mg magnesium; 400 iu vitamin D; 7 mcg vitamin K$_2$; 18 g protein

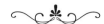

Meat with Sunchokes
SERVES 4–6

Sunchokes—which are crisp, delicious tubers that are nutritious raw or cooked—have many aliases. For a long time the crop was known in America as Jerusalem artichoke though there is no known association with Jerusalem and no botanical relation to artichokes.

We're guessing that the sunchoke has so many names because so many people want to claim it as their own, given its many benefits including to bone health. In particular, this prize find is nearly 50 percent inulin. So for those of us who welcome prebiotics to help with calcium absorption, the sunchoke is a star.

Here's a prebiotics powerhouse recipe we like a lot. This is so easy it's hardly a recipe.

24–32 oz. (680–905 g) meat, preferably pastured but hormone-free, broiled or grilled: pork chops or boneless ribs, shoulder or loin lamb chops, rib beef or buffalo steak

MARINADE

2 medium cloves garlic, chopped
1 Tbsp. dried rosemary
¼ cup (60 ml) olive oil
4 drops freshly squeezed lemon juice or balsamic vinegar, or more to taste

SUNCHOKE SAUTÉ

2 large cloves garlic, minced
1 cup (55 g) sliced mushrooms, such as baby portobello, maitake, or shiitake, washed and dried
1 lb. (455 g) sunchokes, peeled (optional: skin on) and cut into ¼-inch-thick slices
2 Tbsp. olive oil

½ cup (45 g) sliced leeks, white and
  pale green parts
2 tsp. gravy flour or cornstarch
1 tsp. dried rosemary
Salt and pepper to taste
Chopped parsley, for garnish

Prepare the garlic cloves and leave them to develop for 10 minutes. Holding the dried rosemary between your palms, rub it over a small bowl. Rubbing the herb releases the oils. Add the remaining marinade ingredients and lightly whip to incorporate the oil. Pour over the meat. Using tongs or a fork, make sure each piece is covered. Marinate at room temperature for 1 hour.

Sunchoke Sauté: Prepare the garlic cloves and leave them to develop for 10 minutes. If you're using shiitake mushrooms, remove the stems, cut off ground end of each, chop the stems, and slice the mushrooms in half. If you're using baby portobello, slice in ¼-inch (.6 cm) slices. For other mushrooms, you can slice as you wish.

Boil a pan of water large enough to cover the sunchoke slices and still leave room for them to move around. Add the sunchoke slices and boil for 2 minutes. Drain and dry the slices on paper towels.

Steam the leek slices using a steamer on the stovetop or quick-cook them in the microwave on the fresh vegetable setting in a covered dish.

Put the olive oil into a frying pan. Sauté the mushrooms and garlic until the mushrooms are limp and releasing some juice. Turn off the heat. Season to taste.

Broil or grill the marinated meat. Season to taste.

Mix the gravy flour or cornstarch with ¼ cup cold water. When the meat is ready to turn, add the leeks and sunchokes to the mushroom pan, cover, and heat through. You may need to add a drop of boiling water to make a bit of gravy. Mix in half the thickener (gravy flour or cornstarch water), stir, and allow to thicken. Season to taste. If you prefer a thicker gravy, add more of the remaining thickener water. Let this heat right through—but don't let it boil down or burn.

When the meat is ready, cover with vegetables. Serve with steamed or roasted asparagus (page 206).

Nutrition Information per Serving: 45 mg calcium; 50 mg magnesium; 400 iu vitamin D; 28 g protein; prebiotics

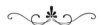

Meatballs and Collard Ribbons

SERVES 2

On the principle that for purposes of bone health, carbohydrates and protein aren't the friendliest pairing (see "Food Combining," page 58, to find out why), here's a dish so delish you may not miss the spaghetti.

COLLARD RIBBONS

1 bunch large fresh crisp collard greens (6–8 leaves)

MEATBALLS

½ lb. (225 g) grass-fed lean (85 percent)
  ground beef
2 tsp. dried Mexican oregano, or more to taste
1 Tbsp. dried parsley
5 basil leaves, torn or scissor-cut into pieces
1 egg
Pinch of red pepper flakes
Pinch of freshly ground black pepper
5 fat cloves garlic, minced
¼ cup (40 g) very finely minced onion
3 Tbsp. olive oil
4 small peeled whole tomatoes

2 cups (470 ml) Grandma Doris's Homemade Spaghetti Sauce (page 166) or ½ jar commercial pasta sauce (page 121)

¼ cup (25 g) freshly grated raw milk Parmesan, or half Parmesan and half Romano, for serving

Collard Ribbons: Carefully remove each half leaf from its stem. Be careful not to tear the leaves. Pile half the leaf halves one on top of another. Roll up like a jelly roll. Keep the roll tight. Using a very sharp knife, cut across the roll to make very fine ribbons. Repeat with remaining leaf halves. Place all the ribbons into a colander. Wash thoroughly to eliminate any microorganisms that might be hiding in the leaves. If you have a water filter, wash the ribbons in filtered water. Place the ribbons in a saucepan and add water until they're just covered; cover the pan with a lid. When you're ready to serve, steam for 4 minutes. Do not cook ahead, as you'll need them piping hot.

Meatballs: Combine the ground beef, oregano, parsley, basil, egg, red pepper flakes, and black pepper. Shape the meat mixture into 8 balls. Sauté the garlic and minced onion in the olive oil until the flavor rises, the onion begins to look soft, and the garlic around the edge of the pan begins to brown. Turn off the heat immediately and, using a slotted spoon, allow the oil to drain from the vegetables. Set them aside in a small dish.

Reheat the oil over medium heat. Place the meatballs in the pan with space between so they do not steam. Turn gently to brown on all sides.

If you are going to freeze the meatballs and reheat later, cook until just done and slightly pink inside. Or you can put the just-done meatballs into the sauce and freeze.

If you are going to use the meatballs immediately, cook until they are as you like to eat them—medium and still pink or brown all the way through. Drain and set in a bowl.

Heat the sauce to just under a boil, put in the meatballs and the whole tomatoes, and leave until just heated through—4 or 5 minutes.

To serve, place a heap of very hot collard greens on each plate, cover with sauce and meatballs, and pass a grater and a chunk of raw milk Parmesan or Romano.

Variation: Cut a fresh buffalo mozzarella into tiny chunks. Mix with the collards before adding the sauce and meatballs or sprinkle on top of the sauce and meatballs and mix in immediately. The mozzarella melts to add a creaminess and the classic stringy texture.

Nutrition Information per Serving: 300 mg calcium; 110 mg magnesium; 20 mcg vitamin K$_2$; 45 g protein; prebiotics

❧ Herbs for Grilled Meat ❧

There's some cause for concern that cooking meat by any means at very high temperatures produces heterocyclic amines (HCAs) and polycyclic aromatic hydrocarbons (PAHs), compounds linked with some cancers. It seems that when rubbed on meat, rosemary and probably oregano inhibit production of these compounds and reduce the potential for inflammation that grilling meat can induce.[1]

Mediterranean oregano and Mexican oregano are two different plants. The Mexican leaf is even higher in polyphenols and powerful antioxidants than the Mediterranean leaf, though both offer a world of health benefit in one.

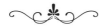

Monkfish Provençale

SERVES 4

Monkfish, also known as seadevils, goosefish, and anglerfish, live just above the ocean floor. They hide in sand awaiting prey and can devour one whole. Their tail flesh is firm and tasty, and it retains its texture and shape during cooking; it is often likened to lobster. Monkfish is not as well known in the United States as it is in Europe, so in the United States typically it is relatively inexpensive compared with halibut and lobster. Monkfish makes a quick delicious dinner, high in protein and minerals.

¼ cup (60 ml) olive oil

2 lb. (905 g) monkfish fillet, cut to 2-inch
  (5 cm) lengths

2 Tbsp. salt-preserved capers

5 olive-oil-preserved anchovies

½ cup (120 ml) cooking sherry or
  dry white wine

2 small cloves garlic, crushed

¼ cup (55 g) crème fraîche

1 Tbsp. crushed dried oregano

4 pieces preserved lemon rind

Heat the olive oil in a stovetop stew pot with a lid. Wash and dry the monkfish pieces, and put them into the pot. Let cook for 5 minutes.

Wash the capers of their salt. Mash the anchovies into a paste in a small bowl. Add the cooking sherry and capers and blend. Put the mixture into the pot, along with the smashed garlic. Cover and cook for 20 minutes.

Mix the crème fraîche with a heavy dose of dried oregano.

The dish will have a thin broth not a thick coating broth, so serve it in small bowls or in cedar wood. The cedar essence works beautifully with the flavors.

Top with a dollop of crème fraîche and grate a bit of preserved lemon on top.

Note: Monkfish has a rich taste, and we like it with a heavier cooking wine. Some, however, may prefer a lighter complement; if so, use a drier white wine for cooking.

Nutrition Information per Serving: 18 g protein; 40 mcg selenium; 218 g phosphorus

Plum All-Around Dinner Salad with Roast Pork Tenderloin and Plum Sauce

SERVES 2

Commercial plum sauce is super sweet, and the base is too often high-fructose corn syrup. This version is a taste treat with the meat as well as the plum salad.

Serve the pork tenderloin hot with boiled sweet potato and the salad for a cold-weather meal or chilled and sliced with salad and corn on the cob for a warmer-weather meal.

DINNER SALAD

2 big handfuls baby arugula or equivalent

1 baby bok choy, sliced or shredded

⅓ cucumber, julienned

½ cup (35 g) red cabbage, sliced very thin
  or shredded

½ cup (75 g) purple or black grapes,
  halved and seeded

DINNER SALAD DRESSING

½ cup (120 ml) pistachio oil

¼ cup (60 ml) well-aged Italian balsamic vinegar

2 Tbsp. wild thyme honey

½ tsp. finely ground red pepper flakes

Sea salt and freshly ground black pepper to taste

ROAST PORK TENDERLOIN

1 pork tenderloin, hormone- and antibiotic-free

1 Tbsp. oil (pistachio oil tastes great with pork)

⅛ tsp. garlic powder

4 cloves garlic, crushed and chopped

2 Tbsp. chopped fresh rosemary

1 clove garlic, slivered (optional)

PLUM SAUCE

4 purple plums, pitted and cut into small cubes

1 Tbsp. honey, preferably wild thyme or sage

2 tsp. raw turbinado sugar

3 Tbsp. balsamic vinegar or 1 Tbsp. bone vinegar

1 large clove garlic, smashed and chopped fine

Dinner Salad: Prepare the ingredients and toss. Dress the salad or set the sauce on the table for individual dressing. The sauce graces hot or cold meat but is especially delicious when you've marinated the pork for 6 hours or more and serve the meat cold.

Dressing: In a small bowl, whisk the oil, vinegar, and honey until it forms a thick sauce. Add the pepper flakes, salt, and pepper to taste.

Roast Pork Tenderloin: Wash the meat and dry in paper towels. Rub oil all over it, then sprinkle with garlic powder and/or make small slits into the meat every 5 or 6 inches (12.5–15 cm) and insert a garlic sliver into each slit. Holding the rosemary in your palms over the meat, rub to release the oils and cover the surface of the meat. Let it sit for an hour or, covered, up to overnight in the fridge.

When you are ready to cook, preheat the oven to 350°F (177°C) and bring the meat to room temperature. Set it in a pan fat-side down. Insert a meat thermometer.

In general roast at 350°F (177°C) for 25 minutes to the pound—for the most tender meat, calculate closely—but oven temperatures vary and it is the internal temperature you're after. The thermometer should read at least 145–150°F (63–66°C). After the first 30 minutes turn the meat over to fat-side up. Turn off the oven and allow the meat to sit until the internal temperature reaches 160°F (71°C). Serve immediately. The center should be just barely pink and the juices should run virtually clear.

Plum Sauce: Put all the ingredients into a saucepan. Bring to a boil then cook on low for about 20 minutes. Blend with an immersion stick blender or mash into uniform sauce.

> **Nutrition Information per Serving:** 80 mg calcium; 40 mg magnesium; 25 g protein; probiotics; trace minerals

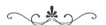

Fresh Sardines: Plated or Sandwiched
SERVES 1

Napoleon was the first to can fish, and the fish he chose for feeding masses of hungry people was the sardine. The skeleton is calcium-rich, and each fish is a pellet of vitamins, minerals, nutrients, and healthy fats. Sardines are low on the food chain, which makes them low in mercury. But if you despair of the canned ones, as Helen does, we think you'll be delightfully surprised by how good fresh sardines are. Prepare these tasty gems with first-press olive oil and freshly scissored herbs along with sea salt and ground pepper. And unlike mackerel, whose cooking smells invade the house, you'll never know the sardines were there.

3 fresh sardines

¼ cup (60 ml) cold-press olive oil or
 coconut oil, divided

1–2 slices lemon

Coarse salt and black pepper to taste

2 rings Vidalia or sweet onion (or substitute
 red onion, but do not sauté it)

1 Tbsp. rough-chopped garlic

1 Tbsp. freshly snipped dill

Sprinkling of dried thyme

1–2 slices fresh sourdough bread

A few capers

Additional lemon, for garnish

1 tsp. chopped parsley

Wash the fish in cold running water. Rub the outside lightly. Run water inside each fish to make sure the cavity is clean and the water runs clear. Lay the fish on paper towels. Turn to dry both sides. Dry the inside gently with additional towels. Rub the inside with a bit of the olive oil and put half a slice of lemon in the cavity of each fish. Lay the fish on a jelly roll pan, square baking dish, or flat plate. Brush the fish on both sides with half the olive oil. Sprinkle inside and out with freshly-ground black pepper and a grind of coarse salt. Leave to marinate in the fridge for 10 minutes or up to an hour.

When you are ready to cook and serve, place the remaining half of the olive oil in a small frying pan. Place a small piece of onion in the pan. When it starts to sizzle, add the remaining onion and the garlic. Adjust the heat so the garlic sautés but does not brown. When the onion becomes translucent yet is still firm and crunchy, and the garlic is turning at the edges, turn off the heat and sprinkle the dill and thyme over the vegetables. Cover and allow to sit covered while you grill the fish.

Place the fish on a hot grill. Cook on each side for 4 to 6 minutes, depending on size. Warm the bread on the grill. Spoon the onion and garlic on one side of the bread. If you like more oil (we do), dip the second slice of bread into the frying pan to take up the remaining oil.

Plate the bread slices on either side of the three fish and garnish with capers, additional lemon and/or a side salad of arugula and cherry tomatoes. Invite each diner to fillet the fish, place the fish onto the bread, and sprinkle with parsley. Enjoy as open- or closed-faced sandwiches.

Note: Sardines are delicate creatures. They stay fresh for a few hours in the fridge, but any longer than that and they need a temperature of between 28° and 32°F (-2° and 0°C). So cover fresh sardines in a bowl of ice cubes. Cook sardines on a grill or in a cast-iron frying pan on the stove.

Nutrition Information per Serving: 180 mg calcium;
40 mg magnesium; 94 iu vitamin D; 18 g protein;
prebiotics

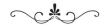

Super-Basic Stir-Fry
SERVES 2

This is richly bone-friendly, quick and easy, and can be adapted many ways to suit your tastes. This is enough to serve two, but you may want to eat it all by yourself. To make this dish vegan, just eliminate the dried shrimp.

1 Tbsp. ghee or coconut oil

3 cloves garlic, smashed

¼ cup (32 g) crumbled salted shrimp

2 peeled and chopped carrots

1 thinly sliced white or yellow onion

2 cups (175 g) Chinese or regular broccoli
 (Chinese broccoli is higher in calcium)

¼ cup (60 ml) shoyu

¼ cup (60 ml) mirin

1 splash plum vinegar

2 cups (505 g) homemade tofu (see "How to Make Tofu" on page 247)

1 cup (70 g) shredded napa cabbage

1 cup (70 g) shredded red cabbage

2 cups (250 g) fresh mung bean sprouts

½ cup (100 g) sprouted adzuki beans

Roasted sunflower seeds or sesame seeds, preferably sprouted, or homemade furikake (see Spice Shake on page 164)

Shredded toasted nori seaweed

Wild yam soba noodles or ramen noodles

Heat the ghee or coconut oil in a large skillet or wok on high heat. Add the smashed garlic and crumbled salted shrimp, moving around so they don't burn. Cook for 2 minutes. Add the carrots, onion, broccoli, shoyu, mirin, plum vinegar, and tofu. Cook for another 4 minutes. Add the napa cabbage, red cabbage, and mung and adzuki bean sprouts; cook for another 3 minutes. Sprinkle with sprouted roasted sunflower seeds or sesame seeds and shredded toasted nori seaweed. Or you can use your own Spice Shake (page 164).

Serve over noodles or just as it comes from the pan.

Notes: There are lots of soybean sprouts around and they're typically from genetically modified soybeans, so make sure you choose organic mung bean sprouts. To increase phytoestrogen content, substitute ½ cup (35 g) organic soy sprouts.

We think the best soba noodles are from Eden Organics. You can find those or others online.

> **Nutrition Information per Serving:** 280 mg calcium; 150 mg magnesium; 26 g protein; phytoestrogen; prebiotics; probiotics; trace minerals; silica; boron

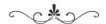

Sweet Potato Enchiladas with Mole Sauce

SERVES 6–12

Spice of life isn't just a throwaway cliché. Herbs and spices contain some of the most condensed and beneficial nutrients in the whole plant kingdom. Add in calcium-rich herbs and your bones profit right along with the rest of you. Recipes for mole, a complex Mexican sauce rich in herbs and spices, are numerous and vary by region and the cook preparing it. There can be more than 30 ingredients in a mole, and the preparation can be time- and labor-intensive. Jennifer Bryman, co-founder and president of HEART Creative Culinary Agency, a Portland-based recipe design and food marketing firm, has shared with us her simplified yet delicious and complex version of mole, which she serves over sweet potato enchiladas. Notice that it is made with rich dark chocolate—a boon to bones.

You'll find the aromatic spices cumin, coriander, chipotle powder, cloves, cinnamon, anise, allspice, and annatto seeds used generously in Mexican cooking. Other distinct ingredients found in the cuisine include garlic, yellow and white onions, green onions or scallions, limes, and queso fresco and Cotija cheeses.

MOLE

2.5 oz. (70 g) ancho chilies (about 5–6 medium), stemmed and seeded

2 Tbsp. lard or coconut oil

½ cup (60 g) chopped white onion

1 tsp. fine sea salt

¼ cup (37 g) blanched, slivered almonds

2 Tbsp. sesame seeds

2 Tbsp. raisins

½ tsp. cinnamon (preferably Ceylon cinnamon)

½ tsp. anise seed

¼ tsp. dried Mexican oregano or thyme

1 corn tortilla, torn into 8–10 small pieces

2.5 oz. (70 g) Mexican or bittersweet chocolate, roughly chopped

3–3½ cups (720–840 ml) chicken stock or broth

ENCHILADAS

2 lb. (905 g) sweet potatoes (about 2 large)

1 Tbsp. coconut oil

¾ cup (85 g) diced white or yellow onion

2 cloves garlic, minced

1 tsp. ground cumin

1 tsp. fine sea salt

2 cups mole (400 g)

12 small tortillas

1 cup (120 g) crumbled queso fresco such as Cotija cheese (optional)

Mole: Stem and seed the ancho chilies, then roughly chop them. Warm the lard or oil in a heavy-bottomed cast-iron pot or Dutch oven over medium heat. Add the chilies, onion, and salt. Fry for 3 minutes, stirring constantly; don't allow the mixture to burn.

Stir in the almonds, sesame seeds, raisins, and spices (cinnamon, anise seed, and oregano). Fry for an additional 3 minutes, stirring constantly until fragrant. Add the tortilla pieces and cook for an additional 1 minute.

Add the chocolate and 3 cups (720 ml) of the chicken broth. Mix and gently simmer for 15 minutes. Remove from the heat, cover, and let steep for 30 minutes or until the chilies are completely softened.

Puree the mixture in a blender or food processor until smooth. Add additional broth as needed to achieve your desired consistency. Use immediately or store in an airtight container in the refrigerator for up to 2 weeks, or in the freezer for 6 months.

Enchiladas: Peel and cut the sweet potatoes into ½-inch (1.25 cm) cubes.

Preheat the oven to 350°F (177°C).

Place the potatoes in a large pot and fill it with just enough water to cover. Bring to a boil and cook for 15 to 20 minutes or until tender. Drain and set aside.

In a large skillet, warm the oil over medium-low heat. Sauté the onion, garlic, and cumin for about 5 minutes, until the onion is soft and translucent. Stir in the sweet potatoes and salt, gently mash with the back of a wooden spoon.

Lightly grease a 9 × 13-inch baking dish. Evenly spread ¾ cup (180 g) of the mole across the bottom of the pan.

Place the tortillas on a baking sheet and bake for 4 minutes. Remove and immediately fill each tortilla with about ⅓ cup (85 g) of the mashed sweet potato mixture. Tightly roll and place seam-side down in the prepared baking dish. Evenly spread the remaining mole over the enchiladas, making sure to cover all corners. Cover with foil and bake for 15 minutes. Remove the pan from the oven and let it sit, still covered, for at least 5 minutes. If desired, sprinkle with crumbled queso fresco.

Note: Cotija cheese, el queso Cotija de Montaña—the cheese of the mountain—originated in Cotija in the Mexican state of Michoacán. It is made in small batches during the summer rainy season when the cows graze and produce rich milk. Cotija is a salty crumbly cow's-milk cheese that adds texture and taste. It is sometimes available grated.

Nutrition Information per Serving: 60 mg calcium; 100 mg magnesium; 12 g protein; 8,000 iu vitamin A; prebiotics

❧ About Mexican ❧ Culinary Herbs

Jennifer Bryman's maternal Mexican heritage makes her an expert in this arena, too. Commonly used Mexican herbs include cilantro (coriander), Mexican oregano—a more pungent flavor than that ordinarily available in the United States—thyme, parsley, mint, marjoram, and epazote. Epazote is a strong, pungent herb with a citrus flavor and is excellent for bone health. It is rich in calcium and offers a rare boost of magnesium, with 100 grams supplying 50 percent of a day's requirement for folate and more than a full day's requirement for manganese. Jen tells us the aroma and taste are not comparable to any single traditional European or American herb; it can be found growing wild in the United States and Mexico. Note: You can find it in many a simmering pot of beans because of its anti-flatulence effects, but it is also used as a vegetable, herb, and tea.

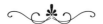

Steamed Whole Fish

SERVES 2

This is the simplest way to cook fish, satisfying and clean. You'll feel calm when you eat this dish because it is so simple yet so tasty. This is the traditional Thai way, and makes a great light dinner for two.

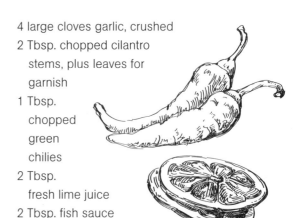

4 large cloves garlic, crushed
2 Tbsp. chopped cilantro stems, plus leaves for garnish
1 Tbsp. chopped green chilies
2 Tbsp. fresh lime juice
2 Tbsp. fish sauce (nam pla)
1 Tbsp. sugar
Pinch of freshly ground pepper
1 whole head-on black bass or rainbow trout (1½–2 lb. [680–905 g]), cleaned and scored to the bone on both sides in 1-inch (2.5 cm) intervals
1 lime, cut into thin slices

Using a mortar and pestle, pound the garlic, cilantro stems, and chilies to a coarse paste. Unless the mortar is wood, leave the paste right there. If the mortar is wood, transfer the paste to a small bowl or a mini processor. Add the lime juice, fish sauce, sugar, and pepper. Mix to a loose paste. Set aside.

Put the fish on a plate that fits inside your steamer; pour the paste over the fish. In a wide pot, add 1 inch (2.5 cm) of water, boil, and put the steamer over the pot. Cover and steam the fish until it's cooked through, 12 to 15 minutes.

Using two large spatulas, transfer the fish to a serving platter. Spoon the fish juices over it. Drizzle with lime juice, then decorate with lime slices and cilantro leaves. Serve with steamed rice.

Nutrition Information per Serving: 125 mg calcium; 50 mg magnesium; 32 g protein; trace minerals

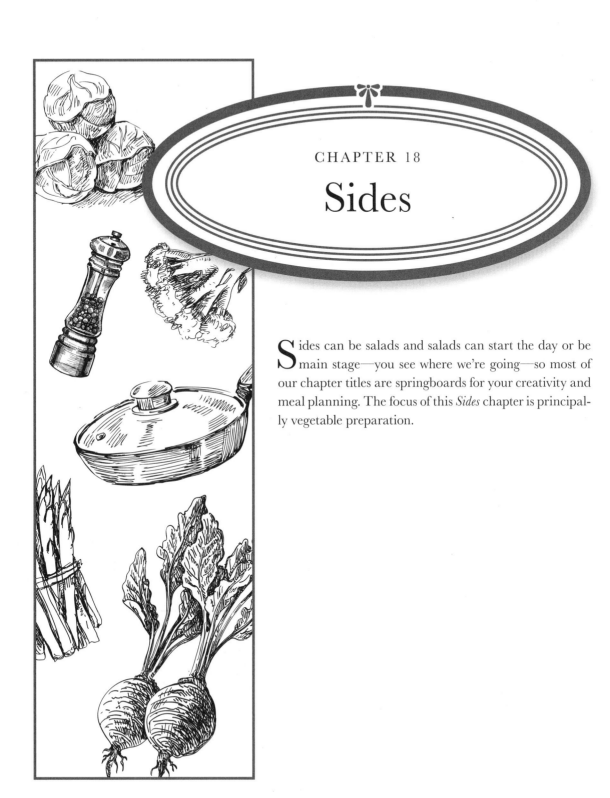

CHAPTER 18

Sides

Sides can be salads and salads can start the day or be main stage—you see where we're going—so most of our chapter titles are springboards for your creativity and meal planning. The focus of this *Sides* chapter is principally vegetable preparation.

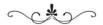

Homemade Nettle Pasta

SERVES 8

Nettle is a group of common and garden herbs—some sting, some don't—widely available in the ground, online, and sometimes at local markets. Nutritionally nettle is even denser than blue-green algae with calcium and also boron, protein, vitamin A, and B vitamins, which help the body make best use of calcium.

Serve nettle pasta simply by combining it with garlic and chili oil. Add cooked vegetables to make Pasta Primavera. Try zucchini or egg-plant—salted, drained, then sautéed—or florets of lightly steamed broccoli and cauliflower.

5 oz. (140 g) fresh nettles (not dried)
2 eggs, room temperature
6½–7 cups (890–955 g) all-purpose flour
(not self-rising)

Put a 2-quart (1.9 L) saucepan of water on to boil for blanching the nettles. Set out a bowl of ice water, which you will use to quickly cool the blanched nettles. Using the tines of a fork, mix the eggs only enough to break up yolks.

Don puncture-resistant gloves, and add the nettles to the boiling water. Blanch the nettles for about 30 seconds, then plunge them immediately into ice water to cool.

Using tongs (and still wearing gloves), remove the nettles from the ice water, squeeze them dry, and puree.

Sprinkle ½ to 1 cup (70–135 g) of the flour onto a clean work surface. Sift 4½ cups (615 g) flour into a large bowl. Make a well in the center. Add the eggs and nettles. Mix gently to incorporate. Add additional flour—up to 1½ cups (205 g) (or as much as needed). Work in

small batches and incorporate well before adding the next batch.

When the dough holds together as a ball, place it on the work surface. Knead for 8 to 10 minutes until the dough is smooth. Boiling often takes out the sting but we prefer to take no chances, so we keep the gloves on. Sprinkle with additional flour, then wrap in waxed, parchment, or freezer paper or BPA/BPS-free plastic wrap. Leave for half an hour.

Roll out the dough on a clean, dry flour-dusted work surface, stretch it a bit (you can wrap it around the rolling pin), lay it flat, and cut into any pasta shapes you like—or use a pasta machine.

Place in a large quantity of water at a rolling boil for 2–3 minutes or until al dente.

Note: To make chili oil, put ¾ cup (180 ml) of olive oil in a pan over low heat with a dried cayenne pepper or a dried red chili and 6–8 cloves garlic (previously minced and allowed to sit for 10 minutes). Infuse for 2 minutes or until the garlic aroma rises.

Nutrition Information per Serving: 50 mcg vitamin K_2; protein; vitamin A; phytoestrogens; trace minerals; trace boron; B vitamins

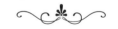

Vitamin A Galette

SERVES 8

This is our bone-friendly version of a traditional French potato pancake. Radish sprouts contain 2.4 times the calcium, 4.9 times the magnesium, 6.3 times the protein, and 39 times the vitamin A of radish roots. Yes, that vitamin A figure is right. A Japanese sweet potato has purple or red skin with pale white or yellow flesh; it tastes like a yam but sweeter.

2 lb. (908 g) Japanese sweet potato, or your
favorite sweet potato

3 Tbsp. ghee (page 243), divided

¼ tsp. salt

½ tsp. black pepper

1 Tbsp. virgin coconut oil

1 yellow or sweet or Vidalia onion, sliced

2 strips unsmoked nitrite- and nitrate-free bacon,
cut into 2-inch (5 cm) pieces

3 small beefsteak or 4 Compari tomatoes

12 oz. (340 g) fresh mung bean sprouts, lightly
chopped (page 48)

¼ cup (10 g) radish sprouts

Greek yogurt or crème fraîche (optional)

Preheat the oven to 400°F (204°C).

Boil the potatoes until the point of a sharp paring knife lets you know the potato is tender right through. Peel while still hot: Holding the potato with a fork, slit the skin with the paring knife and gently scrape away the skin and cushion. Chop into 2-inch (5 cm) cubes and mash with 2 Tbsp. of the ghee, as well as the salt and pepper.

In a cast-iron skillet, heat the coconut oil on medium-high. Fry the onion. After a minute add the bacon and cook until onion is just starting to brown. Add the tomatoes and bean sprouts and cook for 2 minutes more. Add the third tablespoon of ghee and the potatoes to the skillet. Mix with the ingredients already in the skillet. Cook for 5 minutes more until the mix begins to crisp and brown on the bottom of the skillet.

Bake for 15 minutes.

Cut into pie-shaped wedges. Decorate each slice with radish sprouts. Top with a dollop of yogurt or crème fraîche if desired.

> **Nutrition Information per Serving:** 60 mg calcium;
> 100 mg magnesium; 10,000 iu vitamin A; prebiotics;
> probiotics; trace minerals

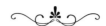

Russian Tzimmes

SERVES 4

Here's a less-sweet meatless variation on a traditional Tzimmes, which combines sweet potatoes, carrots, and dried fruit. Legend has it that the recipe originated in old-world Russia—it is called русский цимес—and today graces many American holiday tables.

Prunes and Medjool dates share the number 2 spot in the list of the top 10 calcium-rich fruits. Experiment with a couple of kumquats, number 4 on that list, if you like a hint of bitter orange. Beta-carotene is fat-soluble. So don't skip the butter.

We adapted this recipe from *Purnell's Complete Cookery*, from the Homemakers Research Institute.

6 oz. (179 g) prunes

6 whole plumped stoned prunes

2 oz. (55 g) Medjool dates or 2 oz. (55 g)
dried apricots

2 medium-sized sweet potatoes or 4 small ones

2 carrots

¼ tsp. salt

½ tsp. nutmeg

¼ cup (½ stick [55 g]) butter

1 Tbsp. natural honey (optional)

Boil just about enough water to cover the prunes and dates—and apricots if you are using them. Cut up all but the 6 prunes into chunks, retaining any juice that chopping produces. Add the chopped prunes, dates, and apricots to the water; boil until the fruit is soft.

Wash the sweet potatoes. Scrape, top, and tail the carrots. Boil both until soft. The carrots will be ready before the sweet potatoes, so remove them when they're fork-tender. Use a wooden skewer to test the sweet potatoes. When they are soft right through, remove and cool slightly.

Slip the skins and the inner cushion off the sweet potatoes and set into a medium-sized bowl with the carrots, salt, nutmeg, and butter. Cut into the vegetables with a fork, folding them all together but keeping the vegetable identities separate. Pour the chopped prunes, dates, and apricots into the carrot-potato mixture with any liquid the chopping produced; blend gently. Spoon into a baking dish and flatten. Cut the remaining 6 plumped prunes in half and space the halves out over the dish. If you want a sweeter taste, drizzle the honey over all.

Reheat to piping hot for serving. Baking at 350°F (177°C) for 15 minutes should do it unless you've doubled the recipe.

Nutrition Information per Serving: 18,000 iu vitamin A

❧ About Sweet Potatoes ❧

Boiled sweet potato with natural butter is one of life's gustatory joys. The potato is cosseted inside a protective layer that slips off with the skin and leaves a smooth, soft, luxurious tuber. We've tried to replicate the texture using conventionally grown sweet potatoes, but the results just aren't the same.

Boiling or steaming sweet potatoes versus roasting or baking seems to have bone- and general-health benefits. The beta-carotene is most available when boiled or steamed, and boiled yields half the glycemic load of baked.

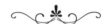

Chopped Raw Broccolini
SERVES 1

This is Helen's go-to lunch and part of her cholesterol-lowering regimen. Raw vegetables contain natural enzymes that help your body digest, so adding a raw dish to a heavier meal is a great way to help your body absorb nutrients.

Broccoli, broccolini, and broccoli raab look alike, and they are nutritionally similar but not the same. Broccolini is a hybrid of broccoli and gai-lin (a.k.a. Chinese broccoli, a.k.a. Chinese kale). Broccolini is sweeter and the stalks are more tender than broccoli. Broccoli raab/rabe (a.k.a. rapini), a favorite in Italian dishes, is a nutritious, characteristically bitter delicious look-alike in the turnip family.

1 bunch raw broccolini, washed, dried, and chopped fine
2 small cloves garlic, smashed and chopped fine
2 Tbsp. olive oil, avocado oil, or coconut oil
Shaves of red onion (optional)
1 scant tsp. apple cider vinegar
¼ cup (35 g) sprouted toasted sunflower seeds

Put the broccolini, garlic, and oil—and red onion if you're using it—into a big bowl. Sprinkle with the vinegar and toss. Cover with a towel and let it rest for 10 minutes. This gives the garlic and onion a chance to develop the health benefits of allium vegetables and the vinegar a chance to release minerals.

Sprinkle on the sunflower seeds.

Note: The sunflower seeds add a bonus boost. A quarter cup (35 g) of them has nearly all your daily vitamin E and copper, half your B_1, and a third of your phosphorus and magnesium. Vinegar to release the minerals and a healthy fat to assist with the absorption make all the ingredients even more bone-friendly. Helen likes her salad with a shaving of red onion. The outer red onion layers provide high levels of quercetin, a potent plant pigment that in most people helps reduce inflammation and treat a number of serious conditions.

> **Nutrition Information per Serving:** 130 mg calcium; 100 mg magnesium; prebiotics; probiotics

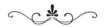

Guacamole

SERVES 6

This marvelous recipe is from Robert Budwig's best seller, *The Vegetable Market Cookbook*. Helen has given this cookbook as a wedding gift to each of her children and to many other people she loves. Every recipe is a gem.

Robert says he first tasted guacamole in the market of Antigua. Just mashed, ripe avocado mixed with a little salt and lemon juice and used as a tortilla topping, which he says was simply delicious. His own recipe includes chili—which he advises you use to taste—and coriander.

Guacamole is best served the day you prepare it. Reserve 1 avocado pit. You will put it into the guacamole before chilling. The pit keeps the mixture from discoloring.

2 large ripe avocados, halved and stoned (pitted)
½ small red onion, very finely chopped
1 clove garlic, crushed
1 Tbsp. finely chopped fresh coriander
1 fresh jalapeño chili pepper, seeded and finely chopped
2 medium-sized ripe tomatoes, peeled, seeded, drained, and chopped
Juice of 1 lime or lemon
1 tsp. salt
½ tsp. freshly ground black pepper

Scoop out the avocado flesh into a bowl and mash until fairly smooth, retaining a little texture. Add the onion, garlic, coriander, chili pepper, tomatoes, lime or lemon juice, salt, and pepper. Mix well, add the reserved avocado stone, cover with plastic wrap, and chill. Remove the stone before serving.

Note: We like to keep the avocados in chunks rather than mashing them smooth. See what you like.

> **Nutrition Information per Serving:** 19 mcg vitamin K; 15 g vitamin C; trace minerals

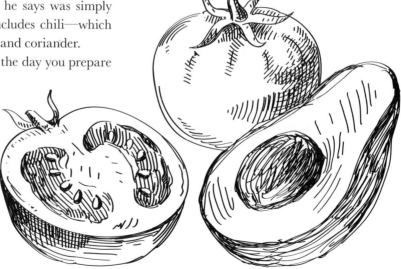

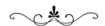

Daikon Kimchi

SERVES 2

Daikon—the word is Japanese for "big root"—is a long white radish the Chinese sometimes call white carrot that is usually available in natural foods stores. Across Asia and India, the versatile daikon is available in many shapes and taste varieties. Daikon features in pickles and other ferments and in a popular citrus soy sauce, ponzu.

This recipe comes from a Korean friend and is the most delicious kimchi we have had. Use it in The Mix-Up Poke Bowl (page 126) or as a snack. Full of probiotics and a delicious pick-me-up. Korean kimchi is typically hot and spicy. Adjust the amount of chili pepper to suit your taste.

4 medium daikon radishes cut into 1- to 2-inch
    (2.5–5 cm) cubes
1½ Tbsp. kosher salt
¼ cup (60 ml) beef bone broth (page 141)
2 cloves garlic, finely chopped
½ tsp. grated or chopped ginger
6 anchovies (canned in olive oil is fine)
1½ tsp. sugar
2 Tbsp. salted shrimp (optional)
1 small sliced onion
4 green onions
2 Tbsp.–½ cup (4–18 g) chopped dried chili
    pepper, or flakes

Mix the cubed daikon and kosher salt in a big bowl and set aside for an hour.

In a blender or food processor, blend the beef broth, chopped garlic, chopped ginger, anchovies, sugar, and, if you're using it, the salted shrimp.

When the daikon is ready, pour the anchovy-shrimp mixture over the daikon, and add the sliced onion, green onions, and dried chili pepper

or flakes. Mix well. Pack into two mason jars. Use a kraut pounder or wooden spoon to pack in the veggies nice and tight. Cover and let sit for 2 days in a pantry or dark cupboard. It is ready to eat in 2 days though you can allow further ferment in the fridge. It keeps for a long time. Laura is testing one for maximum storage time, and it is still fine a year later.

Note: Dried shrimp is available bagged in supermarket frozen food departments.

Nutrition Information per Serving: 30 mg calcium; 15 mg magnesium; 2 g protein; excellent probiotics

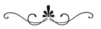

Glazed Beets

SERVES 2–4

Beets and the other members of the chenopod family—including chard, spinach, and quinoa—apparently have a unique ability to strengthen the nervous system and play a powerful part in lessening tumor growth and inflammation. Yellow beets are a deliciously sweet source of the rare chenopod phytonutrients.

Cutting beets into wedges before boiling means a shorter cooking time and more phytonutrients remaining intact. Beet juice makes a natural food coloring and is readily absorbed by a porous surface, so cut boiled red beets on a glazed rather than on a porous surface. Serve these beets as a starter on a bed of watercress or as a vegetable side dish.

4 yellow (or yellow and red) unpeeled beets,
    each cut into 4–6 wedges depending on
    your preference
½ cup (120 ml) balsamic vinegar
3 Tbsp. brown sugar

Boil the beet wedges in water in a large saucepan for 15 minutes. Drain.

In a saucepan, mix the vinegar and brown sugar. Bring to the boil then immediately reduce to low/simmer and continue to cook for about 15 minutes. Stir with a wooden spoon to keep the sugar from sticking. If you're unsure, add a few drops of water. Slip the beet wedges out of their skins, and put into the hot glaze. Mix over high heat for 1 minute.

> **Nutrition Information per Serving:** 2 g protein; trace minerals; 0.8 mg boron; 0.3 mg manganese; B vitamins

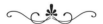

Honeyed Cabbage with Mission Fig Slivers and Toasted Sesame Seed

SERVES 2–4

This side dish is a perfect accompaniment to serve with Chicken Stuffed with Lavender and Figs (page 181) or some steamed broccoli raab.

2 Tbsp. cold-press coconut oil

2 Tbsp. virgin olive oil

6 cloves garlic, sliced in medium slices at least 15 minutes before cooking

1 large or 2 small yellow onions cut in half and prepared in thick slices at least 15 minutes before cooking

½ head green cabbage, sliced very thin almost to a shred

6–8 dried Mission figs, sliced thin

1 scant Tbsp. honey

Sea salt

Freshly ground black pepper

2 Tbsp. sesame seeds, raw or toasted

Put the oils and 1 slice of the garlic into a large frying pan with high sides or a broad-based stir-fry pan. Turn the heat to moderate until the oil around the garlic bubbles. Then add the rest of the garlic and the onion. Cook until the garlic gives off perfume and the onion is translucent. Do not allow the garlic to burn, although browned around the edges is good.

Add the cabbage, stirring until all the cabbage is coated with oil and the garlic and onion are well mixed with the vegetable. Heat until steaming hot and the cabbage is cooked al dente. Toss in the fig slivers, pour the honey over all, and mix well until the honey and cabbage are well blended and the fig slices are just heated to lukewarm.

Fold in salt and pepper to taste. Sprinkle the sesame seed over all.

> **Nutrition Information per Serving:** 60 mg magnesium; 60 mg vitamin C; rare phytonutrients; trace minerals

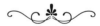

Raw Kale Slaw

SERVES 2–3

Creamy with a kick of garlic, this raw slaw contains ideal ratios of the heavy hitters—calcium, protein, vitamin D, vitamin A, and vitamin K_2 (if you use the egg). It's simply delicious. Laura eats this every other day and never tires of it. It is a solid nutritional base: One large serving contains nearly half of all the daily requirements for building bone.

¾ cup (185 g) tahini (page 234)

½ cup (70 g) sunflower seeds

Juice of ½ lemon

3 Tbsp. olive oil

¼ tsp. sea salt (or to taste)

4 cloves garlic

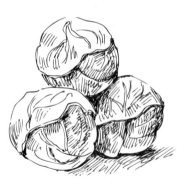

7 sprigs fresh parsley

1 bunch raw emerald or lacinato
kale, shredded or cut small

½ cup (35 g) raw shredded
maitake mushrooms
(hen of the woods)

Combine all the ingredients except the kale and mushrooms in a blender and blend until smooth. If the mixture is too thick, add a little water until it is the texture of a thick soup.

Combine the kale and mushrooms. Pour the soupy mixture over the kale and mushrooms and mix.

Note: Maitake mushrooms are higher in vitamin D content than all other mushroom types, so they are ideal. If you cannot find fresh, look for dried online; soak before use.

Nutrition Information per Serving: 400 mg calcium; 60 iu vitamin D; 37 mcg vitamin K₂; 46 g protein; 1,500 mcg vitamin A

❧ About Brussels Sprouts ☙

Brussels sprouts are at the top of the list in glucosinolates, one of the plant nutrients in cruciferous vegetables known to assist body cells to expunge cancer-causing substances. These mighty mini cruciferous vegetables contribute to the second phase of detoxification system in the liver by supplying one of the required substances, sulfur. Brussels sprouts appear to stabilize DNA in white blood cells.[1]

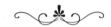

Perfect Roasted Brussels Sprouts

SERVES 4

If you don't like brussels sprouts and wish you did because of their outstanding nutritional profile, make these. Among the attractions: Roasting caramelizes the sprouts' natural sugars, which makes them sweet and delicious. On the nutrition side, preparing your sprouts this way retains the vitamin D and folate, which in turn help regulate inflammation and provide cardiovascular support. And since a good surprise is nice, here's one: Brussels sprouts contain omega-3 fatty acids—1½ cups (132 g) provide a full third of the daily recommendation.

1 lb. (455 g) brussels sprouts

1 Tbsp. olive oil

1 Tbsp. virgin coconut oil

Sea salt to taste

Preheat the oven to 350°F (177°C). Set a rack second from the top.

Wash the sprouts. Pull off any yellow leaves, cut off any brown stem ends, and cut the sprouts in half. Mound them on a cookie sheet. Pour the oils over and through. Make sure they are all coated as you spread them out flat. Salt liberally. Bake for 15 minutes. Some leaves should be browned (they are crunchy and delicious). If no leaves have browned after 15 minutes, turn the oven to broil and broil for 3 minutes.

Nutrition Information per Serving: 100 mg vitamin C; trace minerals; indole; sulfur

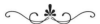

Pickled Savoy and Fennel

SERVES 2–3

This calcium-rich recipe features fennel and cumin, two star members of a powerful family of plants whose lovely flora include coriander, parsley, dill, anise, parsnip, ginseng, carrots, and caraway. Each has a distinctive robust flavor not easily overcome by competing ingredients. Among these, Helen and Chris take any chance to use cumin. Chris says cumin creates a heady suggestion of exotic flavors and faraway places—and transforms the Mexican food he prepares often. Among the many fennel varieties, the one with an edible, celery-like anise-flavored bulb is finocchio.

½ head savoy cabbage, finely shredded
2–3 purple kale leaves, rough-chopped or shredded (optional)
½ bulb finocchio, finely shredded
1½ Tbsp. sea salt
1 tsp. cumin seeds
Pinch of chili pepper (optional)

Mix the vegetables and salt in a big bowl. Massage the salt into the vegetables. Let the mixture rest for 45 minutes loosely covered with a dishcloth, then put it into a quart-sized, widemouthed mason jar. Use a kraut pounder or wooden spoon to pack in the veggies nice and tight.

If there isn't enough liquid released from the cabbage to cover the top of the vegetables by 1 inch, (2.5 cm) top off with brine made from 1 teaspoon sea salt dissolved in 1 cup filtered water. Close up the jar and ferment for at least 7 days, up to 2 weeks in a dark area of your kitchen or pantry.

Nutrition Information per Serving: 85 mg calcium; 35 mg magnesium; probiotics

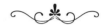

Raw Beef Laab/Larb Lettuce Wraps

SERVES 2–4

This traditional dish from Thailand is spicy, pungent, and delectable. Use very fresh meat from a butcher you know and trust—freshly ground is best—and organic limes. Raw meat is easily digestible. Lime juice denatures the meat, which has the same effect as cooking by heat: It begins to break down the protein structure yet does keep the enzymes and water-soluble vitamins intact and does not oxidize the fat. The chilies will be very hot unless you take out the seeds. It's up to you. You can find good clean fish sauce at an Asian market.

1 Tbsp. raw white rice
4 small dried red chilies
1 lb. (455 g) pasture-raised beef, ground
Juice of 2 limes
3 stalks lemongrass, chopped
1 small red onion, chopped
10 mint leaves, plus 6 for garnish
2 Tbsp. fish sauce
1 head romaine lettuce

Dry-fry the rice and chilies in a small frying pan until the rice grains are brown. Grind in a mortar and pestle or grinder to the consistency of rough sand.

Add the beef and lime juice to a large bowl and mix well. Then add the chili-rice powder and all the other ingredients. Place one heaping tablespoon of the meat mixture on a crisp romaine lettuce leaf, roll up, and garnish with mint leaves.

Nutrition Information per Serving: 30 mg calcium; 30 mg magnesium; 28 g protein; prebiotics

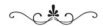

Roasted Asparagus

SERVES 2

This prebiotic vegetable is temperamental. It loses flavor more quickly than other vegetables, so use the freshest you can find and treat it as you do lettuce: Tie a paper towel around the ends and keep in waxed paper or plastic, or stand the bunch in a bit of cold water in a small jug.

Asparagus tests in the nearly safe level for pesticide residue, so when we can't find organic asparagus, we buy conventionally grown.

1 bunch asparagus
2 Tbsp. olive oil
Grated sea salt and freshly ground black pepper
½ lemon, sliced in rounds
¼ cup (20 g) freshly grated Parmesan cheese, made of unpasteurized milk if possible

Break or cut off the inedible ends of the asparagus stalks and discard them. Asparagus purists

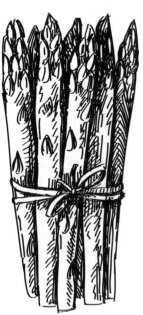

scrape off the leaf sheaths, or bracts—those small red triangular leaves that run randomly up the stalk. Rumor has it that Julia Child always peeled asparagus from just below the tip to make sure no woody fibers remained. If you buy thick asparagus stalks, we advise peeling.

Preheat the oven to 325°F (163°C).

Set the prepared asparagus in a single layer in a baking pan. Rub each asparagus spear all over with olive oil. To do that, drizzle a drop over a spear and use your fingers to coat it overall. Sprinkle with grated sea salt and ground black pepper. Distribute the lemon rounds over the asparagus.

Roast for 15 minutes or until the point of a sharp knife—or a fork with sharp tines—tells you the vegetables are al dente. Turn the oven off. Set the lemon slices to one side. Sprinkle the asparagus with Parmesan and leave it to sit in the oven for a few minutes until the cheese has begun to melt. Serve with 1 lemon slice atop each portion.

Nutrition Information per Serving: high levels of phytonutrients; trace minerals; B vitamins

---

❧ Fish Egg Nutrition ❧

According to an analysis carried out by the Weston A. Price Foundation, a single tablespoon of fish roe contains approximately 17,000 international units of vitamin D along with vitamin A, vitamin K_2, zinc, iodine, and the brain-supporting omega-3 fatty acid DHA in ample amounts.

One tablespoon of fish eggs supplies a dose of vitamin D equivalent to a midday dose on the skin. Vitamins A and K_2 work synergistically with vitamin D to prevent toxicity and overcalcification of the soft tissues.

Smoked Salmon with Fish Roe and Zesty Yogurt Dressing

SERVES 4

Fish eggs, typically called roe, were highly prized by mountain-dwelling South American natives, who sometimes traveled hundreds of miles to the sea to procure dried roe for women of childbearing age to ensure healthy and robust babies and children. The Inuit also consumed roe, particularly that of salmon. They dried roe for consumption during winter months and for special feeding to pregnant women. Smoked salmon contains high levels of vitamin D. Greek yogurt offers protein and calcium with less sugar than most other commercial yogurts. Dill adds a calcium boost, and the dish affords a measure of K_2.

8 slices packaged smoked salmon
¼ cup fish roe
12–16 whole chives
Thin slices of rye or sourdough bread (optional)
8 sprigs fresh dill
6 cloves garlic, finely chopped
12 oz. (340 g) full-fat Greek yogurt
½ tsp. sea salt

Make the dressing by mixing the dill, garlic, yogurt, and salt.

Arrange 2 slices of smoked salmon on a plate. Dollop on the yogurt artfully. Place 1 tablespoon of the roe on the yogurt, then set three chive threads over the top. If you prefer, serve the salmon placed on a slice of bread.

Nutrition Information per Serving: 130 mg calcium; 17,000 iu vitamin D; 11 g protein; high omega-3

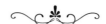

Sourdough Sunday

SERVES 4–6

To many people around the globe, Sunday means pancakes or waffles, English muffins, croissants, brioche, or bagels along with butter and other traditional toppings. Food customs are central to family life, and Helen likes to maintain hers while she feeds her bones. Since Helen is a New Yorker by birth and breeding, Chris is working on a sourdough version of bagels, famously a Sunday brunch icon. Shape sourdough sponge into rolls, croissants, brioche, or baguettes.

8 oz. (225 g) homemade cream cheese or fine-quality Brie, preferably made from natural (raw) milk
1–2 cups (20–30 g) baby arugula
1 cucumber, unpeeled and thinly sliced
8–12 thin slices smoked salmon
1 tsp. capers
1 medium red onion, thinly sliced
1–2 pastured eggs per person, poached
Homemade sourdough or rye bread

On a large platter, set out the cream cheese, arugula, and cucumber. Place the smoked salmon atop the arugula and sprinkle the capers over all.

Slice the bread. Toast and top each slice with some of each platter ingredient along with 1 poached egg. Repeat for a second egg or use two pieces of bread and make a sandwich. Delicious.

Nutrition Information per Serving: 222 mg calcium; 74 mg magnesium; 200 iu vitamin D; 40 mcg vitamin K_2; 37 g protein; probiotics

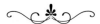

Sunned Mushrooms and Oregano with Kale

SERVES 2–4

You will feel great after eating a serving of this. Not many other food sources are so rich in nutrients and phytochemicals, so we hope you will incorporate them into your diet often. They will take you a long way toward healthy bones.

1 Tbsp. virgin coconut oil
1 tsp. ghee
10 sprigs fresh oregano
1–2 cloves garlic, smashed
1 lb. (455 g) mixed sunned mushrooms
  (page 129)
1 yellow onion, chopped
10 kale leaves
Pinch of truffle salt

Heat the oil and ghee in a large saucepan. Pull the leaves from the oregano sprigs and drop into the pan along with the garlic. Let cook for a minute, then add the mushrooms, onion, truffle salt, and kale. Cook for 10 minutes, stirring occasionally so nothing sticks.

Nutrition Information per Serving: 120 mg calcium; 60 mg magnesium; 4,000 iu vitamin D; 6 g protein; phytoestrogen

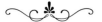

Sweet and Purple Potato Fries

SERVES 2–3

Laura says: "I like to dip mine in Greek yogurt with dill and garlic. Can't say much about these because my mouth is full. Deliciousness."

Helen says: "I roast mine without salt and sprinkle with sea salt and freshly ground black pepper at the table. Delectable."

3 purple-flesh sweet potatoes, cut into wedges
¼ cup (60 ml) virgin coconut oil,
  room temperature
Salt to taste

Preheat the oven to 375°F (191°C).

Put the wedges in a bowl, then rub them with the oil and salt until they're covered. Spread in one layer on a cookie sheet. Bake for 30 minutes, turning over halfway through.

Nutrition Information per Serving: 40 mg magnesium; 18,000 iu vitamin A; trace minerals

✄ About Coconut Oil ✄

Coconut oil is looking more and more like a go-to food for bone health. Not only does the rich, readily available fat enhance and assist nutrient absorption, but preliminary studies suggest it actually increases bone density. Add virgin coconut oil to your diet any way you use vegetable oil: 3½ tablespoons a day for a 150-pound person. Adjust for your weight.

Researchers in Southeast Asia were able to maintain bone structure and prevent bone loss in estrogen-deficient rats through coconut oil. Additionally they were able to actually reverse the effects of estrogen deficiency on bone structure. Rats are widely accepted in this context as a model for human osteoporosis.

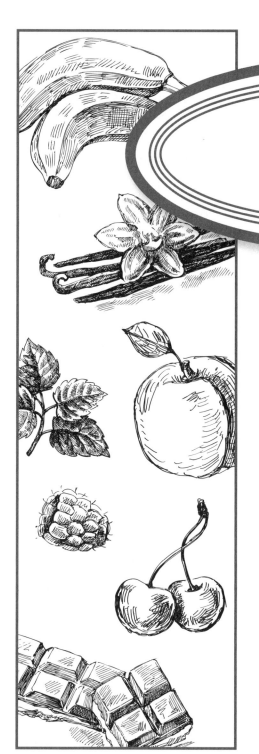

CHAPTER 19

Desserts

Helen's husband, Chris—a retired, small business owner who grew up in the north of England—says afters (desserts) are the perfect finish to a traditional Sunday lunch. That does not mean daily assaults by refined sugar, however; nor does it mean falling headlong into the guilty pleasure trap. It does mean eating sweets in moderation and enjoying them immensely and for the most part preparing them with natural ingredients.

Among the dessert recipes in this chapter, each of us has a favorite, yet we've received praise from friends and family for them all.

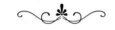

Berry Ice Cream

SERVES 2

If you love ice cream, you're in luck. This confection does not have sugar and does have the lovely texture of homemade. It takes a minute to prepare and both our husbands, who are on diets for weight loss and metabolic syndrome respectively, ask for it several times a week.

Blackberries are the most nutrient-dense among the berries, but blueberries and raspberries are nutrient bullets, too, and perform well in this dish. Use them in combination as you wish. Try just-thawed blackberries. When frozen, strawberries don't chop properly in the mini processor, so we save them for an attractive garnish.

1 cup (240 ml) whole natural milk
1 cup (140 g) frozen blueberries, raspberries, or a mix of the two to make up 1 cup

OPTIONAL INGREDIENTS

1 Tbsp. cacao nibs
Strawberries or cacao nibs, for garnish
Tiny snippet of stevia leaf or ⅓–½ packet coconut sugar

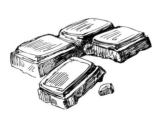

Put all the ingredients into the food chopper attachment of a stick blender (a.k.a. immersion blender). Whir until it turns to ice cream. Take out the blade and dish out, scraping the bowl—you won't want to leave any behind.

If you don't have an immersion blender with a chopper attachment, a small food processor or even a regular blender will turn up good results,

though you won't get all the ice cream out of a regular-sized blender jug.

Nutrition Information per Serving: 150 mg calcium; 150 mg magnesium

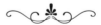

World's Best Milk Shake

SERVES 1

This is a fully customizable recipe. The key is quality ingredients. With those as a starting point, get ready to design your own perfect breakfast, snack, light dinner, whatever, whenever you want to feel just plain happy. And don't forget to thank the chocolate for your shot of magnesium.

Cacao nibs are raw, unfermented cocoa beans and carry high levels of a compound that traps calcium. Roasting the nibs weakens the compound's grip on minerals.

2–3 Tbsp. unsweetened dark chocolate powder (or small chunks)
2 tsp. raw sugar (or to taste; we don't like it too sweet)
2 tsp. boiling water
1½ (360 ml) cups raw milk
1 banana
2 tsp. roasted cacao nibs
2 ice cubes

In a small cup, make a thick paste of the chocolate powder, sugar, and boiling water. Put the paste and the remaining ingredients into a blender and blend on high for 40 seconds. Drink and smile.

Nutrition Information per Serving: 450 mg calcium; 135 mg magnesium; 150 iu vitamin D; 15 mcg vitamin K₂; 16 g protein

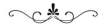

Mint Chocolate Milk Shake

SERVES 1

This is a minty version of the world's best milk shake. Still the world's best.

1 tsp. mint syrup
3 sprigs mint leaves
1½ cups (360 ml) coconut milk
2 ice cubes
2–3 Tbsp. dark chocolate powder
2 tsp. roasted cacao nibs
Add 1 tsp. green powder for an extra vitamin/ mineral boost (optional)
Add 1 tsp. maca and/or reishi mushroom powder, for opening to new ideas and for relaxation (optional)

Place the ingredients into a blender and blend on high for 40 seconds.

Nutrition Information per Serving: 450 mg calcium; 160 mg magnesium; 150 iu vitamin D; 15 mcg vitamin K₂; 16 g protein

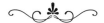

Chocolate Dipped Frozen Bananas

SERVES 8

This variation from Carlota Cassou on a popular dessert recipe feeds gut bugs and bones and happily satisfies a sweet tooth. Dark chocolate, coconut oil, hemp seeds, and the many variations on this traditional recipe make it a treat. Is this really a dessert? Okay then, enjoy it anytime. You can't make enough.

Here's a quick party trick. Once the dark chocolate has hardened, put some white chocolate sauce into an icing bag—or one you make with several layers of waxed paper—and draw to your heart's content.

4 bananas

DARK CHOCOLATE COATING

4 Tbsp. coconut oil (melted)
4 Tbsp. cacao powder
3 Tbsp. agave

WHITE CHOCOLATE COATING

½ cup (115 g) cacao butter
½ cup (60 g) powdered sugar
½ tsp. vanilla extract
¼ cup (35 g) cashews, previously soaked overnight, preferably in filtered water

WHITE CHOCOLATE STRAWBERRY COATING

⅓ cup (55 g) white chocolate mixture (see the recipe above)
½ cup (83 g) strawberries

SUGGESTED TOPPINGS

Shredded coconut
Hemp seeds
Chopped nuts
Tiny currents
Sprinkles
Goji berries
Granola
Cardamom
Keep going . . . enjoy!

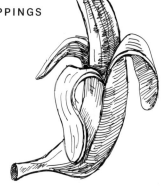

Peel and cut bananas in half. Insert a Popsicle stick into the banana pieces. Place the bananas on a baking sheet and freeze for about 15 to 20 minutes. Remove the bananas from the freezer

and dip each into the chocolate sauce of your choice. The sauce will harden almost immediately. Place the bananas back on the baking sheet and freeze for about 10 minutes more. Enjoy right from the freezer or let the pop stand for a minute or two.

Dark Chocolate Coating: Place the melted coconut oil in a bowl and add the cacao powder. Mix well with a spoon or a whisk until well incorporated. Then add the agave and mix to combine.

White Chocolate Coating: Using a wire whisk, blend the cacao butter, sugar, and vanilla. Add the cashews and mix with a large spoon to coat the nuts.

White Chocolate Strawberry Coating: Blend the white chocolate and strawberries until smooth.

Nutrition Information per Serving: 40 mg magnesium; prebiotics

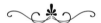

Four Seasons Strawberry Parfait

SERVES 2

Given disputed fillers like carrageenan and overheated dairy in a lot of commercially available ice cream—and the artificial ingredients plus refined sugar and calories—you may imagine that ice cream sundaes and parfaits are a long way off the bone health list.

But take heart. Here's one Helen created in the early days of recipe development to make the most of the local strawberry season, and she's been loving it ever since.

Hull and freeze fresh organic strawberries in season, sourced as locally as possible. Since Helen lives in a four-season climate, she freezes half a dozen baskets of strawberries at a time.

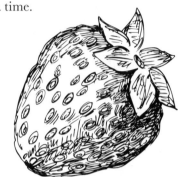

1 fresh ½-gallon (1.9 L) glass bottle of very cold natural milk with the cream still at the top
16 strawberries, hulled and previously frozen by you
2 cups ice cream (homemade, page 213)
1 Tbsp. unsulfured blackstrap molasses

If you are taking cream from your raw milk, use a baster to siphon off 4 tablespoons (¼ cup) of the cream. Then siphon off ½ cup (120 ml) of milk. These amounts are for both servings.

Defrost the frozen strawberries in the fridge. Time it so the berries are just defrosted and still very cold when you are ready to start making the dessert. If you put frozen berries into the fridge first thing in the morning or even overnight, by dinnertime, they should be perfect.

Place 8 strawberries in a stemless red wine glass or a parfait or sundae dish. Add the cream and milk. Top with a scoop of homemade berry ice cream or vanilla bean ice cream. Let it rest for a minute. Using a spoon, scoop the berries, cream, milk, and ice cream into a mix. Drizzle on the molasses.

This is sublime.

Nutrition Information per Serving: 270 mg calcium; 50 mg magnesium; 6 g protein

---

❧ About Ice Cream ❧

If you use commercial ice cream, choose one whose ingredients list shows milk and cream *before* sugar, and does not show other ingredients except natural flavoring such as ground vanilla beans. Ice cream often contains tara gum to improve creaminess and hold the texture during shipment; at this time tara gum is controversial, though investigation is ongoing.

You have to read the labels. To check the amount of sugar, look at the carbohydrate percentage. There is a lot of variation in sugar content, and some of the high-end brands are the sweetest.

Reading labels does become automatic after a while. It's always worth it for the time, savings, and health benefits.

And often you save money, too: It surprised us to find that one of the great-value ice creams fits our ingredients requirements to a T.

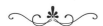

No Cream Ice Cream

SERVES 2 4

Don't worry; this isn't a lackluster substitute you have to endure for the sake of your bones. You'll find all the smooth creaminess that makes eating ice cream so rewarding. The secret is in the soy.

1 cup (120 g) confectioner's (powdered) sugar with tapioca as the only added ingredient
4 pastured egg yolks
1 tsp. cornstarch

2 cups (480 ml) homemade soymilk (See "How to Make Soymilk," page 246)
1 tsp. vanilla extract

Put the sugar, eggs yolks, and cornstarch into a bowl; whisk the mixture.

Heat the soymilk in a saucepan; slowly pour the hot soymilk into the mixture while continuing to whisk briskly. Add the vanilla extract. Gently heat the mixture until it thickens.

Let the mixture cool in the refrigerator for 3 or 4 hours. Pour the mixture into an ice cream maker; mix for 20 minutes—just about when you'll see your ice cream.

> **Nutrition Information per Serving:** 200 mg calcium; 28 mg magnesium; 93 iu vitamin D; 7 g protein; phytoestrogen

---

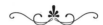

Coconut Milk Ice Cream

SERVES 4

This wonderful ice cream is best served immediately after you make it. If you store it in the freezer, put it back into the ice cream maker to restore the smooth, creamy consistency just before serving. Follow the instructions on your ice cream maker for timing.

1 can full-fat coconut milk (13.5 oz. [400 ml])
3 frozen bananas or ½ cup (60 g) coconut palm sugar
Pinch of sea salt

FOR ALMOND PISTACHIO FLAVOR

1½ tsp. almond extract
1 vanilla bean, seeded, or 1 tsp. vanilla extract
½ cup (73 g) toasted and chopped almonds and pistachios

FOR MINT CHOCOLATE CHIP FLAVOR

2 tsp. peppermint extract

⅓ cup (60 g) raw cacao nibs, or chocolate chips
 of your choice

FOR COOKIES & CREAM FLAVOR

1 Tbsp. vanilla extract

10 cookies broken into pieces

Combine the base ingredients in a blender and blend until smooth. Add the liquid flavorings (extracts) into the blender and blend again. If you are using sugar and/or salt, add them with the liquid flavorings. Pour the mixture into an ice cream machine and turn on. Mix for at least 20 minutes, or until the mix has the consistency of ice cream.

 Stir in the dry ingredients—such as nuts or cookies—and serve.

> **Nutrition Information per Serving:** 35 mg calcium;
> 90 mg magnesium; 4 g protein; prebiotic

Refrigerator Cream Cheese Cake with Lemon Shortbread Crust

SERVES 8

It's always surprising when something good is good for you, especially when it comes to bone health and desserts. But here's one your bones will thank you for, as cream cheese is one of the few foods with a reasonable amount of the MK4 type of vitamin K_2.

 This recipe starts with homemade cream cheese, which in the United States is deemed about 55 percent fat but in different European countries has a higher fat content. You can substitute commercial full-fat cream cheese but avoid those with stabilizers such as carrageenan. Read the label.

Lemon Shortbread Crust

This recipe is perfect for two different and delightful cheesecakes: fresh figs and chocolate.

1½ cups (190 g) shortbread crumbs or flour

⅓ cup (75 g) melted unsalted butter

1 tsp. lemon extract

⅓ cup (65 g) coconut sugar, loosely packed

Mix all of the crust ingredients well in a bowl.

 Pat into a square or rectangular baking pan and bake at 350°F (177°C) for 15 minutes. The crust should be golden. Allow the pan and crust to cool completely on a wire rack.

> **Nutrition Information per Serving:** 100 mg calcium;
> 120 mg magnesium; 10 g protein

No-Bake Cream Cheese Cake with Fresh Fig Topping

16 oz. (455 g) cream cheese at room temperature

½ cup (100 g) sugar or ½–1 tsp. stevia

1 tsp. pure vanilla extract or half and half vanilla
 and lemon extract

1 cup (240 ml) cream

1 Tbsp. lemon zest

4–6 ripe fresh figs, stem ends removed and
 then sliced

Make the shortbread crust. While the crust is cooling, put a mixing bowl and beaters into the fridge (for 20 minutes) or the freezer (for 5 minutes) to chill.

 When the crust is completely cooled, put the cream cheese in a room-temperature bowl. Using a hand mixer with beaters at room temperature, whip the cheese until integrated and spreadable—somewhat like the consistency of soft ice cream. Add the stevia and extract.

Put the cream into the chilled bowl and use the chilled beaters to whip it until it thickens into traditional whipped cream. Using a rubber spatula, fold the whipped cream into the cream cheese very gently until just incorporated. Using the spatula, scoop the mixture gently onto the crust. Even out the top. Sprinkle the lemon zest on top. Refrigerate for at least 1 hour before serving.

To serve, top either the cake or individual portions with fresh fig slices.

> **Nutrition Information per Serving:** 160 mg calcium; 25 mg magnesium; 17 mcg vitamin K$_2$; 8 g protein

No-Bake Chocolate Cheesecake with 85% Chocolate Flakes

This version is excellent served with Fresh Cherry Sauce.

2 dozen pitted cherries
2 oz. (55 g) 85% dark chocolate, melted
　over water with 2 Tbsp. raw butter
16 oz. (455 g) cream cheese at
　room temperature
½ cup (100 g) sugar
1 tsp. pure vanilla extract
2 cups (480ml) cream
8 fresh mint leaves (optional)
Shaves of a sweeter chocolate or a dusting
　of stevia (optional)

Pit the cherries and cut them into halves or quarters.

Make the shortbread crust. Melt the chocolate with the butter and let the mixture stand until it reaches room temperature but has not hardened.

Follow the instructions above for making the filling. When the cream cheese has the consistency of soft ice cream, add the chocolate and whip until fully integrated.

While the cake is in the refrigerator, make the Fresh Cherry Sauce (page 164).

Cover the top with shaved chocolate or a dusting of stevia. To serve, top either the cake or the individual portions with cherries and a mint leaf.

> **Nutrition Information per Serving:** 100 mg calcium; 60 mg magnesium; 17 mcg vitamin K$_2$; 8 g protein

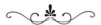

Rosy Summertime Rhubarb Compote or Crumble
SERVES 2

Cooked rhubarb turns a rosy pink that makes for a lovely tart compote on its own, perhaps with a scoop of ice cream—or in a crumble like this one. It offers 105 mg calcium a cup, it's full of fiber and red-fruit goodness, and it's ultra simple to prepare. But there are caveats. Rhubarb roots and leaves are not edible. If you grow it you must twist the stems off several inches from the root—and whether you grow it or buy locally, cut the leaves and stem off completely. Worth the trouble? Ask anyone British what's for dessert with traditional Sunday lunch . . .

2–4 Tbsp. castor (a.k.a. ultrafine and
　superfine) sugar
4 stalks mature rhubarb or 6 smaller stalks
½–1 cup (70–145 g) blackberries or very ripe
　clingstone peaches, halved and pitted, unpeeled
1 cup (240 ml) water

Like celery, to which it is not related, rhubarb stems may have fibrous strings best removed before cooking. To take off the toughest cords, at the root end place the knife blade at the underside of the stalk and slice almost all the way through. Bend the slice toward the top and pull. The fibers will come free. Discard them. Cut the stalks into 1-inch (2.5 cm) chunks.

Put the sugar in a pan with water and boil. Add the rhubarb. Boil for 15 minutes or until the rhubarb is tender. Drain, saving the syrup.

Note: For topping, a syrup of your clingstone peaches, a few clingstone peach slices, blackberries, and/or a generous scoop of vanilla bean ice cream all make perfect counterpoint to the flavorsome rhubarb tartness.

For a richer syrup, add 1 or 2 tablespoons of pure fruit spread—sweetened with apple or pear juice, not sugar—to the cooking water before adding the rhubarb.

Traditional British Crumble

Crumble is a fruit compote assembled and baked with a crunchy topping over all. It is a British favorite, especially for Sunday lunch afters. The topping is almost always some combination of sugar, flour, or ground nuts made rich with an aromatic spice and unsalted butter.

Chris's favorite topping is demerara sugar, some flour, pulverized almonds, and cinnamon, but people substitute oats for flour, allspice or ginger for cinnamon. . . . Best to make it up as you like.

8 oz. (225 g) flour or ground oats
½ cup (1 stick [115 g]) butter—
  no margarine here ever
2–4 oz. (55–115 g) brown or white sugar
1 teaspoon spice

Place the prepared compote in an 8-inch-square (20 cm) baking dish.

To prepare the crumble topping, work the flour, butter, and sugar with your fingers until the mixture resembles crumbs. Add 1 teaspoon of a spice such as cinnamon, or more to taste. Sprinkle the crumble evenly over the compote. If you want a bit more color, sprinkle additional cinnamon lightly over the top. Bake in a 350°F (180°C) oven until the topping is browned and crunchy, about 20 minutes. Serve the crumble warm or cold with dairy or soy ice cream (page 213), or if you want to follow the British tradition, with cold heavy cream.

Note: Helen likes to use half flour and half ground almonds and lots of cinnamon, which works exceptionally well when the fruit is stewed apples and blackberries, the British all-time favorite.

> **Nutrition Information per Serving:** 140 mg calcium; 40 mg magnesium; 19 mg vitamin C

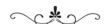

Tahini Chocolate Cakes
MAKES 6 CAKES; SERVES 3–6

These luxurious tahini chocolate cakes from the cookbook *Smashing Plates* by Maria Elia are served with crème fraîche dusted with lime zest. Use dark chocolate: The higher the cocoa bean content, the more magnesium you'll consume. A 6-ounce bar of dark chocolate supplies you with nearly all the magnesium you need in a day. In fact, dark chocolate is so nutritious, Japanese physicians have been prescribing it.

10 Tbsp. (150 g) unsalted butter,
  plus more for greasing pans
⅓ cup (25 g) unsweetened cocoa,
  plus more for pans

3 Tbsp. (27 g) sesame seeds

½ cup (60 g) all-purpose flour

Pinch of salt

5½ oz. (165 g) 70% dark chocolate, in pieces

3 large eggs

1 cup (200 g) superfine sugar

5 Tbsp. (100 g) tahini

Zest of 1 lime

Crème fraîche or ice cream, for serving

Heat oven to 350°F (177°C). Use butter to grease 6 half-cup muffin molds; or you can use smaller molds. Dust the molds with cocoa and sprinkle the sesame seeds in the bottom of each. Sift together remaining ⅓ cup (30 g) cocoa with the flour and a pinch of salt. Set aside.

Melt the chocolate and remaining 10 tablespoons butter in a heatproof bowl over simmering water, or in a small, heavy saucepan on very low heat. (Watch carefully if using a saucepan.) When almost completely melted, remove from the heat and stir until smooth. Set aside.

Using a whisk or electric beater, whisk the eggs and sugar together until pale and fluffy, about 5 minutes. Stir a little of this mixture into the tahini to lighten it, then stir the tahini into the egg mixture. Stir in the cooled chocolate mixture. Fold in the cocoa mixture.

Pour the batter into the molds and set the molds on a baking sheet. Place in the oven and bake 12 to 14 minutes, less for smaller molds. A skewer or toothpick inserted in the middle should not come out clean.

Cool 20 minutes or more before unmolding. Dust the tops with lime zest and serve with crème fraîche or ice cream.

Nutrition Information per Serving: 190 mg calcium; 138 mg magnesium; 20 mcg K$_2$; 12 g protein

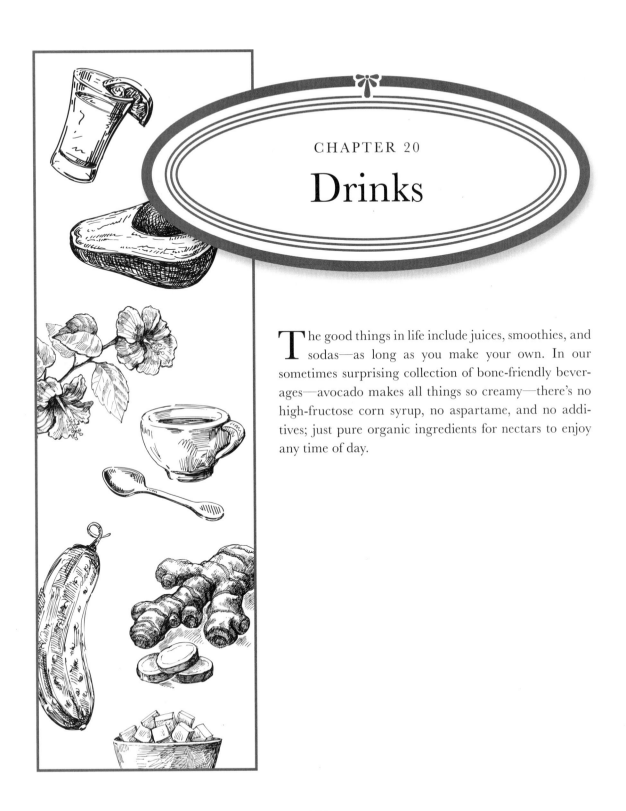

CHAPTER 20
Drinks

The good things in life include juices, smoothies, and sodas—as long as you make your own. In our sometimes surprising collection of bone-friendly beverages—avocado makes all things so creamy—there's no high-fructose corn syrup, no aspartame, and no additives; just pure organic ingredients for nectars to enjoy any time of day.

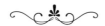

Avocado Shake

SERVES 1

Avocado is a fruit. It's rich in potassium, beneficial fats, and most of the amino acids that make up a complete protein—and everything is bio-available. Among avocados Hass is the creamiest; it is our choice here.

Make the shake savory or sweet. Either is luscious and fit for royal bones. It becomes smooth and creamy when buzzed in a blender with ice cubes. The savory shake is less well known than the sweet one though no less delicious. Ours is dairy-free.

Savory Shake

1 Haas avocado

2 cloves garlic, chopped

1 cup (240 ml) unpasteurized coconut water

½ cup (120 ml) filtered water

1 big sprig cilantro

Juice of ¼ lemon or to taste

Pinch of salt

2 ice cubes

2 shakes cayenne pepper

Nutrition Information per Serving: 80 mg calcium; 100 mg magnesium; 5 g protein

Sweet Shake

The Vietnamese use condensed sweetened milk when they make this drink, and the Indonesians add espresso and/or sweet chocolate.

1 medium Haas avocado

1 cup (240 ml) raw milk or coconut milk

2 Tbsp. raw sugar (or to taste)

¼ tsp. vanilla extract

1–2 tsp. cacao nibs

2 ice cubes

For the savory shake, chop the garlic 10 minutes before making the shake.

Then, for either type of shake, halve the avocado, remove the seed, and scoop the flesh into a blender. Add all of the remaining ingredients and pulse for 40 seconds. If the result is too thick for

---

❧ About Lemon ❧

A squeeze of lemon juice leaves an alkaline residue, which contributes toward a neutral pH balance. pH in balance means the body has exactly the levels of acid and alkaline it needs to operate metabolic machinery at maximum efficiency. Enzymes catalyze reactions at the right speed; electrical charges keep communication going through the nerve network.

Why does this matter here? The body has an exquisitely sensitive sensing mechanism. If the balance just begins to tip, the body rectifies that right away. And if it's looking like an acid overload, the body immediately pulls alkaline material from the richest source at its disposal, which is your bones.

The lemon—and the other ingredients in this shake—leave mostly alkaline residue. Since Western diets are typically high in food that leaves acid residue (protein is the key actor on that stage), a solid hit of food that leaves an alkaline residue offsets the acids, maintains the balance, and leaves the bones intact.

your taste, add a bit more coconut water and mix for a few seconds more.

To serve the shake, pour it into a chilled glass. Best to drink it right away.

Nutrition Information per Serving: 300 mg calcium; 100 mg magnesium; 12 g protein

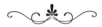

Homemade Sodas

SERVES 16

Commercial sodas are a no-go for bone health. In fact, an orthopedist told us that due to their high levels of phosphate, colas were the worst offender for bone health; he was terrified thinking about the extra-large-sized soda generation getting older. Let's get them tasting our sodas, which are more delicious than almost any commercial soda you can find. Oh, and they use live yeast, so they're probiotic to boot.

You'll need bottles or jars with a metal bail that clamps tightly in place to bottle your soda. Use fresh herbs. Reduce the sugar content to suit your taste.

Ginger Beer

1 oz. (28 g) fresh gingerroot, coarsely chopped
1 lemon, thinly sliced
1 gallon (3.8 L) water
2 cups (400 g) sugar
⅛ tsp. active yeast, or ½ cup (120 ml) ginger bug (page 222)
8 sprigs fresh rosemary

Mash the gingerroot and lemon slices at the bottom of a pot. Add the water, bring to a boil, and simmer for 30 minutes. Remove from the heat,

strain out the solids, and stir in the sugar until it's dissolved.

Cool to lukewarm. Stir in the yeast or ginger bug and let stand for 1 hour. Put a sprig of fresh rosemary in each bottle or jar, then funnel in the ginger beer. Cap tightly. Store in the pantry for 3 to 4 days, then refrigerate for 2 days more.

Carbon dioxide buildup in this soda can be powerful, so be cautious when opening.

Root Beer

Root beer is a fizzy drink made from fermented roots. Most of the herbs in this recipe are also used medicinally. If you have herbal knowledge, you can add or subtract herbs as you like to create your own custom drink. The variety of root beer recipes available is very broad, with ingredients lists that reflect what's locally available where the root beer is made. Better-quality commercial sodas use sassafras and wintergreen roots.

1 gallon (3.8 L) water
¼ oz. (7 g) hops
¼ oz. (7 g) dried burdock root
½ oz. (14 g) dried sarsaparilla root
½ oz. (14 g) dried sassafras root
¼ cup (14 g) wintergreen leaf
½ oz. (14 g) dried licorice root
1 tsp. juniper berries
1 cinnamon stick
½ oz. (14 g) wild cherry tree bark
1 Tbsp. dried ginger
1 Tbsp. birch bark
1–1½ cups (200–300 g) sugar (depending on taste)
⅛ tsp. active yeast or ½ cup (120 ml) Ginger Bug (page 222)

Follow the instructions for Ginger Beer above, except for the mashing of gingerroot. (There is no ginger in this recipe.)

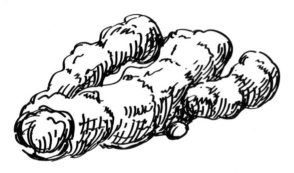

Ginger Bug

Ginger bug is a mix of fermented ginger and sugar. It is a bacterial starter for homemade sodas.

The ingredients list for this recipe is a base amount of ingredients that you will add to the Bug each day. Since you repeat adding those ingredients over a period of several days, start out with a big piece of gingerroot in the refrigerator (or freezer), and grate only the amount you need each day.

2 Tbsp. freshly grated ginger
1 Tbsp. whole unrefined cane sugar
2 Tbsp. filtered water
Additional quantities of each ingredient to add
over a 5-day period

Put the three ingredients into a 16-ounce mason jar, set the screw top lid on loosely, and put the jar in the pantry or a warm spot in the kitchen.

Starting the next day, every day for 5 days mix an additional 2 tablespoons grated ginger, 1 tablespoon sugar, and 2 tablespoons water into your jar. The mixture will bubble as it ferments. It is ready to use on day 6. Keep it in the fridge and feed it the same three ingredients in the same ratio once a week. If you keep using it, you can keep it indefinitely.

Nutrition Information per Serving: phytoestrogens; phytonutrients; high in trace minerals

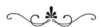

Golden Milk
SERVES 2

You hear a lot about golden milk lately, and that's a good thing. It is delicious, comforting, beautiful to behold, and a nutritional inspiration. You can adjust the proportions to make it sweet enough for dessert. In our houses it is very often an evening tonic.

Turmeric is a powerful anti-inflammatory, which is important for bone health because inflammation can increase bone loss, as explained in chapter 2. However, turmeric is difficult for the body to absorb. Here's where the black pepper's piperine rides to the rescue. Piperine is an alkaloid—a compound derived from plants that helps cells absorb nutrients. Piperine helps boost turmeric absorption by 2,000 percent.

2 cups (480 ml) natural milk or homemade
soymilk (page 246)
5 tsp. skinned and finely chopped fresh
turmeric root, or 1 Tbsp. turmeric
root powder
1½ tsp. freshly ground black pepper
2–3 tsp. raw honey
Pinch of cayenne, ½ tsp. ghee, 1 basil leaf
(optional)

Slowly warm the milk, turmeric root, and pepper in a small saucepan. Do not allow the milk to boil, because boiling would destroy enzymes that help the body digest the milk.

If you use turmeric powder instead of fresh root, mix the powder in a teaspoon of hot water in a small cup, and then add that mixture to the milk in the saucepan.

When steam starts to rise, pour the milk into small cups and stir in honey to taste. If you wish, top with cayenne or turmeric powder, or—if you have not gotten enough good fats today—a bit of ghee. The sight and scent of a fresh basil leaf on top adds to the pleasure.

Nutrition Information per Serving: 276 mg calcium; 30 mg magnesium; 9 g protein; phytonutrients; prebiotics

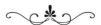

Good Bones Low-Oxalate Green Juice

SERVES 2

The lore about green juice is that you feel the nutritional boost the minute you drink it, and it's probably true because green juice is so readily absorbed. The downside can be using greens that are high in oxalic acid, which blocks mineral absorption by the body.

Spinach, chard, and beet greens are highest in oxalic acid, so we use other greens when we make juice. If you want to make juice from the three high-oxalate greens, time your consumption of foods containing calcium for a couple of hours before or after drinking a high-oxalate juice (see chapter 4 for more about oxalic acid).

If you are consuming the juice for benefits other than calcium absorption, then the only caveat is for people who have, have had, or easily form kidney stones, which are formed from calcium and oxalic acid.

½ cucumber
4 sprigs parsley
½ head romaine
5 leaves kale
2 stalks celery

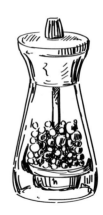

Pinch of salt
Pinch of spirulina powder
¼ tsp. chia seeds
1 tsp. dulse (dried seaweed)
4 savoy cabbage leaves
2 heads baby bok choy
Pinch of turmeric
Pinch of black pepper

Put all the ingredients through a juicer.

Nutrition Information per Serving: 600 mg calcium; 190 mg magnesium; 6 g protein; phytoestrogen

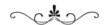

Green Dream Fruit and Spirulina Powder Smoothie

SERVES 2

Spirulina are blue-green algae that grow principally in salty seawater and warm alkaline lakes. They contain as much iron as equivalent weights of beef. Spirulina can absorb contaminants from a natural water environment, so we prefer a powder form sourced naturally yet warranted free from harmful bacteria and heavy metals.

Laura loves this smoothie for breakfast or for post-workout. It contains complete protein, vitamin C from strawberries for tissue repair, and phytoestrogens for hormone balance as well as B vitamins, iron, potassium, magnesium, calcium, zinc, and trace minerals.

2 bananas
1 Tbsp. spirulina powder
1 cup (150 g) frozen strawberries or strawberries with raspberries and/or blueberries

1 cup (240 ml) vanilla or plain homemade (or
  Eden brand) soymilk
1 cup (240 ml) raw milk
2 ice cubes

Place all the ingredients in a blender and blend until smooth.

Nutrition Information per Serving: 210 mg calcium;
85 mg magnesium; 10 g protein; trace minerals

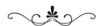

Sweet Hibiscus Tea

SERVES 4–8

Hibiscus is a large, beautiful edible flower. The blossoms are very rich in daidzein, a phytoestrogen, and in quercetin—a plant pigment called a flavonoid that among other metabolic activities boosts immunity.

The many hibiscus species are a common ingredient in food cultures from Mexico to Iran. The flower's brightly colored petals support cardiovascular and respiratory health. Because of its extremely high iron content, it is considered a tonic for the blood in traditional medicines.

Though it does not directly influence bone turnover, this tea is a terrific, safe herbal support for basic metabolic functions. When ice cold it is so light, refreshing, and delicious, it is our go-to choice for making shrub (page 130), or to enjoy on its own.

2 cups (80 g) dried hibiscus flowers
2-inch-thick (5 cm) piece of ginger, peeled,
  halved, and sliced
Cinnamon stick (optional)
8 cups (1.9 L) water
½–1 cup (170–340 g) honey
Basil leaves (optional, for garnish)
Lemon or lime wedges (optional, for garnish)

Place the flowers into a large bowl.

In a saucepan, add the ginger and cinnamon (if you're using it) to the water and boil. Put the hibiscus flowers in a large bowl and pour the flavored water over the flowers. Let the tea steep for 20 minutes.

At this point the tea is not ready to drink. It is strong and tart. Strain the tea through a strainer or colander into a jug and mix in honey to taste. Honey gives a delightful sweet-tart experience.

Decorate with a basil leaf or a wedge of lemon or lime. Use in shrub or ice it for a beautiful summer drink.

Note: Hibiscus flowers are often sold in local farmers markets and open-air markets, or you can order online from Mountain Rose Herbs.

Nutrition Information per Serving: 50 mg vitamin C;
8.6 mg iron; antioxidants; trace minerals;
phytonutrients

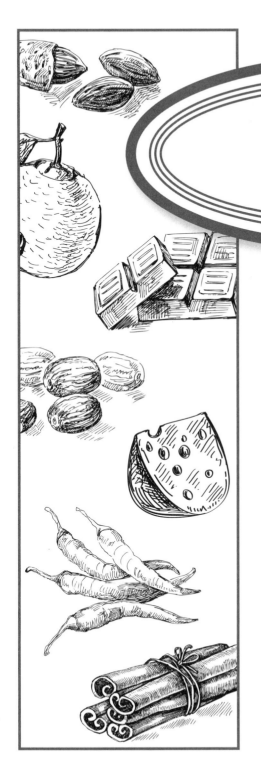

CHAPTER 21

Snacks

S nacks are compact helpings of nutrients to sustain you on the go. Lots of people like snacks, and some people keep their blood sugar up with smaller, more frequent meals. All of our snacks are bone-friendly and good for health in general.

Dried mulberries are so good for you they are used in traditional medicines, though from the super-sweet flavor you will have no thoughts of medicine. Three tablespoons provide just 90 calories, gram for gram as much iron as steak, a power plant of vitamin C, and 8 percent RDA of calcium. See the rest in *Easy On-the-Go Snacking* below.

Inevitably, we all pick up packaged snacks now and then. Our advice about packaged snacks is this: Strive for contents that are as unprocessed as possible (like nuts and dried fruit), and analyze the snack packaging along with the ingredients list. Sustainable packaging such as from plant starch is much less likely to contain endocrine disruptors like BPA and other chemicals that can be harmful to health or the environment.

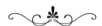

Fig Jam and Gouda

SERVES 4–8

The combination of figs and cheese is a bone bonanza. A 2-ounce serving of Gouda or Brie plus about three figs will provide about a third of the average daily calcium requirement and half the K₂. Enjoy alongside a dish of sprouted sunflower or pumpkin seeds, and you are adding a real boost to your bone health efforts.

Raw milk Brie is not ordinarily available in the United States, but it is widely available in Europe and other countries where people are free to enjoy the health benefits of raw dairy. More good news: Early testing for K₂ shows Brie as a likely candidate.

15 fresh ripe figs
2 cups (405 g) organic turbinado sugar
¾ tsp. (3g) powdered pectin
1 Tbsp. butter

Puree the figs and put into a saucepan with the sugar and the pectin. Stir over medium heat until the sugar dissolves. Simmer, stirring occasionally, for 20 to 30 minutes until the mix becomes a paste.

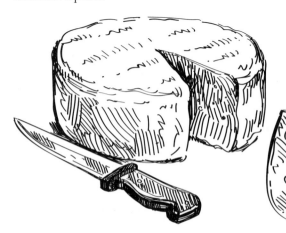

Grease the base and sides of six ramekins with butter and divide the paste evenly among them. Smooth the surface and loosely cover with parchment paper. Let sit overnight at room temperature.

Remove the jam from the ramekins, and refrigerate in a covered glass storage container.

Serve the jam treats with 3-inch (7.5 cm) cuts of brick Gouda cheese, big slices of Brie, fresh figs, or on crackers such as Parmesan and Basil Crisps (page 176).

Decorate with sprigs of fresh rosemary.

Variation: For a more savory taste, reduce the sugar to ½–1 cup (100–200 g) and add a tiny pinch of rubbed fresh rosemary.

Note: We prefer turbinado sugar because among sugars it is minimally processed.

Nutrition Information per Serving: 300 mg calcium; 20 mg magnesium; 75 mcg vitamin K₂

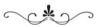

Date Night

MAKES 12–18 PIECES; SERVES 6–12

Dates, tahini, seed oil, and spices make up these satisfying, delicious, chewy raw desserts that resemble chewy caramels. Cardamom and cinnamon bring out the flavors.

Cardamom is the seed of one plant in the ginger family, which includes about 1,300 species. When people describe cardamom, you might think it's a wine when they describe it as a mix of ginger and grapefruit, with floral notes and menthol undertones. But the flavor does seem to float by with a hint of sweetness, subtle and aromatic, and the chews

❧ About Tamarind ❧

If you can find it, you may wish to use sweet tamarind in place of some dates. Tamarind has a long history in traditional medicine acting against inflammation and lowering low-density lipoprotein. In addition, of particular interest here, the pulp has a date-like consistency, is particularly rich in thiamine, and is a rare source of magnesium. Other nutrients include calcium, copper, potassium, iron, selenium, and zinc. You'll need to scrape the tamarind pulp and soak it before using it for this or other dishes.

are memorable. If you use cardamom, grind your own from seeds. They're costly, but you only need a little.

1 cup (145 g) Medjool dates, pitted
½ cup (120 g) tahini (page 234)
Zest of 1 orange
½ tsp. ground cinnamon, cardamom, or cumin
2 Tbsp. coconut oil
⅛ tsp. sea salt

Place all the ingredients except the salt in a food processor. Process until the ingredients form a paste. Line a pan with parchment paper.

Roll the paste into balls, and as you go, roll each ball in lightly ground sea salt. Place the balls on the parchment paper. Place the tray of balls in the freezer for an hour. Store in the freezer for up to a month.

Nutrition Information per Serving: 40 mg magnesium; phytonutrients

❧ Easy ❧ On-the-Go Snacking

Lots of people like snacks, and some people keep blood sugar up with smaller, more frequent meals. All of these snacks are bone-friendly and good for health in general.

Especially if you have bone health issues, use sprouted nuts and seeds. You can sprout your own (see "Sprouting Beans," page 48, for more information), or buy already sprouted. Many Whole Foods Markets sell sprouted almonds and pumpkin seeds. Blue Mountain Organics (bluemountainorganics.com) has a wider selection.

Here are some of our favorite snacks for eating when we're on the run:

- Dried mulberries.
- Prunes.
- Dried unsulfured apricot halves.
- Dried Mission or Turkish figs.
- Dried goji berries: A medicinal staple, these are chewy, satisfying and nutritious, but not sweet.
- Bone health trail mix: dried mulberries, chopped dried Mission figs, dried sour cherries, sprouted almonds, pecans, macadamia nuts, Brazil nuts, dark chocolate bits.
- Dark chocolate: 85 percent cocoa solids in moderation (really).
- Crudités with tahini (page 234).

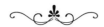

Phyto Granola Energy Bar

SERVES 10

Most granola and energy bars are sold as health foods, but read the labels: Most contain highly processed unsprouted grains, and many are loaded with refined sugar. So most do not promote health and some may impair it.

Here is a snack bar you can count on as a health food. It is full of protein, magnesium, phosphorus, and phytoestrogens. It has been found that estrogen—or phytoestrogens in high enough amounts in the diet—delays the progression of Alzheimer's as well as bone loss.[1]

1 cup (110 g) sprouted cereal

½ cup (75 g) crushed sprouted almonds

¼ cup (35 g) sprouted sunflower seeds

1 Tbsp. sprouted flaxseeds

1 Tbsp. sprouted sesame seeds

1 Tbsp. hemp seeds

⅓ cup (55 g) dried sour cherries

½ cup (65 g) dried apricots

½ cup (165 g) brown rice syrup

½ tsp. vanilla extract

1 tsp. cinnamon

⅛ tsp. salt

¼ cup (65 g) sprouted nut butter

1 cup (155 g) soaked rolled oats

½ cup (75 g) chopped sprouted nuts of your choice (optional)

Heat the oven to 225°F (107°C).

Line an 11 × 7 × 1½-inch baking pan with parchment paper. Coat the paper lightly with ghee.

Mix the dry ingredients in a bowl: cereal, almonds, seeds, and dried fruit. Set aside.

In a small pot, heat the brown rice syrup to liquid, and add the vanilla, salt and spices, and nut butter. Mix and heat until the mixture is liquid enough to pour. Put the soaked oats in a large bowl and pour the hot brown rice syrup over. Mix until the syrup is incorporated into the oats. Add the dry ingredients (including the optional chopped sprouted nuts) to the oats and mix the whole thing well. Transfer the mixture to the baking pan and press with lightly oiled hands or a spatula to flatten.

Bake for an hour, or until the oats are dried. Cut into squares. Store in an airtight jar.

Note: We use Ezekiel brand sprouted cereal. You can use this same ingredients list to make a tasty granola. Just bake the mixture without forming it into bars.

Nutrition Information per Serving: 50 mg calcium; 80 mg magnesium; 4 g protein; phytoestrogens; phytonutrients

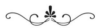

Roasted Sprouted Tamari Almonds

SERVES 12–24

Almonds are a great addition to a bone health diet as long as they are sprouted and you don't eat them by the pound—the very high omega-6 fatty acid level in almonds is the only limiting factor to this otherwise super-bone-healthy food.

3 cups (435 g) raw sprouted almonds

¼ cup (60 ml) tamari

½ tsp. sugar

Preheat the oven to 300°F (149°C).

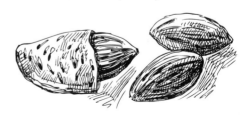

❧ About Hemp Seeds ☙

Hemp hearts are so rich in beneficial nutrients, they are tagged by some as a whole food. So why has the public been reluctant to embrace hemp in a balanced diet?

There are several species of cannabis, and one has buds dense with tetrahydrocannabinol (THC), which has intense psychoactive properties. But a different species can be used to produce hemp seeds (for consumption), fiber, and oil. There are trace amounts of THC in hemp seed shells, virtually none in the shelled seed, and overall hemp seeds do not have psychoactive properties. This is widely confirmed in employment drug tests.

That put to rest, let's go on to celebrate hemp seeds.

Hemp seed is a rich source of magnesium and phosphorus as well as iron, zinc, beta-carotene, potassium, riboflavin, niacin, and thiamin among other nutrients required for good health.

Hemp seeds contain all amino acids required to make protein, which is remarkable in a plant. Two tablespoons of hemp hearts supply about the same amount of protein as two egg whites or 2 ounces of cooked meat. And while hemp seeds contain phytates that inhibit mineral absorption, hemp protein does not contain phytates, so using hemp hearts in place of factory meat is a very sound choice.

Oh, did we mention that they're delicious? Roasted seasoned hemp seeds are marvelous snacks though they're hard to come by, and hemp hearts, which you can find in most good food stores, go well with everything from salads to smoothies and can make hummus one of the most nutritious party dips around.

Spread the almonds in one layer on a baking sheet and bake for 15 minutes.

Mix the tamari and sugar in a large bowl until sugar dissolves. Add the hot almonds to the bowl and stir to coat. Let the mixture sit in the bowl for 10 minutes.

Put the wet almonds back on the cookie sheet and bake for 12 minutes more. Flip the almonds and bake another 12 minutes, until they are dark brown. Remove from the oven; allow to cool completely.

Nutrition Information per Serving: 75 mg calcium; 6 mg protein

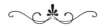

Spiced Pepitas
Or, How to Roast Pumpkin (and Squash) Seeds

We Westerners tend to discard pumpkin and squash skins and seeds, even though they are among the most nutritious parts of the vegetable. Next time you make a squash dish (such as Butternut Squash and Natto Powder Soup, page 145) or a pumpkin pie or carve a pumpkin for Halloween, save the seeds for this super easy bone-friendly snack. You can use the seeds of any edible squash. Caution:

This is a very spicy recipe. If you prefer snacks with less heat, reduce the quantities of cayenne pepper and chili powder. You can also dilute the spiciness by sprinkling the seeds as a garnish on a salad rather than eating them straight out of hand.

Tip: After opening a pumpkin, reach in and pull the seeds out. Typically they slip off the pulp and that way save you a lot of seed cleaning.

2 cups (260 g) seeds from a pumpkin or a squash

1 Tbsp. olive oil

1 tsp. black pepper

1 tsp. cayenne pepper

1 tsp. ground cumin

1 tsp. ground Ancho or Chimayo chilies
  or chili powder

2 tsp. lime juice

1 tsp. salt

OPTION FOR SPICY SWEET PEPITAS

⅓ cup sugar

1 large egg white, beaten until frothy

1 tsp. ground cinnamon

Soak 2 cups of fresh seeds in salt water for 8 hours. Hull the seeds; that is, remove the outer skin.

Preheat the oven to 350 F.

Drain and dry hulled seeds in paper towel.

Put the seeds into a bowl. Mix with the rest of the ingredients.

Spread on cookie sheet in one layer. Bake for 20 minutes.

Devour.

Option for Spicy Sweet Pepitas: Omit the lime juice and add these to the mix before baking.

Unhulled Seeds: Depending on the size/age of your squash or pumpkin you can use unhulled seeds. The result is crunchier and the fibrous shell is good for intestines.

Nutrition Information per Serving: Magnesium 300 mg; phytonutrients; trace minerals; iron

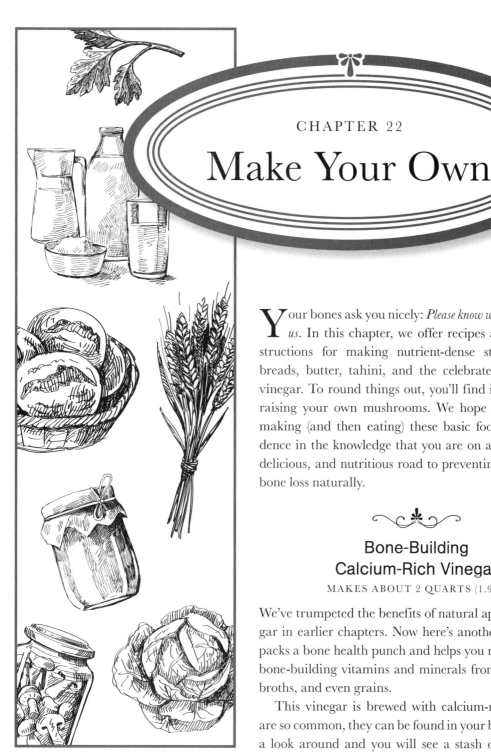

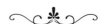

CHAPTER 22
Make Your Own

Your bones ask you nicely: *Please know what you're feeding us.* In this chapter, we offer recipes and how-to instructions for making nutrient-dense staples such as breads, butter, tahini, and the celebrated bone health vinegar. To round things out, you'll find instructions for raising your own mushrooms. We hope you will enjoy making (and then eating) these basic foods with confidence in the knowledge that you are on a safe, effective, delicious, and nutritious road to preventing and treating bone loss naturally.

Bone-Building Calcium-Rich Vinegar
MAKES ABOUT 2 QUARTS (1.9 L)

We've trumpeted the benefits of natural apple cider vinegar in earlier chapters. Now here's another vinegar that packs a bone health punch and helps you reap even more bone-building vitamins and minerals from greens, bone broths, and even grains.

This vinegar is brewed with calcium-rich herbs that are so common, they can be found in your backyard. Take a look around and you will see a stash of calcium-rich herbs—suddenly you will see these weeds in a new light!

Just one tablespoon of Bone-Building Vinegar equals 350 to 400 mg of calcium (1,000 to 1,200 mg is recommended for menopausal and post-menopausal women). To get that much calcium from food, you'd need to eat: 1 tablespoon of blackstrap molasses; 1 cup (144 g) of cooked turnip greens, kale, broccoli, bok choy, or mustard greens; 2 cups (180 g) of cooked collard greens; 2 tablespoons of almond butter or tahini. This vinegar is one of bone health's closest friends.

Organic apple cider vinegar is the base for infusing the bone-building herbs. Use ingredients that are available near you and in season. You can find fresh herbs at your local farmers market, or you can order from the suppliers listed in the resources section. We do not recommend foraging for yourself unless you have certified professional training in and knowledge of herbology.

INGREDIENTS

You will need a selection of any five of these bone-building herbs:

Dandelion leaves	Alfalfa
Stinging nettle	Parsley
Horsetail	Comfrey
Red clover	Raspberry leaves
Hound's-tongue	Blackberry leaves
Motherwort	Thimbleberry leaves
Mugwort	Sage
Mint	Amaranth leaves
Wild arugula	Lamb's-quarter
Chickweed	Kale
Shepherd's purse	Cabbage
Oatstraw	

If you want to boost the bone-building properties, add 0.35 ounce (10 g) of each of a few specific Chinese herbs: Gu Sui Bu and Xu Duan work together to build healthy bone. Bu Gu Zhi and Du Zhong also assist in bone building and repair. These herbs are available without a prescription from Chinese herbal pharmacies or from some of the suppliers listed in the resources section. All can be safely added to your bone-building brew.

MAKING THE VINEGAR

Fill a jar with fresh well-snipped herbs—you'll need a lot. Pour in apple cider to cover the herbs. Seal and label the jar with the date. Put the jar in a dark cupboard well away from any exposure to direct sunlight. Wait 6 weeks.

Aim for at least a tablespoon per day. Put on salads or in stir-fries; season beans or grains. A good preventive home remedy is drinking a teaspoon of bone-building vinegar in any amount of filtered water in the morning. Not only does it provide a substantial calcium supplement in fully natural form, but grandmothers past have said it relieves conditions from minor arthritic pain to acid reflux.

LAURA'S PREFERRED INGREDIENTS LIST

Dandelion (*Taraxacum officinale*). Dandelion leaves (dandelion greens) are a good source of silicon, magnesium, calcium, and boron. Not only does dandelion contain calcium, but it also increases calcium absorption. Additionally, it promotes digestive health by stimulating bile production, resulting in a gentle laxative effect. Inulin, a naturally occurring soluble fiber in dandelion, further aids digestion by feeding the healthy probiotic bacteria in the intestines, and it has a beneficial effect on blood sugar levels.

Horsetail (*Equisetum arvense*). Bone growth involves the process of adding calcium for hardness, plus increasing collagen. Silicon is essential for both of these processes. An important study conducted at the School of Public Health at the University of California–Los Angeles (UCLA) shows that silicon-supplemented bones have a 100 percent increase in collagen when compared with low-silicon bones. Silicon works by chemically binding the structures of surface tissues and those that connect the bones. Silicon not only promotes growth, bone formation, and tooth formation, but also has inhibitory effects on coronary heart disease and arteriosclerosis. Horsetail's predominant constituent, silicon, is responsible for the majority of the plant's healing properties. Organic silicon should be distinguished from nonorganic silicone. Organic silicon (as found in horsetail) will recalcify; inorganic silicone will not. In many cases horsetail has also been found to ease the pain of rheumatism and to stimulate the healing of torn ligaments.

Red clover (*Trifolium pratense*) contains high amounts of isoflavone compounds, such as genistein, which are phytoestrogens (see page 75). Research on both red clover and soy isoflavones is currently looking at their action as potential alternatives to estrogen in menopausal women. A double-blind study found that menopausal women had improved function of their arteries while taking red clover extract compared with placebo. This could mean menopausal women would have less trouble with high blood pressure and/or atherosclerosis. This herb is also considered a valuable tonic to assist the body in recovering from various diseases including cancer of the bowels, breast cysts, liver congestion, tuberculosis, and herpes simplex, as well as for rebuilding energy levels after long and lingering illnesses. Red clover works well with other herbs, often boosting their healing powers.

Hound's-tongue (*Cynoglossum officinalis*). Hound's-tongue's constituent allantoin speeds the healing of connective tissue and bone. The leaves also contain many minerals helpful in the building and strengthening of bone.

Mugwort (*Artemisia vulgaris*) is used in most traditional medicines, as it grows well all over the world. It has also been used as a culinary herb since the Iron Age, when it was used to flavor drinks—before hops, mugwort was used to flavor beer. It has many medicinal qualities, including maintaining general health and strong bones. It is also used to assist with dreaming.

Stinging nettle (*Urtica* spp.) is a very good source of digestible iron and the rare vitamin K_2, which makes it a valuable herb in not only bone building but also treating anemia as well as fatigue and many other health issues. It invigorates as well as heals.

Gu Sui Bu (*Drynaria fortunei*) is used in Traditional Chinese Medicine specifically for its ability to assist the bone absorption of calcium. It is used for mending bone as well as preventing and treating osteoporosis by increasing bone mass density.

Xu Duan (*Dipsacus asper*) is a complement to Gu Sui Bu in Traditional Chinese Medicine. Plants work together to propagate effect. It has similar properties as above. Roughly translated from the Chinese, its name means "restore what is broken."

Bu Gu Zhi (*Psoralea corylifolia*) means "tonify bone fat" and is used as a catalyst for bone deposition in Traditional Chinese Medicine.

Du Zhong (*Eucommia ulmoides*) also complements Gu Sui Bu and Xu Duan in bone formation; consider it an assistant.

Yin Yang Huo (*Epimedium*) is shown to stimulate bone growth through safe plant hormones.

Laura's Advice:
❧ Foraging ❧

In my garden I can find dandelion, red clover, stinging nettle, all growing wild. If I look a little farther afield there is celeriac, sage, mugwort, and shepherd's purse. I planted some mint and now it grows wild as it pleases.

Going out to find these plants, harvesting them, and using them to promote good health are a deeply satisfying, entirely sustainable acts of care for me and the planet. So I don't get stuck in traffic; I don't spend hard-earned money. There is no packaging and no waste. I just go out into the sun, absorb vitamin D, pick flowers, and later unlock the minerals. Then I have a natural source of calcium, vitamins, and minerals and the joy of creating something myself—something that has the power to help my patients live a healthier, longer life and develop stronger bones. And the plant? It will simply regrow what I pick, happy to contribute.

Helen does not yet know how to recognize the various plants she might otherwise collect herself to make bone health vinegar, so she, perhaps like you, will source her herbs elsewhere. I have encouraged her, and I encourage you, to search out and work with a local gardener or herbalist. See the resources section for a list of herbal suppliers we trust.

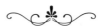

Tahini
MAKES ABOUT 1 CUP (240 ML)

Tahini is famously a base for hummus, the dip typically made of chickpeas and tahini and seasoned with lemon and cumin, though roasted eggplant-and-tahini dip also makes a marvelous change.

Tahini is a welcome source of calcium as well as zinc and selenium, and is the starting point for mainstay dishes around the world. If you're skeptical about tahini's versatility, taste Maria Elia's Tahini Chocolate Cakes (page 216).

Tahini is ground toasted sesame seed thinned with a bit of olive oil. Buy the seeds in bulk and sprout by the batch for individual recipes.

1 cup (145 g) white sesame seed, preferably
　soaked and sprouted
2–4 Tbsp. olive oil

Toast the sesame seeds over low heat in an iron pan until they are golden. Don't rush it by raising the heat; if you do, some will go dark and taste bitter.

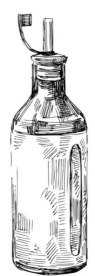

Put the slightly golden toasted seeds into a small food processor. If you whiz the seeds in a big processor, it's a job to scrape it all off the sides, and inevitably you leave more than you'd like. Many immersion/stick blenders come with a small food processor fit perfectly for this task.

Put 1 tablespoon of olive oil in with the seed paste and mix around with a small spoon or a wooden skewer to loosen it a bit. Then add a bit more olive oil and blend again. It will be very thick rather than a creamy liquid. Tahini thins out and becomes creamy when you mix it with other ingredients. Store in an airtight container in a cold fridge for several weeks at least. The sesame oil will rise to the top. Stir up a bit before taking what you need for a recipe.

> **Nutrition Information per Serving:** 88 mg calcium; 35 mg magnesium; zinc trace; copper trace

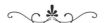

Natto, Because We Must

MAKES 1 QUART (.9 L)

Natto is the cultured soybean staple in the Japanese diet, often served at breakfast. You make it by mixing soybeans with *Bacillus subtilis* var. *natto* and allowing it to culture. Natto is the main source of vitamin K_2 worldwide. However, it is an acquired taste. Some would say a *very* acquired taste. (Helen isn't alone in describing it as slimy and foul smelling.) If you are lucky and you either like or come to like the taste of natto, then you will have a constant source of vitamin K_2 in your diet, and you will rarely need supplementation.

You can buy natto starter spores—nattomoto powder—at CulturesForHealth.com and make your own natto. New on the market is natto powder, which is dehydrated and ground natto. It is much easier to eat.

If you are bold and wish to make your own natto, here's how. The information is available at Cultures for Health online. The fermentation process requires the natto be kept at about 100°F (38°C) degrees for 22 to 24 hours. Ovens with a low temperature setting or a dehydrator oven will work. Natto has a strong odor while fermenting, so you may want to isolate it.

2 lb. (905 g) soybeans (about 4 cups)
2 tsp. water, boiled 5–10 minutes to sterilize
1 spoonful (0.1 g) nattomoto powder—use the special spoon that comes with the natto spores)

Sterilize all equipment in very hot water before using. Wash the soybeans and soak for 12 hours. Be sure to use three times as much water as soybeans for soaking. You will end up with 8 to 12 cups (1.4–2 kg) of beans.

Drain the beans from the soaking water. Fill a nonreactive (such as stainless steel or enameled) pot with water and boil the beans for 9 hours—again, using 3 times the amount of water to beans. Let them cool for an hour.

Dissolve 1 special spoonful of natto spores into 2 teaspoons of sterilized water measured with a sterilized stainless-steel spoon. Pour the natto spore solution over the beans while the beans are still warm. Stir the bean-water mixture using a spoon that has been sterilized in hot water.

Put a thin layer of beans in each of three or four ovenproof glass containers with lids. Discard any beans that spill as you work—do not pick them up and put them into a container. Place cheesecloth or butter muslin over the containers and then the tight-fitting lids.

Preheat an oven, food dehydrator, or Japanese warmer to 100°F (38°C). Put the covered containers in the oven for 22 to 24 hours, keeping the temperature steady. At the end of the fermentation period, let the natto cool for 2 hours then remove the cloth, replace the lid, and store the containers in the refrigerator overnight.

The natto can be consumed the next morning. Natto can be aged in the refrigerator for 3 days.

> **Nutrition Information per Serving:** 775 mcg vitamin K_2; approx. 450 mcg per Tbsp.

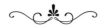

Fermented Vegetables

MAKES APPROXIMATELY 1 QUART (.9 L)

This is a basic recipe that accommodates just about any vegetable. Here we use green beans. The nutritional content per serving will vary depending on what type of vegetable you ferment.

1 lb. (455 g) fresh green beans, topped or
　topped and tailed
1 large clove garlic, thinly sliced
Pinch of red pepper flakes
1 tsp. dried dill or 3–4 sprigs fresh dill
2 cups (480 ml) filtered water
1½ Tbsp. unrefined sea salt

Sterilize a quart-sized widemouthed canning jar in a dishwasher or rinse it in boiling water, and set aside.

Blanch the beans in boiling water for 2 minutes. Drain the beans and plunge them immediately into a bowl of ice water (cold enough so ice cubes remain). Leave until the beans are no longer hot. Drain the cooled beans well in a colander or strainer and pat dry with paper towels.

Place half of the sliced garlic into the jar. Add the red pepper flakes and dill. Add the beans to your jar, stem-end down, packing them close together. Fill the jar completely with the green beans. Sprinkle the remaining garlic slices on top of the beans in the jar.

Mix together the water and salt to form a brine. Pour the brine into the jar of beans to cover. Be sure to leave a 1-inch (2.5 cm) space from the top of the jar for expansion. If the brine does not cover the beans, simply make up another batch using the same ratio of salt to water. It is important that the brine cover the vegetables to prevent mold from forming.

Cover the jar and close tightly. If you're using air lock, fill with water according to instructions.

Allow the vegetable to ferment for 3 days at room temperature, maintaining the temperature ideally between 68° and 72.5°F (20° and 24°C). Check after day 2 to make sure there is no mold and the water is not cloudy. On day 3 the vegetables should taste fermented but still be crunchy. You can extend or shorten the fermentation time depending on your taste.

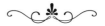

Chris's Sourdough Everyday Bread

MAKES 2 LOAVES

Chris says: "I first ate sourdough two years ago and wondered why I'd waited so long. It makes great sandwiches and terrific toast. When Helen learned that sourdough and rye were her practical choices for daily bread, I decided to make our own.

"You make the bread in two stages over 2 days. First make the sponge, the initial mix of starter, the rising agent: It's starter, flour, and water. Make it in the evening as it must rest for 12 hours. Next morning you make the dough."

This is Laura's favorite sourdough, too, and there's a great rye recipe on page 240.

This recipe calls for a stand mixer with a paddle attachment and a dough hook.

SPONGE

1 cup (230 g) cold starter (inactive)
3 cups (375 g) bread flour
3 cups (720 ml) water

DOUGH

2-plus cups (250 g) flour
1–2 tsp. finely ground sea salt
Full-cream milk, cream or 1 egg mixed with water
　to make a glazing wash

Sponge: Put the cold starter into a medium-sized bowl. Add the flour and water and whisk into a smooth, thick paste. Cover with a small kitchen towel or unbleached parchment paper and leave at room temperature for 12 hours.

Note: Whenever there is a call for stretch film, you'll want to put a light spray of olive, hemp, or avocado oil on the underside. Then you can use this same piece throughout.

Dough: Fit the paddle attachment onto the stand mixer.

Uncover the sponge. It will be active and frothing on top. (This is why I prefer to use plastic wrap rather than a towel to cover the sponge.) Using a spatula, put half the sponge into the stand mixer bowl. Turn the mixer to its slowest speed, add about 1 cup of the flour, and mix until all the flour is incorporated—2 or 3 minutes. Let it rest for an hour.

Remove the paddle attachment and fit the dough hook.

Add the rest of the flour a little at a time, and finally the salt.

Knead for about 5 minutes. The dough will be firm; it should be still moist but should not be sticky.

Spray oil to coat the inside of a large bowl. Put the dough into the bowl, scraping and blending anything left in the mixer bowl.

For the first rise, spray oil over the top of the dough to prevent it from forming a dry skin, then cover the bowl loosely. Set in a warm-room-temperature place to rise. You're looking for it to increase in volume to nearly double. If you push gently on the

top and it springs back, it's still working on the rise. If you press gently and the indentation stays, it's done. This could take a few hours, but you can check periodically. If you push gently, you won't affect the dough. While it's rising, spray a bit of oil onto a clean counter space.

When it's finished the first rise, punch down the dough. It's best if you make a fist and spray it with the oil, then punch down right through to the bottom of the risen dough. Gather the dough and put it onto the oiled counter space. Cover the dough and let it rest for 15 minutes.

While it's resting, spray a coating of oil onto the baking sheet or loaf pans you will use.

Shape your loaf. Using two well-oiled hands, run your hands around as you turn the dough to make it smooth and round for baking. Make sure any breaks in the dough are on the underside.

For the second rise, leave the loaf on the baking tray or in the loaf pan to rise again. Cover loosely. Let it rise until nearly double, again for several hours.

Toward the end of the second rise, preheat the oven to 400°F (204°C).

Use a small sharp knife to make three diagonal cuts across the top of the loaf. Glaze the top with the cream or egg wash applied with a pastry brush and set the dough into the oven.

Spray water into the oven top, bottom, and sides. Some spray will fall onto the bread. This helps to form the wonderful chewy crust.

Bake at 400°F for 10 minutes, then reduce the temperature to 375°F (191°C) and bake for an additional 30 minutes. Use the food thermometer

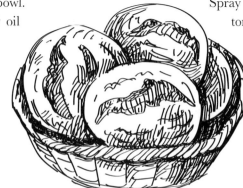

to check the internal temperature; bake until the internal temperature reaches 200° to 210°F (93°–99°C).

LOAF TWO

Wondering what happened to the other half of the sponge? While the first loaf is enjoying its first rise, you can start the process with the second half of the sponge.

Nutrition Information Per Serving: 8 g calcium; 12 g magnesium; 8 g protein; trace minerals

Artisan Whole-Grain Sourdough

MAKES 1 LOAF

Eric Rusch of Breadtopia.com created this sourdough recipe and the rye bread recipe on page 240. Eric says this whole-grain sourdough is the best (mostly) whole-grain bread he's baked and on par with some of the best whole-grain bread he's had anywhere. Eric's videos at the Breadtopia website help explain the ins and outs of making many and varied breads.

EVENING OF DAY 1

7 oz. or ⅞ cup (200 g) water
4 oz. or ½ cup (120 g) sourdough starter
8⅓ oz. or 2 cups (236 g) whole wheat flour

MORNING OF DAY 2

9⅔ oz. or about 1¼ cups (274 g) water
3 oz. or ⅞ cup (85 g) rye flour
8¾ oz. or 2 cups (250 g) white bread flour
6 oz. or a tad over 1¾ cups (170 g) spelt flour
scant Tbsp. (13 g) salt

Evening of Day 1: Mix all the ingredients together. Ferment (let sit out at room temperature covered loosely) at 69°F (21°C) for 12 hours.

Morning of Day 2: Add the day 2 ingredients to the day 1 ingredients. Knead, place in a covered bowl, and refrigerate for 24 hours.

Morning of Day 3: Form a boule (round loaf) and ferment it (let it sit out on counter) for 5 hours at 69°F. Bake at 485°F (252°C) for 40 to 45 minutes.

Notes: The recipe was created using grams for measurement. For those without a kitchen scale, Eric has translated to ounces and cups.

Eric says that you needn't be overly concerned about the 69°F proofing temperature. If you come close, great, but go with whatever your house temperature is at the time. If it's summer and your house is very warm, find the coolest spot you can. Temperature does impact results, but unless you are running a bakery, you may enjoy the varying outcomes.

The original recipe calls for 20 grams/0.7 ounce of salt. We'd like to see no more than 13 grams—just under ½ ounce—which Eric says works just fine. Feel free to experiment.

Regarding baking time and temperature, all ovens vary somewhat, and you might have to make some adjustments here. After the first couple of times with this recipe, Laura found that the bread baked just right with her La Cloche (a clay baking dome) at 485°F for the first 30 minutes, then 10 more minutes at 450°F (232°C) with the lid off.

If you treasure big holes in the crumb, experiment with increasing the hydration. You'll get a flatter loaf with a more open crumb.

Nutrition Information per Serving: 10 g calcium; 15 g magnesium; 12 g protein; trace minerals

❧ About Flour ❧

Nicky Giusto is a fifth-generation miller and baker at Central Milling, a 148-year-old family-owned flour supplier based in Logan, Utah.

"Central Milling flours were organic, local, and sustainable before those words were ever used in relation to food," Nicky says. "And nothing has changed, even as demand for our flours grew and they scaled up. Know the farmers and the farming practices of the local farmers and work with them to produce high-quality, nutritious grains. Know and work with the bakers who buy the flour, so we can create the flavors and balances artisanal bakers require. The only change for us has been one of scale—that is, knowing and working with farmers and bakers in many states."

Central Milling does not purchase grains that have been stored in grain elevators, Nicky says, because elevators commingle grains and you can't know exactly what's in there. "It is paramount for us to know that the grains we provide are of the highest, purest quality and free of starkly dangerous pesticides like Roundup."

Central Milling produces a large variety of flours including white; however, since white flour is less nutritious, they retooled their white-flour mills to mill the naked grain and then return some germ and bran.

The company also makes flour using sprouted grain. "Non-whole-grain flours remove the bran and germ through the refining process; whole grains retain all three parts of the kernel," Nicky explains. "Under properly controlled variables—including time, tempera-ture, and moisture—whole grains can be 'sprouted' from the kernel, producing a state between seed and new plant. When the kernel's sprout growth pushes through its bran layer, the process triggers enzymatic activity that breaks down the grain's starch into simpler, easier-to-digest molecules and releases nutrients for better absorption. At this point, sprouted grain is often dried and ground into flour for use in baking. But we take the newly sprouted grain and mill it into a living mash, preserving the enzymatic activity that began during sprouting. Then we bake breads from the sprouted grains.

"Longer fermentation is more important with flour containing less bran and germ. In other words, the whiter the flour, the longer you should ferment it. But all flour benefits from long fermentation," Nicky continues. "The key to bread that is good for bone health—and also easy on digestion—is a long fermentation process that breaks down gluten, increases nutrients, and weakens phytic acid." For sourdough, Nicky recommends their flour types 110, 85, and 70.

Central Milling offers a course titled Baking with the Ancients. Participants learn how to use whole grains properly to make a satisfying loaf, and explore the ideas dear to our bone health hearts—souring of grains, fermenting with starters, and sprouting.

Nicky's advice to home bakers? "Be patient, and don't rush bread. Good bread takes time. It's an experience, not a chore. Relish every step. It's a live being that transforms and grows and makes you happy when you pull it out of the oven."

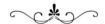

Artisan Sourdough Rye Bread

MAKES 1 LOAF

"This is my favorite rye bread recipe of all time," Eric Rusch says. (Of course, he says that about all his creations.) This one includes both sourdough and instant yeast versions.

70 grams (⅓ cup) Sourdough Starter
   (omit if making the instant yeast version)
1 tsp. instant yeast (omit if making sourdough
   leavened version)
400 grams (1¾ cups) water
44 grams (2 Tbsp.) molasses
8 grams (1 Tbsp.) fennel seed
2 grams (1 tsp.) anise seed
3 grams, (1 tsp.) caraway seed
Zest of 1 orange
245 grams (1¾ cups) rye flour
245 grams (1¾ cups) bread flour
12 grams (1¾ tsp.) salt

Sourdough Version: In a mixing bowl, mix the starter into the water. Add the molasses, all the seeds, and the orange zest.

In a separate bowl, combine the flours and salt.

Gradually stir the dry ingredients into the wet using a dough whisk or spoon until the flour is well incorporated. Cover with plastic and let rest for 15 minutes. After about 15 minutes, mix again for a minute or two. Again let rest for 15 minutes and mix one more time as before. Now cover the bowl with plastic wrap and let sit at room temperature for roughly 12 to 14 hours.

Instant Yeast Version: Don't use sourdough starter. Instead mix the instant yeast into the dry ingredients before combining with the wet ingredients.

For Both Versions: After the long 12-to-14-hour proof, stretch and fold the dough and shape into boule or batard (round or oblong) shape for baking.

Nutrition Information per Serving: 8 g calcium; 12 g magnesium; 8 g protein; phytoestrogen; trace minerals

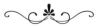

Traditional Chickpea Flatbread

SERVES 4

Gluten-free, vegan-delicious Italian flatbread: It goes with everything, and it's good for bones. Top with white bean hummus or Gouda cheese. Dip in soup or enjoy the naked flavor with just a drizzle of good olive oil. Chickpea flour is sprouted garbanzo flour; it's also called gram flour. We use a standard half-sheet cookie sheet (18 × 13) when making this recipe.

3½ cups (840 ml) cold water
2½ cups (230 g) sprouted chickpea flour
1 tsp. salt
½ tsp. black pepper
¼ cup (60 ml) extra-virgin olive oil

OPTIONAL INGREDIENTS

2 Tbsp. chopped fresh herbs—oregano,
   rosemary, thyme, marjoram
2 cloves minced garlic
½–1 tsp. spices: za'atar (page 156), chili, or
   ground cumin

Preheat the oven to 350°F (177°C).

Put the water into a large mixing bowl. Add the flour in three batches of roughly equal size, incorporating the flour thoroughly into the water after adding each batch. Whisk until smooth. Add the seasonings.

Let the mixture stand on the counter for 3 hours.

Pour the olive oil onto the cookie sheet. If there is foam on top of the chickpea mixture, skim it off and discard. Pour the mixture onto cookie sheet. The layer should be about ¼ inch (.6 cm) deep. Bake for 30 minutes, until golden. Let set for 15 minutes after removing from the oven.

Note: Blue Mountain Organics carries good sprouted bean and grain flours that make your job much easier. You can find them in the resources section.

> **Nutrition Information per Serving:** 70 mg calcium; 70 mg magnesium; 12 g protein; trace minerals; 1.7 mg zinc; B vitamins; 172 mcg folate

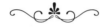

Ezekiel Bread

SERVES 8–12

This bread starts with sprouted beans and sprouted fermented grains that are dried and ground into flour—or you can use organic commercial sprouted bean and grain flours with good results. See chapter 3 for information on sprouting beans and grains. You can substitute sprouted garbanzo bean flour and sprouted black bean flour for any of the beans.

Our Ezekiel Bread is a complete protein, so if you are vegan or vegetarian this is an ideal addition to your diet. It is a batter bread, so it will become less elastic during kneading from traditional wheat-based bread dough, and it requires only one rise.

2½ cups (315 g) hard red wheat or milled
    sprouted flour
1½ cups (190 g) spelt, rye, or milled sprouted flour

½ cup (65 g) barley or milled sprouted flour
¼ cup (30 g) millet or milled sprouted flour
¼ cup (50 g) lentils (green are best) or milled
    sprouted flour
2 Tbsp. great northern beans or milled
    sprouted flour
2 Tbsp. red kidney beans or milled sprouted flour
2 Tbsp. pinto beans or milled sprouted flour
4 cups (960 ml) lukewarm water
1 cup (340 g) honey
½ cup (120 ml) ghee, plus more for
    greasing the pans
2 tsp. salt
2 Tbsp. yeast

If you are starting with whole grains and beans, your first step is sprout them as described in "Sprouting Beans" on page 48. When they're sprouted and dry, mix them all in a big bowl and grind them into flour.

If you are using already milled flours, simply mix all the flours together in a large bowl.

In a separate large bowl, mix the lukewarm water, honey, and ½ cup (120 ml) ghee. Then add the grain-legume flour, salt, and yeast.

Knead for 10 minutes. As this is batter bread, it will not form the kind of smooth elastic ball that wheat-based bread dough does. Instead, it is decidedly sticky. Be prepared with some extra flour for your hands and knead this dough right in the bowl.

Pour the dough into ghee-greased 10 × 5 × 3-inch or equivalent pans. Turn to coat with ghee. Let rise in a warm place for 1 hour covered with a damp cloth.

Bake at 350°F (177°C) for 45 to 50 minutes.

> **Nutrition Information per Serving:** 20 mg calcium; 30 mg magnesium; 4 g protein; phytoestrogen; all trace minerals

Natural Milk Butter

Helen's husband, Chris, makes their household butter using the cream that rises in natural milk. "The milkman arriving each day is a great childhood memory," Chris says. "There was a big urn with a metal cup at the end of a long handle. The milk came to us straight from the cow and it was truly delicious.

When milk is churned to make butter, the membranes surrounding the milk fat globules rupture, and clumps of milk fat gather together. The air from the churning traps liquid, and this runs off the fat. The naturally occurring lactic acid bacteria gently ferment this in the process. This is traditional buttermilk.

Some people prefer the taste of cultured butter and cultured buttermilk. Both are tangier than the uncultured varieties. To culture buttermilk, you add lactobacillus bacteria. Here's how.

Ingredients

You will need 3 cups (720 ml) of cream. If you are fortunate enough to live near a farm approved to sell natural milk, buy the milk in glass bottles rather than plastic. It is easy to see the cream level, so when you are taking it off you pull the least possible amount of milk with it. You may need four bottles of milk in order to skim off a full 3 cups (720 ml) of cream. Of course, if you are fortunate enough to live where the farmer is permitted to sell raw cream, your cup runneth over.

Readying the Cream

Stand fresh-bought milk in the fridge at 34° to 35°F (1°–2°C) for at least twenty-four hours. This allows virtually all the cream to rise. Using a baster, siphon the cream off to within ½ inch (1.25 cm) of the milk. Put the cream into a tall jar.

Leave the cream to settle in the fridge for 24 hours and siphon again, leaving as much milk as possible in the bottom of the jar. The leftover milk will contain 1 percent or less butterfat; use as you use any milk.

Pulsing the Cream

The average time from cream to butter/buttermilk is about 4 minutes of pulsing in a blender. Pour the 3 cups of cream into the blender jug. Pulse on the CHOP setting for 30 to 45 seconds. Using a spatula, push down the air pockets that form around the blades.

Continue to pulse in 30-second bursts. As the cream whips, poke it down from the sides. Early butter sticks to the sides; the buttermilk will wash it down, or you can poke it down with the spatula.

Now it is time to check in with your butter. After a slow start, the cream moves quickly to become butter, much as egg white suddenly becomes meringue or cream thickens into whipped cream. The change in the sound of the blender motor will let you know when the cream is fast becoming butter. Continue on short pulses—10 seconds or so—for about a minute. This helps the butter to bind.

Put a strainer or cheesecloth over the top of a large jar (or use a deep bowl). Using a spatula to restrain the butter, gently pour buttermilk from the blender jug into the jar (or bowl).

Tip the butter into a second bowl. Harvest as much butter as you can from the blades and jug.

Washing the Butter

Butter keeps well if you wash it. To wash butter, cover it with fresh, clear, cold water. Mash the butter against the sides of the bowl with the back of a spoon. Rotate the bowl and process the butter evenly all around. Probably the water will become a bit cloudy. Keep changing the water and pressing on the butter until the water remains perfectly clear even when you press.

Pour off all the water. Keep pressing on the butter and draining until no more water runs off.

"The more fastidious you are about washing the butter, the better the taste," Chris says. "And the taste truly is sensational. Sometimes I add a bit of sea salt, chives, very finely chopped garlic—whatever herbs we have fresh in the garden. If you want feel like a king, put some of your own butter on your own homemade sourdough bread."

Ghee

Ghee is the Indian name for clarified butter. Butter contains milk solids and oil. *Clarifying* refers to separating the milk solids from the butter oil.

The structure of this cooking oil is such that it passes easily through the lipid membranes of cells, and therefore vitamins and minerals from food cooked in ghee are well transported into the cells. This food comprises short-, medium-, and long-chain fatty acids, both unsaturated and saturated (see page 82 for more on fatty acids). Ghee contains omega-3 essential fatty acids along with the fat-soluble vitamins A, D, E, and K_2. Ghee made from organic butter of pastured cows is one of the best natural sources of CLA (conjugated linoleic acid). CLA is produced in large amounts by grass-fed animals (as opposed to grain-fed/factory-farmed animals). CLA improves the action of insulin; it also protects against cardiovascular disease, high blood pressure, high cholesterol and triglycerides, and osteoporosis.

Ghee has been used for centuries to help with digestion and elimination, for energy, sexual vitality, healthy skin, hair, and joints.

Only make ghee from pasture-raised butter. Ghee's superior ability to transport nutrients makes it even more important that you ensure the purity of the butter.

The smoke point of ghee is nearly 500°F (260°C), so it is ideal for high-heat cooking.

How to Make Ghee

Melt 1 pound (450 g) unsalted butter in a medium-sized heavy saucepan on medium heat until it just starts to boil. Turn down the heat to low and continue to cook at this heat. Do not cover. The butter will foam and sputter. Curds will begin to form on the bottom of the pot and the butter will turn a warm golden color. The butter can suddenly burn, so keep your eye on the heat and lower as needed. The oil will separate and move away some of the foam; the ghee should be clear to the bottom. When it is clear and has stopped sputtering, take it off the heat. Let it cool a bit and pour it through a fine sieve or layers of cheesecloth into a clean, dry glass container with a tight lid. The liquid will be a warm golden color. Discard the curds. If the oil is dark brown, the ghee has burned and is no good.

A pound of butter requires about 15 minutes of cooking time.

Ghee can be kept on the kitchen shelf, covered. It does not need refrigeration. The medicinal properties improve with age as beneficial bacteria populate.

Two pounds (900 g) of butter will fill a quart jar with ghee.

Calcium Supplements from Eggshells

The richest source of calcium from food is a pastured egg's shell. To make a calcium supplement from eggshells, you will need a collection of 12 boiled shells.[1] To harvest a whole shell, boil an egg for 5 minutes, run it under cold water, peel, and enjoy; or you can boil (for 5 minutes) shells from eggs you have used for other purposes. Allow the shells to air-dry. Keep your collection of clean, dry eggshells in a covered jar until you have 12.

This supplement will be most productive if you take it with complex carbohydrates, and have sufficient vitamin D and vitamin K_2 in your diet. Vitamin D lasts a long time in the body, as does vitamin K_2 in the form of MK7, so they don't need to be taken at the same time as the calcium.

One eggshell contains about 800 mg of calcium, depending on size, so it's enough supplement for about two days, if you are eating about half your daily intake in calcium. Most of us will take in enough calcium through food alone.

Eggshell calcium is very absorbable and contains traces of many additional elements: silicon, boron, magnesium, copper, iron, strontium, and zinc, among others that are necessary for bone health. Use eggshells from naturally pasture-raised chickens, hens, ducks, or geese, as the natural diet of the animal will provide the right natural balance of minerals in the shells.

How to Make the Supplement

As you collect shells, wash them gently. You want to thoroughly rinse out the white and leave the membrane intact. Leave on a paper towel to air-dry. You can save dry eggshells in the jar until you have 12 of them collected.

Baking the shells makes them break down more easily in the vinegar. Spread all 12 shells on a baking sheet. Bake at 250°F (121°C) degrees for 10 minutes, which also fully dehydrates them and will kill any lurking pathogens.

Break up the eggshells and put them in a sealable jar with 2 cups (480 ml) of raw apple cider vinegar. Let sit for about 3 days, or until the eggshells are dissolved. The mixture will bubble. During this time the vinegar degrades the shell and releases the calcium.

Shake gently. Take about 4 teaspoons a day. This will give you about 400 mg of calcium.

Use on grains or greens to release minerals—on fresh salad greens or lightly boiled leafy green vegetables, and if you soak oats overnight to reduce phytic acid for examples—or in any hot or cold dish that calls for vinegar. You can mix it with honey and water or mix honey into the jar.

Of course you can take it straight, but we favor combining the calcium with food. That will make the calcium much more absorbable and provide the additional nutrients it needs for absorption and transport to bones.

Alternative Method

Grind baked eggshells in a coffee or seed grinder until powdered. Put into a jar with a good seal (to keep out moisture).

When you are ready to take, mix ⅓ teaspoon of the powder with 1 teaspoon of lemon juice or vinegar, let it sit for 2 hours, and then mix with a few teaspoons of water and swallow the supplement. Take this two to three times a day, depending on your supplement needs.

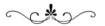

Apple Cider Vinegar

MAKES ABOUT 1½ QUARTS (1.4 L)

Apple cider vinegar is a mainstay of bone health life. It brings out the minerals in plant-based food, which aids mineral absorption. We cannot overestimate the contribution of apple cider vinegar to Helen's success, or the enthusiasm with which she is adding shrub to her routine.

Here's the recipe for a small batch of apple cider vinegar. You may like to experiment with combinations of sweet and tart apples. If the apples are conventionally grown, remove pesticide residues by dipping the apples in a wash of diluted natural apple cider vinegar and rinsing. It only takes a moment and can remove pesticides that stick even after a water wash. Or you may wish to peel and discard the skin.

Do not substitute non-nutritive or artificial sweeteners. Sugar starts the conversion of the apple water to alcohol. And that's in addition to the others reasons we avoid them.

3 apples, everything but the stem

1 Tbsp. unrefined muscovado sugar

Filtered water to cover the chunked apples (a reverse-osmosis filter is best; use a carbon filter if you have nothing else)

Chunk the apples. Discard the stems. Place in a wide-neck sterilized 2-quart jar.

Mix the sugar or sweetener of your choice with 1 cup of filtered water. Pour the sugar water into the jar. Pour in enough additional water to cover the apples. Cover the jar with cheesecloth or paper towels. Seal the jar cover with a rubber band.

Leave where no one will knock it over for 1 to 2 weeks. You'll see bubbling begin. This is the start of the water and apples making cider.

Remove the cheesecloth or paper cover and discard. Strain the water. Press on the apples in the strainer. Return the cider to the same jar. Cover the jar with cheesecloth or paper towels. Seal with the rubber band.

Leave for 3 to 6 weeks. Check on the strength by tasting after 3 weeks.

Check occasionally to see that the mother of vinegar is developing nicely. Pour into a sterilized bottle or jar with a cover. Store in the cupboard.

Note: You can make vinegar using the discards after making an apple dish. Use the peel and core from 6 to 8 apples. Also, you may use 1 cup (200 g) of sugar for a gallon jar of vinegar. More sugar hastens the conversion of water to alcohol and shortens the fermentation time.

Soymilk and Tofu

Soymilk is what remains after you soak mature raw soybeans, remove the hulls, grind the beans, and then boil them to produce a slurry bean pulp and a white liquid called soymilk. To make tofu, you coagulate the soymilk and press the curd. The coagulation agent determines the nature of the tofu—silky, medium, firm.

One of the most heavily touted soy products is soymilk. It gives manufacturers a triple-whammy lucky break: They can promote the positive perceived health benefits of soy; capitalize on the mother-and-apple-pie misconception that any and all milk strengthens teeth and bones; and offer an alternative to people who believe they are, or count among the rare individuals who actually are,

245

lactose-intolerant. As is the case with anything soy, the soymilk/tofu debate about nutritional benefit versus absorption and hormones is vigorous.

Here are some facts.

Soy is one of the most adulterated crops in the United States, with perhaps even over 90 percent of the soy grown in the United States now being genetically modified.

If you start with organic soybeans—true organics are never genetically modified and do not carry pesticide residue—and soak them for 16 hours, then remove the hulls and make your soymilk, you have a drink that delivers soy's mineral payload absent a lot of the anti-nutrients oxalic and phytic acids and lectin. Unfortunately commercial companies have been tacking around the regulations, so though it's time consuming, we like to make our own. We are happiest using a reverse-osmosis filter that takes out heavy metals and replaces lost minerals, because the standard jug water filters are apparently just a nod to water purification. But please stick to tap or filter as your water source and avoid water from plastic bottles that may have been heated and reheated in warehouses, releasing plastic hardeners like BPA or BPA substitutes.

The best commercial soymilk makers have developed patented enzyme inhibitors that combat the powerful anti-nutrients found in soy, which becomes a step in their preparation process. We don't have access to these inhibitors, so in order to make the milk as beneficial as possible we must take extra cooking steps.

Just as some agents can cause milk to coagulate, which transforms milk into curds and whey, agents can cause soybean paste to become soymilk and curd, also known as tofu.

To coagulate the milk, one agent we like is magnesium chloride, which in Japanese is *nigari*.

The finest *nigari* is a mineral-rich residue from sea salt. One example is Mitoku brand Bitterns *nigari*. If you can't find *nigari* you can use regular Epsom salt.

How to Make Soymilk

Soak 1½ cups (140 g) of dry soybeans in water for a minimum of 8 and a maximum of 16 hours. Drain and rinse the beans and remove the husks.

Bring 7½ cups (1.8 L) of water to a boil in a big stockpot. In a blender or food processor blend the beans with another 4 cups (960 ml) of water—you will need to do this in batches—and add the puree to the boiling water. The texture of the soybean puree (*go* in Japanese) should be yellow and creamy with flecks of bean fiber.

Heat this on high heat until it boils violently, stirring constantly so it doesn't stick. It is cooked when it froths to four times its original height.

Set up a colander with cheesecloth over another pot. Pour the milk through the cloth. The pulp—in Japanese this is *okara*—will remain in the colander. Milk the pulp, squeezing it as much as possible. Wrap up the cloth and press it with a wooden spoon. Open the cloth and break up the bean fiber. Add 2⅓ cups (510 ml) of cold water to the *okara* in the cloth and mix to a slush. Wrap up the cloth again and squeeze again. Squeeze out until the *okara* is dry and crumbly.

Bring the milk to a boil and let it boil for 7 minutes. At this point the milk is cooked enough to use: This is soymilk. If you are making tofu, this will be your base for the tofu recipe below. If you are going to use it as soymilk, then add sugar to taste and let it cool. Enjoy.

One cup of soymilk has all the potassium, iron, magnesium, and protein you need daily, along with three-quarters of the fiber, copper, and manganese, and half the calcium.

How to Make Tofu

First, you will need a tofu box. Tofu boxes in the home are usually about 14 × 9 inches, with holes in the sides and a top. You can make one yourself, or find one online. Tofu kits are available on Amazon and come with everything you need including the coagulating agent.

Mix 1½ teaspoons *nigari* in 1 cup (240 ml) cold water.

Using freshly made soymilk, while the milk is still hot, add ⅔ cup (160 ml) of the *nigari* solution to the milk, stirring constantly. The curds and whey should begin to separate.

Leave the milk to coagulate for 5 minutes with a lid.

Sprinkle the rest of the *nigari* solution over the curds and spread evenly. Cover and leave for 2 minutes more. The curds are ready for shaping into tofu when the liquid—called whey—is clear of all milky hue.

Prepare a tofu box and line it with cheesecloth or muslin cloth. Drain the whey from the curds, and pour the curds into the box. Put a lid on the box and press down for 20 minutes for softer tofu, 50 minutes for firmer.

Remove the tofu from the box and set it in cold water for 10 minutes to firm.

Grow Your Own Shiitake Mushrooms

Lin Howitt is a retired molecular biologist, but that background didn't bring her to shiitake mushrooms. "During a year off from college working on a farm," Lin told us, "my son Evan discovered a love for all things agricultural—and in particular for hops and shiitakes. We have a stream on our woodland property which is the ideal environment for growing shiitakes, so with

considerable help from his dad, Evan inoculated 60-plus logs with shiitake spawn. Now busy with an acre of hops and a microbrewery, Evan has handed the mushroom raising to his (delighted) parents. Really I never tire of seeing those buttons come out."

We asked Lin whether it's difficult to grow shiitakes; whether they're fragile. "Actually the growing platform is not at all fragile. The hard work comes with inoculating oak, beech, and/or maple branches (logs) with mushroom mycelium.

"Mycelium is the vegetative part of a fungus, consisting of a mass of branching, threadlike hyphae. Fungal colonies composed of mycelia are found in and on soil and many other substrates. A typical single spore germinates into a mycelium, which cannot reproduce sexually; two compatible mycelia join and form a mycelium capable of producing the fruiting bodies we call mushrooms.

"We do this in the fall. The logs are placed in woodland shade, preferably by a stream, and for approximately nine months the mycelial plugs infiltrate the log body. Then in late spring when the temperatures are warming, we submerge the logs in the stream for 24 hours, then return them to the shade. 'Buttons' appear and then maybe a week later, you have lovely full mushrooms, ready for pulling off the log."

Getting Prepared

Here is Lin's summary of how to grow your own shiitake mushrooms. First, she says, gather your tools and material.

Drill. There is a specially designed drill bit for mushroom growers. The tip is about ½ inch (1.25 cm) long. Or use any drill that will approximate the size hole this one makes. Into these holes you'll place the spawn and then paint over each one with hot paraffin wax.

Shiitake spawn. Spawn is the stage between spore and mycelium. You can buy spawn from companies that grow it from spores and sell it as shiitake mushroom starter plugs. They look like blocks of bumpy sawdust.

Paraffin wax. You paint over the spawn-filled holes with melted paraffin wax.

Hot plate and pot. You need to prepare the wax while you are outdoors. We use a hot plate and an old metal pot. No open flames around the extremely flammable wax.

Paintbrush. Dip a thick artist's paintbrush in the warm, melted wax and paint the wax over the spawn-filled hole.

Logs. Beech, oak, and maple make good mushroom logs. We use freshly cut branches, allowed to sit for approximately 2 weeks to deactivate the natural anti-fungal enzymes. The branches should be 6 to 10 inches (15–25 cm) in diameter, about 4 feet long, and straight. This is what we call the log.

Two additional lengths of wood. Two additional logs or even old boards would be good. You need these to stack the seeded logs during the nine-month germination period so that the logs are not resting on the ground. This keeps the many ground fungi from infecting your logs.

Sturdy wire. Stretch a length of sturdy wire between two trees. This is where the inoculated logs rest.

Preparing the Logs

To inoculate the logs, drill holes ½ inch (1.25 cm) deep about 4 inches (10 cm) apart. Make rows that are also about 4 inches (10 cm) apart all the way around the log.

Put a small chunk of mycelial plug into each hole and cover with a thin layer of paraffin wax.

You can make a stack of inoculated logs by layering sets of logs in a perpendicular fashion, up to about four sets tall. The logs need at least 60 percent shade and a water source close by. Allow to remain for nine months.

After nine months, sit the logs in a stream or other water. If the logs are not completely submerged, turn them over the next day to get the air-exposed side into the water. Then remove them the following day. If the logs are completely submerged (not likely, since they want to float and we haven't figured out any way to weight them down) then 24 hours in the water is enough.

Bring the logs up to the bank. Lean them vertically against the bank or a wire stretched between two sturdy trees. Then, depending on the weather, in somewhere around four to eight days you'll see those little button tops popping up all along the log. In another four to seven days you'll have full-sized shiitake mushrooms.

Spoiler alert: The mushrooms don't grow from the plug holes. That's why putting the mycelium into the plug holes is called inoculating the log. The mycelium break down the wood in order to grow, and the mushrooms emerge anywhere within the log that the organism has taken root.

To harvest, pull the mushrooms off the logs by taking hold at the log end of their tough stems.

After harvesting the mushrooms, return the logs to their shaded stack. You can flush them again the following year. Some logs will give you three to four years of harvest.

While we start in the fall, your own best time to start depends on the local climate.

ACKNOWLEDGMENTS

The Healthy Bones Nutrition Plan and Cookbook is a labor of love on so many fronts—mother and daughter, nature and science, and kind people who work unselfishly to make the world a better, safer place. Our warmest thanks to Fern Bradley, whose eagle eye, enduring patience, and editorial talent were invaluable. How lucky we are that Chelsea Green sent Fern our way. Great thanks to the entire team at Chelsea Green, and to Pati Stone for tirelessly helping us refine and perfect.

Great thanks to Ysanne Spevack/The Conscious Cook and Cass Nelson-Dooley for lending a professional eye, and to Dr. Dawn DeSylvia for unceasing encouragement.

We are fortunate to have met so many generous people who contributed freely the fruits of their own culinary arts to support a natural approach to bone health. Thank you.

And thanks to Dr. Sidney Baker for crossing the bridge with Laura.

Restaurants

Andrea Chiaramonte, chef, La Forcola Valencia, Spain
Juan Carlos and Paloma Santos Alvarez La Pilareta
    (Bar Pilar), Valencia, Spain

Cookbook

Alice Waters, *The Art of Simple Food*
Maria Elia, *Smashing Plates*

Company Interview

Nicky Giusto, Central Milling

Academic

Daoshing Ni, L.Ac., MBA, DOM, PhD
Founder, Yo San University, Marina del Rey, California
Founder, Tao of Wellness, Santa Monica, California
Daniel P. Reid, *The Complete Book of Chinese Health
& Healing* (Shambhala)

Advocacy for Nutrition and Health

Lisa Y. Lefferts, senior scientist, Center for Science in the
Public Interest, Washington, DC
Jo Robinson, an investigative journalist who, in books
and at her website Eat Wild, provides vital information about how to restore essential nutrients to fruits,
vegetables, meat, eggs, and dairy products

Recipes from Individuals and Companies

Andy Weir, Reynolds.com
Carlota Esteve de Miguel Cassou, CarlotaEatMeRaw.com
Chobani Yogurt, chobani.com
Clifford A. Wright, CliffordAWright.com
Eric Rusch, Breadtopia.com
Jennifer Bryman, theheartskitchen.com
Jennifer Porteus, HealthyBugs.com
Karen Diggs, KrautSource, krautsource.com
Kresha Faber, NourishingJoy.com
Lauren Rae, InspiredWellness.com
Molly Watson, About.com
PaleoLeap.com
Robert Budwig, cookbook author, illustrator,
and designer, www.robertbudwig.com

Personal Nutrition Plan
Worksheets

Use these worksheets in conjunction with the instructions in chapter 9 to customize a nutrition plan that will optimize your nutrient intake for bone health.

Nutrition Evaluation Results

Doctor's name: _____

Report date: _____

Nutrient Tested	Laboratory Range	My Result
Vitamin D$_3$		
Calcium		
Phosphorus		
Vitamin A		
Magnesium		
Vitamin K*		
Vitamin C		
Protein		
Trace Minerals:		
Zinc		
Copper		
Manganese		
Boron		
Strontium		
Silica		
Vitamin B$_1$		
Vitamin B$_2$		
Vitamin B$_3$		
Vitamin B$_6$		
Vitamin B$_{12}$		

Note: There is a separate testing protocol for gut flora. Testing for probiotics is not part of a standard nutrition evaluation. Likewise, there is currently no standard test for levels of phytoestrogens.

* At the time of this writing, there is no laboratory test for vitamin K$_2$. Current tests measure overall vitamin K status.

Notes:

_____

_____

_____

_____

_____

_____

_____

My Food Preferences

Date: _____

What I bought this week:

_____
_____
_____
_____
_____
_____
_____
_____
_____
_____
_____
_____
_____

The foods I buy that I enjoy most are:

Fresh	Prepared	Processed
_____	_____	_____
_____	_____	_____
_____	_____	_____
_____	_____	_____
_____	_____	_____
_____	_____	_____
_____	_____	_____
_____	_____	_____
_____	_____	_____
_____	_____	_____

Fresh foods include fruits and vegetables, meats and fish, and whole grains (preferable organically raised) that you will wash, prepare, and cook yourself. Prepared foods include premade salads and ready-to-eat meals, including frozen foods. Prepared foods may contain processed ingredients. Processed foods include items such as boxed breakfast cereals, potato chips, instant mashed potatoes, and deli meats.

What I Ate This Week

Week beginning: _____

Note: Circle or highlight the items you cooked.

Monday	Tuesday	Wednesday
Breakfast		
Lunch		
Dinner		
Snacks and Drinks		

What I Ate This Week

Thursday	Friday	Saturday	Sunday

One-Day RDA Calculation

Daily Meal	Vitamin D₃ 5,000 iu or 125 mcg	Calcium 800–1,000 mg	Phosphorus 700 mg	Vitamin A 10,000–15,000 iu (as retinol) or 700 mcg
Breakfast				
Lunch				
Dinner				
Snacks and Drinks				
Total				

One-Day RDA Calculation

Magnesium 600–1,000 mg	Vitamin K$_2$ 80–300 mcg	Vitamin C 400–600 mg	Protein 50–150 g	Trace Minerals						Probiotic	Phytoestrogen >50 mg
				Zn	Ca	Mn	B	Sr	Si		

One-Week RDA Calculation

Week beginning: _____

The shaded lines are for adding RDAs from supplements.

	M	T	W	T	F	S	S	Total
Vitamin D								
Calcium								
Phosphorus								
Vitamin A								
Magnesium								
Vitamin K$_2$								
Vitamin C								
Protein								
Trace Minerals								
Probiotic								
Phytoestrogen								

Number of days I took collagen powder supplement: _____

Plant foods I prepared correctly to weaken anti-nutrients:

_____

_____

_____

Four-Week RDA Calculation

The shaded lines are for adding RDAs from supplements.

	Week 1	Week 2	Week 3	Week 4	Total
Vitamin D					
Calcium					
Phosphorus					
Vitamin A					
Magnesium					
Vitamin K$_2$					
Vitamin C					
Protein					
Trace Minerals					
Probiotic					
Phytoestrogen					

Number of days I took collagen powder supplement: _____

Plant foods I prepared correctly to weaken anti-nutrients:

_____

_____

_____

Gap Analysis

The information about what you eat and how much nutrition your food provides will reveal any dietary gaps in bone health nutrition. The gaps you record below will not be precise; however the data will identify those nutrients in which you're in somewhat short supply and more importantly, it will identify where you may be nutrient deficient. To fill out the chart below, refer back to the information you've compiled in the Four-Week RDA Calculation. Your levels may be somewhere on the continuum from a bit short to extremely deficient. All deficiencies are assessed in the context of your health, bone health, and overall diet. Discuss deficiencies with your health care provider before deciding on a course of action.

Bone Health RDA	Amount My Diet Provides
Vitamin D_3: 5,000 iu	
Calcium: 800–1,000 mg	
Phosphorus: 700–1,000 mg	
Vitamin A (retinol): 10,000–15,000 iu or 700 mcg	
Magnesium: 600–1,000 mg	
Vitamin K_2: 80–300 mcg	
Vitamin C: 400–600mg	
Protein: 50–150 g	
Trace Minerals (Zn, Ca, Mn, B, Sr, Si)	
Probiotic	
Phytoestrogen: ≥50 mg	

If there are nutrient gaps, what are my plans to address them? Do I need to speak with my doctor about them?

_____

Which ingredients, combinations, and recipes will I add to my diet in order to close the gaps?

_____

Name of the Nutrient I Need to Increase: _____

How I will move toward closing the gap . . .
Ingredients:

_____

Combinations:

_____

Recipes:

_____

Personal Nutrition Plan

An Overview of My Personal Nutrition Plan

_____
_____
_____
_____
_____
_____
_____

Ideas for Keeping My Bones Healthy

_____
_____
_____

What I Will Cook

_____
_____
_____

How I Will Measure Progress

_____
_____
_____

Bone Health Recipes I've Made/Modified/Enjoyed

_____
_____
_____

Notes: Things to Discuss with My Doctor, Reminders,
Notes about Progress, and Adjustments to My Plan

_____
_____
_____
_____
_____
_____
_____

Bone Health Improvement Goals and Action Plans

☐ **Goal**

_____
_____
_____

Action Plan

_____
_____

How I Will Know When I Have Achieved This Goal

_____
_____

☐ **Goal**

_____
_____
_____

Action Plan

_____
_____

How I Will Know When I Have Achieved This Goal

_____
_____

☐ **Goal**

_____
_____
_____

Action Plan

_____
_____

How I Will Know When I Have Achieved This Goal

_____
_____

Bone Health Plan and Progress Checklist

Use this worksheet as a record of your accomplishments as you implement your two-year Personal Nutrition Plan. You can track your progress by simply checking boxes as you take each step.

This ☐ is a progress box.
☑ Tick it when you have taken that step.
☒ X it if you decide to skip that step but make a note of why you did so. You may wish to revisit these decisions with your healthcare provider over time.

☐ I have had my first nutrition evaluation and discussion with my healthcare provider.
☐ I have filled in my results on the Nutrition Evaluation Results worksheet.
☐ I have started a food journal.
☐ I feel that I know how to read a one-day RDA calculation worksheet.
☐ I have begun filling out my own one-day RDA calculation worksheets.
☐ I have monitored my RDAs for four consecutive weeks.
☐ I have begun taking any supplementation found necessary.
☐ I have started to cook for bone health.
☐ I am keeping track of the bone health foods I eat.
☐ I am keeping track of recipes used, modified, or created.
☐ I have shared recipes on the Medicine Through Food website.
☐ I have prepared four bone health meals four times a week.

☐ After clearance from my healthcare provider, I exercise each day I include a bone health meal.
☐ I have started making bone health vinegar.
☐ I drink bone shrub daily.
☐ I have had a second nutrition evaluation.
☐ I have eliminated processed foods from my diet.

For those with osteoporosis or osteopenia:

☐ I am making and using bone vinegar shrub daily.
☐ I take a daily supplement of vitamin K_2.
☐ I use collagen powder daily.
☐ I take a vitamin D supplement daily.
☐ I exercise daily.
☐ I take cod liver oil daily.
☐ I avoid all processed food.
☐ I sprout my own grains, seeds, nuts, and beans.
☐ I have made a sourdough bread starter and I'm baking bread.
☐ I primarily choose sourdough, Ezekiel, and rye breads.
☐ I have identified a source of Gouda cheese, preferably made from raw milk, and enjoy it several times a week.
☐ I have started growing some of my own greens and herbs.

Notes: _____

_____

_____

_____

_____

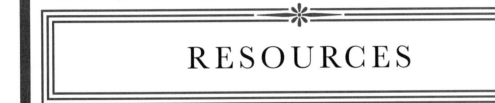

RESOURCES

Food and Herbs

EGGS, ORGANIC AND PASTURED

Organic Egg Scorecard

www.cornucopia.org/organic-egg-scorecard

The Cornucopia Institute has compiled this list. Producers are listed from "5-Eggs" for exemplary to "1-egg." The top tier producers manage diverse, small- to medium-scale family farms. They raise their hens in mobile housing on well-managed and ample pasture or in fixed housing with intensively managed rotated pasture.

FERMENTED CACAO BEANS

Wilderness Family Naturals

wildernessfamilynaturals.com

Excellent source of raw cacao and chocolate products. They also supply great wholesome foods.

FISH, CANNED (SAFELY PACKAGED)

EDF Seafood Selector

seafood.edf.org/tuna

This website lists foods that are offered for sale in BPA-free cans, along with foods you would think are BPA-free, but aren't.

Inspiration Green

www.inspirationgreen.com/bpa-lined-cans?jnf42fc50a=2

Listing of companies and products that use BPA-free cans, and products that don't use BPA-free packaging.

The following companies offer fish in cans that are mostly BPA-free, and a further list of the products they sell—and other major suppliers—whose packaging does contain BPA.

Oregon's Choice, www.oregonschoice.com
Crowne Prince Natural, www.crownprince.com
King Oscar, www.kingoscar.com
Ecofish (Henry and Lisa's), www.ecofish.com
/henryandlisas.htm

GOAT'S CHEESE AND GOAT'S CHEESE GOUDA

Beemster

www.igourmet.com/shoppe/Beemster-Goat-Gouda.asp

Beemster is a Dutch cheese maker whose goat cheese and goat's-milk Gouda are delicious. Beemster is not easy to find in the United States, but you can ask your local market to stock it, or order it online.

HERBS

Sonoma County Herb Exchange
Sonoma, CA
http://www.sonomaherbs.org/herbalexchange.html

Juliet Blankespoor
Chestnut School of Herbal Medicine, Asheville, NC
http://chestnutherbs.com/juliet

Avena Botanicals
Rockport, ME
http://www.avenabotanicals.com

Mountain Rose Herbs
Eugene, OR
www.mountainroseherbs.com

Starwest Botanicals
Sacramento, CA
www.starwest-botanicals.com

Sacred Succulents
Sebastopol, CA
http://sacredsucculents.com
Excellent books and information on plants.

Appalachian Medicinal Herb Growers Consortium
www.brccm.org/ahgc

Chinese Medicinal Herb Farm
Petaluma, CA
www.chinesemedicinalherbfarm.com

Sunpotion Transformational Foods
www.Sunpotion.com

Lotus Blooming Herbs
authenticshilajit.com
Lotuse Blooming Herbs sells excellent quality Shilajit.

NUT BUTTER (FROM SPROUTED NUTS)

Wilderness Family Naturals
www.wildernessfamilynaturals.com/category/nuts
-and-seeds-nut-butters.php
As with cacao, this is a great trusted source.

SPIRULINA AND OTHER SEAWEED POWDERS

Mountain Rose Herbs
Eugene, OR
www.mountainroseherbs.com/products/spirulina
-powder/profile
Mountain Rose Herbs vouches for the strength of its products based on antioxidant activity tests.

SPROUTED FLOURS

Blue Mountain Organics
www.bluemountainorganics.com/by-type/grains-and
-cereals/flours

SPROUTED NUTS AND SEEDS

Blue Mountain Organics
www.bluemountainorganics.com/by-type/seeds-and-nuts

Supplements

COLLAGEN PEPTIDES

Vital Proteins
www.vitalproteins.com

COD LIVER OIL AND COD LIVER OIL WITH HIGH VITAMIN BUTTER OIL

Green Pasture Products
Greenpasture.org

We recommend to patients, and Helen takes, a cod liver oil supplement from Green Pasture Products. The cod liver oil is fermented in the traditional Roman and Viking style. The product provides a clean, whole food form of vitamin D_3. Laura recommends to her patients the fish oil combined with high vitamin butter oil, which supplies vitamin K_2 as well.

Evclo
Evclo.com

Norwegian extra-virgin raw cod liver oil from wild livers.

COCONUT OIL

Living Tree Community Foods
www.livingtreecommunity.com/store2/product
.asp?id=51&catid=30

MAGNESIUM OIL

Ancient Minerals
www.ancient-minerals.com

SILICA

BioSil
Biosilusa.com

Jarrow Formulas
Jarrow.com

VITAMIN D_3

Thorne Research
Thorne.com

Trace Minerals Research
www.traceminerals.com

VITAMIN K_2 (MK4)

Thorne Research
Thorne.com

Jarrow Formulas
Jarrow.com

PROBIOTICS

Dr. Ohhira Probiotics
drohhiraprobiotics.com

ENZYMES

SeraVita Nutraceuticals
seravita.com/supplements.html
Trimazyme

Health and Food Information

FERMENTATION INFORMATION AND RECIPES

Cultures for Health
Culturesforhealth.com
Everything cultured—what, how, and why including make-your-own sourdough starter, yogurt, pickles, probiotics.

Kraut Source
Krautsource.com
Fermentation comes to the modern kitchen.

FOOD SAFETY

Center for Food Safety
centerforfoodsafety.org
Mission to protect human health and the environment.

Center for Science in the Public Interest
cspinet.org
Food safety, food and health, tackling big business.

The Environmental Working Group
ewg.org
Nonprofit, nonpartisan, dedicated to protecting human health and the environment.

NONGMO Project
Nongmoproject.org
Availability of non-GMO foods and products.

Union of Concerned Scientists
csusa.com
Failure to Yield report on GMO crop performance.

RAW MILK

Farm to Consumer Legal Defense Fund
Farmtoconsumer.org
Raw milk defense; cow and goat share.

FRAX

FRAX, World Health Organization Fracture Risk Assessment Tool
http://www.shef.ac.uk/FRAX

The World Health Organization Collaborating Center for Metabolic Bone Diseases at the University of Sheffield, UK has the FRAX tool that you can use to assist with fracture assessment, and discuss with your doctor. Click CALCULATION TOOL, choose your geographic region, and fill in the boxes. There is another calculation tool on the right to assist with weights and measures.

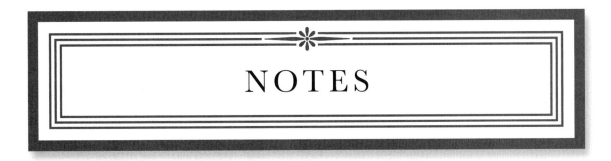

NOTES

Introduction:
Why Supplements Alone Won't Save Us

1. "Osteopenia: When you have weak bones, but not osteoporosis." *Harvard Health Publications*. Published 9 June 2009. http://www.health.harvard.edu/womens-health/osteopenia_when_you_have_weak_bones

2. "Facts and statistics." *International Osteoporosis Foundation*. http://www.iofbonehealth.org/facts-statistics

3. Ibid.

4. Salynn Boyles, "Statins may raise diabetes risk in older women." *WebMD*. 9 January 2012. http://www.webmd.com/cholesterol-management/news/20120109/statins-may-raise-diabetes-risk-in-older-women

5. Henna Cederberg et al., "Increased risk of diabetes with statin treatment is associated with impaired insulin sensitivity and insulin secretion: a 6 year follow-up study of the METSIM cohort." *Diabetologia* 58, no. 5 (May 2015): 1109–1117. http://www.ncbi.nlm.nih.gov/pubmed/25754552; and Naveed Sattar et al., "Statins and risk of incident diabetes: a collaborative meta-analysis of randomised statin trials." *Lancet* 375, no. 9716 (27 February 2010): 735–742. http://www.ncbi.nlm.nih.gov/pubmed/20167359.

6. J. Lazarou, B.H. Pomeranz, and P.N. Corey, "Incidence of adverse drug reactions in hospitalized patients: A meta-analysis of prospective studies." *Journal of the American Medical Association* 279, no. 15 (15 April 1998): 1200–1205. http://www.ncbi.nlm.nih.gov/pubmed/9555760.

7. Jörg Schilcher et al., "Risk of atypical femoral fracture during and after bisphosphonate use." *Acta Orthopaedica* 86, no. 1 (February 2015): 100–107.

http://www.ncbi.nlm.nih.gov/pubmed/25582459; and Jane E. Corrarino, "Bisphosphonates and atypical femoral fractures." *The Journal for Nurse Practitioners* 11, no. 4 (April 2015): 389–396. http://www.npjournal.org/article/S1555-4155(15)00081-1/pdf.

8. "Number of children & adolescents taking psychiatric drugs in the U.S." CCHR International. http://www.cchrint.org/psychiatric-drugs/children-on-psychiatric-drugs/

9. "FDA drug safety communication: ongoing safety review of oral osteoporosis drugs (bisphosphonates) and potential increased risk of esophageal cancer." *U.S. Food and Drug Administration*. 21 July 2011. http://www.fda.gov/Drugs/DrugSafety/ucm263320.htm.

10. Tun-Pin Hsueh and Hsienhsueh Elley Chiu, "Traditional Chinese medicine speeds-up humerus fracture healing: two case reports." *Complementary Therapies in Medicine* 20, no. 6 (December 2012): 431–433. http://www.ncbi.nlm.nih.gov/pubmed/23131374; and L. Chang, "The verification for the efficacy of Jenq Guu Tzyy Jin Dan and Qili San on the treatment of cerebral concussion and body injury." *Taipei Journal of Traditional Chinese Medicine* 9 (2006):102–106.

11. "Low-fat diet not a cure-all." *Harvard T.H. Chan School of Public Health*. http://www.hsph.harvard.edu/nutritionsource/low-fat/; and Dr. Dwight Lundell, "Heart surgeon speaks out on what really causes heart disease." *Signs of the Times*. Published 1 March 2012. http://www.sott.net/article/242516-Heart-Surgeon-Speaks-Out-On-What-Really-Causes-Heart-Disease.

12. Jane E. Brody, "Thinking twice about calcium supplements." *The New York Times.* 8 April 2013. http://well.blogs.nytimes.com/2013/04/08/thinking-twice-about-calcium-supplements-2.

13. "Vitamin D and calcium to prevent fractures: preventive medication." *U.S. Preventive Services Task Force.* February 2013. http://www.uspreventive servicestaskforce.org/Page/Document/Update SummaryFinal/vitamin-d-and-calcium-to-prevent -fractures-preventive-medication

Introduction to Part 1:
Take Charge of Your Bone Health

1. Ellen J. O'Flaherty, "Modeling normal aging bone loss, with consideration of bone loss in osteoporosis." *Toxicological Sciences* 55, no. 1 (2000): 171–188. http://toxsci.oxfordjournals.org/content/55/1/171.full.

Chapter 1: About Your Bones

1. "Introduction to bone biology." *AMGEN.* http://bonebiology.amgen.com/.

2. Takuo Fujita, "Osteoporosis in Japan: factors contributing to the low incidence of hip fracture." *Advances in Food and Nutrition Research* 9 (1994): 89–99. http://www.ncbi.nlm.nih.gov/pubmed/7747676.

3. Liana C. Del Gobbo et al., "Circulating and dietary magnesium and risk of cardiovascular disease: a systematic review and meta-analysis of prospective studies." *American Journal of Clinical Nutrition* 98, no. 1 (May 2013). http://ajcn.nutrition.org/content/early/2013/05/29/ajcn.112.053132.

4. F.H. Nielsen et al., "Effect of dietary boron on mineral, estrogen, and testosterone metabolism in postmenopausal women." *The FASEB Journal* 1, no. 5 (November 1987): 394–397. http://www.ncbi.nlm.nih.gov/pubmed/3678698.

5. Megan Brooks, "Top 100 selling drugs of 2013." *Medscape.* Accessed 9 September 2015. http://www.medscape.com/viewarticle/820011.

6. "Heart attack risk increases 16-21% with use of common antacid." *ScienceDaily.* Published 10 June 2015. Accessed 10 September 2015. www.science daily.com/releases/2015/06/150610143621.htm.

7. L. Gueguen and A. Pointillart, "The bioavailability of dietary calcium." *Journal of the American College of Nutrition* 19, no. 2 (April 2000): 119S–136S. http://www.ncbi.nlm.nih.gov/pubmed/10759138.

8. M. Shiraki et al., "Vitamin K2 (menatetrenone) effectively prevents fractures and sustains lumbar bone mineral density in osteoporosis." *Journal of Bone and Mineral Research* 15, no. 3 (2000): 515–21. http://www.ncbi.nlm.nih.gov/pubmed/10750566.

9. P.J. Caraballo, "Changes in bone density after exposure to oral anticoagulants: a meta-analysis." *Osteoporosis International* 9, no. 5 (1999): 441–448. http://www.ncbi.nlm.nih.gov/pubmed/10550464.

10. L.J. Schurgers et al., "Oral anticoagulant treatment: friend or foe in cardiovascular disease?" *Blood* 104, no. 10 (15 November 2004): 3231–3232. http://www.ncbi.nlm.nih.gov/pubmed/15265793.

11. Kuniko Hara et al., "Interaction of warfarin and vitamin K2 on arterial thrombotic tendency using a rat aorta loop model." *Nihon Yakurigaku Zasshi* 113, no. 3 (1991): 185–92. http://www.ncbi.nlm.nih.gov/pubmed/10347843.

12. Ghada N. Farhat and Jane A. Cauley, "The link between osteoporosis and cardiovascular disease." *Clinical Cases in Mineral and Bone Metabolism* 5, no. 1 (January–April 2008):19–34. http://www.ncbi.nlm.nih.gov/pmc/articles/PMC2781192/; and S.J. Chen et al., "Osteoporosis is associated with high risk for coronary heart disease: a population-based cohort study." *Medicine* 94, no. 27 (July 2015): e1146. http://www.ncbi.nlm.nih.gov/pubmed/26166125.

13. "Vitamin C prevents bone loss in animal models." *ScienceDaily.* Published 9 October 2012. Accessed 10 September 2015. https://www.sciencedaily.com/releases/2012/10/121009151258.htm.

14. Robert P. Heaney and Donald K. Layman, "Amount and type of protein influences bone health." *American Journal of Clinical Nutrition* 87, no. 5 (May 2008): 1567S–1570S. http://www.ncbi.nlm.nih.gov/pubmed/18469289.

Chapter 2:
Systemic Factors That Promote Bone Loss

1. Sheldon Cohen et al., "Chronic stress, glucocorticoid receptor resistance, inflammation, and disease risk." *Proceedings of the National Academy of Sciences* 109, no. 16 (17 April 2012): 5995–5999. http://www.ncbi.nlm.nih.gov/pmc/articles/PMC3341031/.

2. H. Kerbage et al., "Effect of SSRIs on bone metabolism." *L'Encéphale* 40, no. 1 (February 2014): 56–61. http://www.ncbi.nlm.nih.gov /pubmed/23810751.

3. S.J. Warden and E.M. Haney, "Skeletal effects of serotonin (5-hydroxytryptamine) transporter inhibition: evidence from in vitro and animal-based studies." *Journal of Musculoskeletal and Neuronal Interactions* 8, no. 2 (April–June 2008): 121–132. http://www.ncbi.nlm.nih.gov/pubmed/18622081.

4. Linda L. Humphrey et al., "Homocysteine level and coronary heart disease incidence: a systematic review and meta-analysis." *Mayo Clinic Proceedings* 83, no. 11 (November 2008): 1203–1212. http:// www.ncbi.nlm.nih.gov/pubmed/18990318.

5. Robert R. McLean et al., "Homocysteine as a predictive factor for hip fracture in older persons." *The New England Journal of Medicine* 350, no. 20 (13 May 2004): 2042–2049. http://www.ncbi.nlm.nih .gov/pubmed/15141042.

6. "Diets high in salt could deplete calcium in the body." *ScienceDaily*. Published 24 July 2012. Accessed 10 September 2015. www.sciencedaily .com/releases/2012/07/120724131604.htm.

7. Dinesh Kumar Dhanwal, "Thyroid disorders and bone mineral metabolism." *Indian Journal of Endocrinology and Metabolism* 15, suppl. 2 (July 2011): S107–S112. http://www.ncbi.nlm.nih.gov/pmc /articles/PMC3169869/.

8. Jennifer L. Bedford and Susan I. Barr, "Higher urinary sodium, a proxy for intake, is associated with increased calcium excretion and lower hip bone density in healthy young women with lower calcium intakes." *Nutrients* 3, no. 11 (November 2011): 951–961. http://www.ncbi.nlm.nih.gov/pmc /articles/PMC3257722/.

9. J. Teas et al., "Seaweed and soy: companion foods in asian cuisine and their effects on thyroid function in American women." *Journal of Medicinal Food* 10, no.1 (March 2007): 90–100. http://www.ncbi.nlm .nih.gov/pubmed/17472472.

10. P. Amaresh Reddy, C. V. Harinarayan, Alok Sachan, et al., "Bone disease in thyrotoxicosis," *Indian Journal of Medical Research*, March 2012; 135(3): 277–286. http://www.ncbi.nlm.nih.gov /pmc/articles/PMC3361862/

Chapter 3:
Choose Natural Food for Healthy Bones

1. Cheryl Long and Tabitha Alterman, "Meet real free-range eggs." *Mother Earth News*. Published October/November 2007. http://www .motherearthnews.com/real-food/free-range-eggs -zmaz07onzgoe.aspx.

2. A. Bhattacharya et al., "Biological effects of conjugated linoleic acids in health and disease." *Journal of Nutritional Biochemistry* 17, no. 12 (December 2006): 789–810. http://www.ncbi.nlm.nih.gov /pubmed/16650752.

3. F. Beppu et al., "Potent inhibitory effect of trans9, trans11 isomer of conjugated linoleic acid on the growth of human colon cancer cells." *The Journal of Nutritional Biochemistry* 17, no. 12 (December 2006): 830–836. http://www.ncbi.nlm.nih.gov /pubmed/16563722.

4. Karl Michaëlsson et al., "Milk intake and risk of mortality and fractures in women and men: cohort studies." *British Medical Journal* (2014): 349. http:// www.bmj.com/content/349/bmj.g6015.

5. Kimberly Hartke, "Government data proves raw milk safe." *The Weston A. Price Foundation*. Published 1 August 2011. http://www.westonaprice.org/press /government-data-proves-raw-milk-safe/.

6. J. Uribarri et al., "Advanced glycation end products in foods and a practical guide to their reduction in the diet." *Journal of the American Dietetic Association* 110, no. 6 (June 2010): 911–916. http://www.ncbi .nlm.nih.gov/pubmed/20497781.

7. Helen Vlassara, "Identifying advanced glycation end products as a major source of oxidants in aging: implications for the management and/or prevention of reduced renal function in elderly persons." *Seminars in Nephrology* 29, no. 6 (November 2009): 594–603. http://www.ncbi.nlm.nih.gov/pubmed/20006791.

8. Ziqing Li, "Advanced glycation end products biphasically modulate bone resorption in osteoclast-like cells." *American Journal of Physiology—Endocrinology and Metabolism* 310, no. 5 (1 March 2016): E355–E366. http://www.ncbi.nlm.nih.gov/pubmed/26670486.

9. Uribarri et al. 911–16.

10. Ibid. 911–16.

11. "Q&A on the carcinogenicity of the consumption of red meat and processed meat." *World Health*

Organization. Published October 2015. http://www
.who.int/features/qa/cancer-red-meat/en/.

12. "All about cooking & carcinogens." *Precision Nutrition.* http://www.precisionnutrition.com /all-about-cooking-carcinogens.

13. Pon Velayutham Anandh Babu et al., "Effect of green tea extract on advanced glycation and cross-linking of tail tendon collagen in streptozoto-cin induced diabetic rats." *Food and Chemical Toxicology* 46, no. 1 (January 2008): 280–285. http://www.ncbi.nlm.nih.gov/pubmed/17884275.

14. R.A. Waterland, "Post-weaning diet affects genomic imprinting at the insulin-like growth factor 2 (Igf2) locus." *Human Molecular Genetics* 15, no. 5 (1 March 2006): 705–716. http://www.ncbi.nlm.nih.gov /pubmed/16421170.

Chapter 4: Disarm Anti-Nutrients in Plant-Based Foods

1. D. Siegenberg et al., "Ascorbic acid prevents the dose-dependent inhibitory effects of polyphenols and phytates on nonheme-iron absorption." *The American Journal of Clinical Nutrition* 53, no. 2 (February 1991): 537–541. http://www.ncbi.nlm .nih.gov/pubmed/1989423.

2. Heidi Stallman, "Guide to low oxalate greens." *Low Oxalate Info.* Published 7 June 2012. Accessed 10 September 2015. http://lowoxalateinfo.com/guide -to-low-oxalate-greens/.

Chapter 5: Gut Bugs Can Be Bone's Best Friends

1. "Home." *HealthyGutBugs.com.* www.healthygutbugs.com.

2. Anatoly Bezkorovainy, "Probiotics: determinants of survival and growth in the gut." The *American Journal of Clinical Nutrition* 73, suppl. 2 (February 2001): 399S–405S. http://www.ncbi.nlm.nih.gov /pubmed/11157348.

3. International Commission on Microbiological Specifications for Foods (ICMSF), *Microorganisms in Foods 6: Microbial Ecology of Food Commodities.* New York: Springer, 2005.

Chapter 6: Considering Supplements

1. "Dietary guidelines." *Office of Disease Prevention and Health Promotion.* http://health.gov/dietaryguidelines.

2. B.E. Christopher Nordin, "Calcium requirement is a sliding scale." *The American Journal of Clinical Nutrition* 71, no. 6 (June 2000): 1381–1383. http:// www.ncbi.nlm.nih.gov/pubmed/10837273.

3. "Calcium supplements linked to significantly increased heart attack risk, study suggests." *ScienceDaily.* Published 23 May 2012. Accessed 10 September 2015. www.sciencedaily.com/releases /2012/05/120523200752.htm.

4. Paul J. Veugelers and John Ekwaru, "A statistical error in the estimation of the recommended dietary allowance for vitamin D." *Nutrients* 6, no. 10 (October 2014): 4472–4475. http://www.ncbi.nlm .nih.gov/pmc/articles/PMC4210929/.

5. Carolyn Dean, "Magnesium is crucial for bones." *The Huffington Post.* 15 June 2012. 10 September, 2015. http://www.huffingtonpost.com/carolyn -dean-md-nd/bone-health_b_1540931.html.

6. S.L. Booth, "Assessment of dietary phylloquinone intake and vitamin K status in postmenopausal women." *European Journal of Clinical Nutrition* 49, no. 11 (November 1995): 832–841. http://www.ncbi .nlm.nih.gov/pubmed/8557021.

7. Dr. Susan E. Brown. "Protein and bone health: a paradox unraveled." *Better Bones.* http://www.better bones.com/bonenutrition/protein/benefits.aspx.

8. Anitra C. Carr and Balz Frei, "Toward a new recommended dietary allowance for vitamin C based on antioxidant and health effects in humans." *The American Journal of Clinical Nutrition* 69, no. 6 (1999): 1086–1107. http://www.ncbi.nlm.nih.gov /pubmed/10357726; and Jane Higdon, Ph.D., "Vitamin C." *Oregon State University Linus Pauling Institute Micronutrient Information Center.* http://lpi .oregonstate.edu/mic/vitamins/vitamin-C.

9. Karl Michaëlsson, "Long term calcium intake and rates of all cause and cardiovascular mortality: community based prospective longitudinal cohort study." *The British Medical Journal* (2013): 346. http://www.bmj.com/content/346/bmj.f228.

10. M.F. Holick, "Optimal vitamin D status for the prevention and treatment of osteoporosis." *Drugs Aging* 24, no. 12 (2007): 1017–1029. http://www .ncbi.nlm.nih.gov/pubmed/18020534.

11. L.C. Hofbauer, "Vascular calcification and osteoporosis—from clinical observation towards

molecular understanding." *Osteoporosis International* 18, no. 3 (March 2007): 251–259. http://www.ncbi .nlm.nih.gov/pubmed/17151836.

12. L. Plantalech et al., "Impairment of gamma carboxylation of circulating osteocalcin (bone gla protein) in elderly women." *Journal of Bone and Mineral Research* 6, no. 11 (November 1991): 1211–1216. http://www.ncbi.nlm.nih.gov/pubmed/1666807.

13. Kresimir Pucaj et al., "Safety and toxicological evaluation of a synthetic vitamin K2, menaqui-none-7." *Toxicology Mechanisms and Methods* 21, no. 7 (September 2011): 520–532. http://www.ncbi.nlm .nih.gov/pmc/articles/PMC3172146/.

14. Noriko Koitaya et al., "Low-dose vitamin K2 (MK-4) supplementation for 12 months improves bone metabolism and prevents forearm bone loss in postmenopausal japanese women." *Journal of Bone and Mineral Metabolism* 32, no. 2 (March 2014): 142–150. http://www.ncbi.nlm.nih.gov/pubmed/23702931.

15. Ravin Jugdaohsingh, "Silicon and bone health." *The Journal of Nutrition Health and Aging* 11, no. 2 (March–April 2007): 99–110. http://www.ncbi.nlm .nih.gov/pmc/articles/PMC2658806/.

16. Charles T. Price, Kenneth J. Koval, and Joshua R. Langford, "Silicon: A review of its potential role in the prevention and treatment of postmenopausal osteoporosis." *International Journal of Endocrinology* 11 (2013). https://www.researchgate.net/publication /237200455_Silicon_A_Review_of_Its_Potential _Role_in_the_Prevention_and_Treatment_of _Postmenopausal_Osteoporosis.

17. Dr. Roger J. Williams. *The Wonderful World Within You.* Wichita, Kansas: Bio-Communications Press, 1977.

Chapter 7: Phytoestrogens, Cholesterol, and Bone Loss Pharmaceuticals

1. Kenneth D. R. Setchell and Eva Lydeking Olsen, "Dietary phytoestrogens and their effect on bone: evidence from in vitro and in vivo, human observation-al, and dietary intervention studies." *American Journal of Clinical Nutrition* 78, suppl. 3 (2003): 593S–609S. http://www.ncbi.nlm.nih.gov/pubmed/12936954.

2. "Soy phytoestrogens may block estrogen effects." *ScienceDaily*. Published 16 January 2006. Accessed 10 September 2015. https://www.sciencedaily.com /releases/2006/01/060115154340.htm.

3. Marji McCullough, "The bottom line on soy and breast cancer risk." *American Cancer Society*. Published 2 August 2012. http://blogs.cancer.org/expertvoices /2012/08/02/the-bottom-line-on-soy-and-breast -cancer-risk/.

4. S. Yamamoto et al., "Soy, isoflavones, and breast cancer risk in Japan." *Journal of the National Cancer Institute* 95, no. 12 (June 2003): 906–913. http:// www.ncbi.nlm.nih.gov/pubmed/12813174; and E. Zhao and Qing Mu, "Phytoestrogen biological actions on mammalian reproductive system and cancer growth." *Scientia Pharmaceutica* 79, no.1 (2011): 1–20. http://www.ncbi.nlm.nih.gov/pmc /articles/PMC3097497/.

5. L.A. David et al., "Diet rapidly and reproducibly alters the human gut microbiome." *Nature* 505, no. 7484 (23 January 2014): 559–563. http://www.ncbi .nlm.nih.gov/pubmed/24336217.

6. M.D. Gammon et al., "The Long Island Breast Cancer Study Project: description of a multi-institu-tional collaboration to identify environmental risk factors for breast cancer." *Breast Cancer Research and Treatment* 74, no. 3 (June 2002): 235–254. http:// www.ncbi.nlm.nih.gov/pubmed/12206514.

7. "Vitamin D and flavonoids examined for impact on breast and ovarian cancers." *ScienceDaily*. Published 7 April 2006. Accessed 10 September 2015. www .sciencedaily.com/releases/2006/04/060407144100. htm; Neela Guha et al., "Soy isoflavones and risk of cancer recurrence in a cohort of breast cancer survivors: Life After Cancer Epidemiology (LACE) Study." *Breast Cancer Research and Treatment* 118, no.2 (November 2009): 395–405. http://www.ncbi.nlm .nih.gov/pubmed/19221874; and Xiao Ou Shu et al., "Soy food intake and breast cancer survival." *The Journal of the American Medical Association* 302, no.22 (9 December 2009): 2437–43. http://www.ncbi.nlm .nih.gov/pubmed/19996398.

8. John W. Erdman, Jr., "AHA Science Advisory: soy protein and cardiovascular disease: a statement for healthcare professionals from the Nutrition Committee of the AHA." *Circulation* 102, no. 20 (2000): 2555-59. http://www.ncbi.nlm.nih.gov /pubmed/11076833.

9. Ye Won Hwang et al., "Soy food consumption and risk of prostate cancer: a meta-analysis of

observational studies." *Nutrition and Cancer* 61, no. 5 (2009): 598-606. http://www.ncbi.nlm.nih.gov /pubmed/19838933.

10. A Warri et al., "The role of early life genistein exposures in modifying breast cancer risk." *British Journal of Cancer* 98, no. 9 (6 May 2008): 1485–1493. http://www.ncbi.nlm.nih.gov/pubmed/18392054.

11. W. P. Castelli, "Cholesterol and lipids in the risk of coronary artery disease—The Framingham Heart Study." *The Canadian Journal of Cardiology* 4, suppl. A (July 1988): 5A–10A. http://www.ncbi .nlm.nih.gov/pubmed/3179802.

12. Donald J. McNamara, "Dietary fatty acids, lipoproteins, and cardiovascular disease," in *Advances in Food and Nutrition Research*, ed. John E. Kinsella (Academic Press, 1992), 253–351.

13. Juan Antonio Moreno et al., "The effect of dietary fat on LDL size is influenced by apolipoprotein E genotype in healthy subjects." *The Journal of Nutrition* 134, no. 10 (October 2004): 2517-2522. http://www .ncbi.nlm.nih.gov/pubmed/15465740.

14. Robert H Knopp and Barbara M Retzlaff, "Saturated fat prevents coronary artery disease? An American paradox." *The American Journal of Clinical Nutrition* 80, no. 5 (November 2004): 1102–1103. http://www.ncbi.nlm.nih.gov/pubmed/15531654.

15. Zil Hayatullina et al., "Virgin coconut oil supplementation prevents bone loss in osteoporosis rat model." *Evidence-Based Complementary and Alternative Medicine* (2012) http://www.ncbi.nlm.nih .gov/pmc/articles/PMC3457741/.

16. Dennis M. Black et al., "Fracture risk reduction with alendronate in women with osteoporosis: the fracture intervention trial." *The Journal of Clinical Endocrinology & Metabolism* 85, no. 11 (2000): 4118–24. http://www .ncbi.nlm.nih.gov/pubmed/11095442.

17. Tara Parker-Pope, "New cautions about long-term use of bone drugs." *The New York Times* (New York, NY), 9 May 2012.

18. Jun Iwamoto, Tsuyoshi Takeda, and Shoichi Ichimura, "Combined treatment with vitamin K2 and bisphosphonate in postmenopausal women with osteoporosis" *Yonsei Medical Journal* 44, no. 5 (2003): 751–56. http://www.ncbi.nlm.nih.gov/pubmed /14584089.

Chapter 10: Setting the Stage

1. Jenna Bilbrey, "BPA-free plastic containers may be just as hazardous." *Scientific American*. Published 11 August 2015. http://www.scientificamerican.com /article/bpa-free-plastic-containers-may-be-just -as-hazardous/.

2. Zil Hayatullina et al.

Chapter 14: Salads

1. Alice Waters, *The Art of Simple Food* (New York: Clarkson Potter, 2007).

Chapter 17: Main Stage

1. "To block the carcinogens, add a touch of rosemary when grilling meats." *ScienceDaily*. Published 24 May 2008. www.sciencedaily.com/releases /2008/05/080521184129.htm.

Chapter 18: Sides

1. C. Hoelzl et al., "DNA protective effects of Brussels sprouts: Results of a human intervention study." *AACR Meeting Abstracts* (December 2007).

Chapter 21: Snacks

1. Sarah C. Janicki and Nicole Schupf. "Hormonal influences on cognition and risk for Alzheimer disease." *Current Neurology and Neuroscience Reports* 10, no. 5 (September 2010): 359–366. http://www.ncbi .nlm.nih.gov/pmc/articles/PMC3058507/.

Chapter 22: Make Your Own

1. J. Rovenský et al., "Eggshell calcium in the prevention and treatment of osteoporosis." *International Journal of Clinical Pharmacology Research* 23, nos. 2–3 (2003): 83–92. http://www.ncbi.nlm .nih.gov/pubmed/15018022.

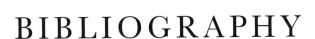

BIBLIOGRAPHY

American Chemical Society. "Solving the Mystery of How Cigarette Smoking Weakens Bones." *ScienceDaily*. www.sciencedaily.com/releases/2012/07/120726153951.htm (accessed September 8, 2015).

Andrews, Ryan. "Phytates and Phytic Acid: Here's What You Need to Know." *PrecisionNutrition*. http://www.precisionnutrition.com/all-about-phytates-phytic-acid.

BBC News. "Adults' Antidepressant Bone Risk." BBC News. http://news.bbc.co.uk/2/hi/health/6286681.stm (accessed September 8, 2015).

———. "Calcium Pills 'Raise Heart Risk.'" BBC News. http://news.bbc.co.uk/2/hi/health/7187265.stm (accessed September 8, 2015).

———. "Osteoporosis Drug Advice Concerns." BBC News. http://news.bbc.co.uk/2/hi/health/5403500.stm (accessed September 8, 2015).

Beth Israel Deaconess Medical Center. "Osteoporosis: Not Just a Woman's Disease." *ScienceDaily*. www.sciencedaily.com/releases/2014/11/141105140708.htm (accessed September 8, 2015).

British Medical Journal. "Risk of Cardiovascular Death Doubled in Women with High Calcium Intake: High Risk Only in Those Taking Supplements as Well." *ScienceDaily*. www.sciencedaily.com/releases/2013/02/130212192030.htm (accessed September 8, 2015).

Cashman, Kevin. "Prebiotics and Calcium Bioavailability." *Current Issues in Intestinal Microbiology* 4, no. 1 (2003): 21–32.

Center for Science in the Public Interest. "Chemical Cuisine." Center for Science in the Public Interest. http://www.cspinet.org/reports/chemcuisine.htm (accessed September 8, 2015).

Dempster, David W. "Osteoporosis and the Burden of Osteoporosis-Related Fractures." *American Journal of Managed Care* 17, suppl. 6, (2011): 164–69.

Flore, R., F. R Ponziani., T. A. Di Rienzo, M. A. Zocco, A. Flex, L. Gerardino, A. Lupascu, L. Santoro, A. Santoliquido, E. Di Stasio, E. Chierici, A. Lanti, P. Tondi, and A. Gasbarrini. "Something More to Say About Calcium Homeostasis: The Role of Vitamin K_2 in Vascular Calcification and Osteoporosis." *European Review for Medical and Pharmacological Sciences* 17, no. 18 (2013): 2433–40.

Gallagher, James. "Calcium Pills Pose 'Heart Risk.'" BBC News. http://www.bbc.com/news/health-18175707 (accessed September 8, 2015).

Gregory, Jesse F. "Denaturation of the Folacin-Binding Protein in Pasteurized Milk Products." *Journal of Nutrition* 112, no. 7 (1982): 1329–38.

Grenham, Sue, Gerard Clarke, John F. Cryan, and Timothy G. Dinan. "Brain-Gut-Microbe Communication in Health and Disease." *Frontiers in Physiology* 2, no. 00094 (2011). http://www.frontiersin.org/Journal/Abstract.aspx?s=465&name=gastrointestinal_sciences&ART_DOI=10.3389/fphys.2011.00094.

Hafner, Katie. "Bracing for the Fall of an Aging Nation." *New York Times*, November 2, 2014, Health section.

Heaney, Robert P., and Donald K. Layman. "Amount and Type of Protein Influences Bone Health." *American Journal of Clinical Nutrition* 87, no. 5 (2008): 1567S–70S.

Huang, Z. B., S. L. Wan, Y. J. Lu, L. Ning, C. Liu, and S. W. Fan. "Does Vitamin K_2 Play a Role in the Prevention and Treatment of Osteoporosis for

Postmenopausal Women: A Meta-Analysis of Randomized Controlled Trials." *Osteoporosis International* 26, no. 3 (2015): 1175–86.

Hubert, Patrice A., Sang Gil Lee, Sun-Kyeong Lee, and Ock K. Chun. "Dietary Polyphenols, Berries, and Age-Related Bone Loss: A Review Based on Human, Animal, and Cell Studies." *Antioxidants* 3 (2014): 144–58.

International Osteoporosis Foundation. "22 Million Women Aged Over 50 Affected by Osteoporosis in European Union." *ScienceDaily*. www.sciencedaily.com/releases/2013/11/131111102425.htm (accessed September 8, 2015).

———. "New Study Quantifies Total Costs of Fragility Fractures in Six Major European Countries." *ScienceDaily*. www.sciencedaily.com/releases/2011/03/110324153511.htm (accessed September 8, 2015).

———. "Osteoporosis-Related Fractures in China Expected to Double by 2035." *ScienceDaily*. www.sciencedaily.com/releases/2015/04/150408102703.htm (accessed September 8, 2015).

———. "Why Men Are the Weaker Sex When It Comes to Bone Health." *ScienceDaily*. www.sciencedaily.com/releases/2014/10/141009091937.htm (accessed September 9, 2015).

Iwamoto, Jun. "Vitamin K_2 Therapy for Postmenopausal Osteoporosis." *Nutrients* 6, no. 5 (2014): 1971–80.

Iwamoto, Jun, Tsuyoshi Takeda, and Yoshihiro Sato. "Role of Vitamin K_2 in the Treatment of Postmenopausal Osteoporosis." *Current Drug Safety* 1, no. 1 (2014): 87–97.

Kanis, J. A., A. Odén, E. V. McCloskey, H. Johansson, D. A. Wahl, and C. Cooper. "A Systematic Review of Hip Fracture Incidence and Probability of Fracture Worldwide." *Osteoporosis International* 23, no. 9 (2012): 2239–56.

Kasukawa, Yuji, Naohisa Miyakoshi, Toshihito Ebina, Toshiaki Aizawa, Michio Hongo, and Koji Nozaka. "Effects of Risedronate Alone or Combined with Vitamin K_2 on Serum Undercarboxylated Osteocalcin and Osteocalcin Levels in Postmenopausal Osteoporosis." *Journal of Bone and Mineral Metabolism* 32, no. 3 (2014): 290–97.

Kawashima, H., Y. Nakajima, Y. Matubara, J. Nakanowatari, T. Fukuta, S. Mizuno, S. Takahashi,

T. Tajima, and T. Nakamura. "Effects of Vitamin K_2 (Menatetrenone) on Atherosclerosis and Blood Coagulation in Hypercholesterolemic Rabbits." *Japanese Journal of Pharmacology* 75, no. 2 (1997): 135–43.

Koitaya, Noriko, Mariko Sekiguchi, Yuko Tousen, Yoriko Nishide, Akemi Morita, Jun Yamauchi, Yuko Gando, Motohiko Miyachi, Mami Aoki, Miho Komatsu, Fumiko Watanabe, Koji Morishita, and Yoshiko Ishimi. "Low-Dose Vitamin K_2 (MK-4) Supplementation for 12 Months Improves Bone Metabolism and Prevents Forearm Bone Loss in Postmenopausal Japanese Women." *Journal of Bone and Mineral Metabolism* 32, no. 2 (2014): 142–50.

Kolirin, Lianne. "Women Risking Heart Disease from Calcium." *Express*. http://www.express.co.uk/life-style/health/377316/Women-risking-heart-disease-from-calcium.

Landecker, Hannah. "Food as Exposure: Nutritional Epigenetics and the New Metabolism." *Biosocieties* 6, no. 2 (2011): 167–94.

Marshall, Deborah, O. Johnell, and H. Wedel. "Meta-Analysis of How Well Measures of Bone Mineral Density Predict Occurrence of Osteoporotic Fractures." *BMJ Clinical Research* 312, no. 7014 (1996): 1254–59.

Massachusetts Institute of Technology. "Engineering Bone Growth: Coated Tissue Scaffolds Help Body Grow New Bone to Repair Injuries or Congenital Defects." *ScienceDaily*. www.sciencedaily.com/releases/2014/08/140819155332.htm (accessed September 8, 2015).

McGruther, Jenny. "GMO-Free Foods: A List for Those Who Are GMO Free." *Nourished Kitchen*. http://nourishedkitchen.com/gmo-free-food/ (accessed September 8, 2015).

Nair, Arun K., Alfonso Gautieri, Shu-Wei Chang, and Markus J. Buehler. "Molecular Mechanics of Mineralized Collagen Fibrils in Bone." *Nature Communications* 4, article number 1724 (2013). http://www.nature.com/ncomms/journal/v4/n4/full/ncomms2720.html.

Plataforma SINC. "Genetic Factor in Osteoporosis Discovered." *ScienceDaily*. www.sciencedaily.com/releases/2010/09/100922082333.htm (accessed September 8, 2015).

Raggatt, Liza J., and Nicola Chennell Partridge. "Cellular and Molecular Mechanisms of Bone Remodeling." *Journal of Biological Chemistry* 285, no. 33 (2010): 25103–08.

Reynaud, Enrique. "Protein Misfolding and Degenerative Diseases." *Scitable.* http://www.nature.com /scitable/topicpage/protein-misfolding-and -degenerative-diseases-14434929 (accessed September 8, 2015).

Robbins J. A., A. M. Schott, P. Garnero, P. D. Delmas, D. Hans, and P. J. Meunier. "Risk Factors for Hip Fracture in Women with High BMD: EPIDOS Study." *Osteoporosis International* 16, no. 2 (2005): 149–54.

Rude, R. K., F. R. Singer, and H. E. Gruber. "Skeletal and Hormonal Effects of Magnesium Deficiency." *Journal of the American College of Nutrition* 28, no. 2 (2009): 131–41.

Scholz-Ahrens, Katharina E., Peter Ade, Berit Marten, Petra Weber, Wolfram Timm, Yahya Asil, Claus C. Glüer, and Jürgen Schrezenmier. "Prebiotics, Probiotics, and Synbiotics Affect Mineral Absorption, Bone Mineral Content, and Bone Structure." *Journal of Nutrition* 137, no. 3 (2007): 838–46.

Schroeder, Lawrence J., Michael Iacobellis, and Arthur H. Smith. "Heat Processing and the Nutritive Value of Milk and Milk Products." *Journal of Nutrition* 49 (1953): 549–61.

Schwartze, E. W., F. J. Murphy, and R. M. Hann. "Studies on the Destruction of Vitamin C in the Boiling of Milk." *Journal of Nutrition* 2 (1930): 325–52.

Seelig, Mildred S. "Skeleletal and Renal Effects of Magnesium Deficiency: Magnesium, Bone Wasting, and Mineralization." In *Magnesium Deficiency in the Pathogenesis of Disease: Early Roots of Cardiovascular, Skeletal and Renal Abnormalities.* New York: Plenum Publishing, 1980.

Smilowitz, Jennifer T., and J. Bruce German. "Mammalian Milk Genomics: Knowledge to Guide Diet and Health in the 21st Century." *NABC (National Agricultural Biotechnology Council) Report 22: Promoting Health by Linking Agriculture, Food, and Nutrition* (2010): 71–79.

Stevenson, M., M. Lloyd-Jones, and D. Papaioannou. "Vitamin K to Prevent Fractures in Older Women: Systematic Review and Economic Evaluation." *Health Technology Assessment* 13, no. 45 (2009): iii–xi, 1–134.

Union of Concerned Scientists. *Failure to Yield: Evaluating the Performance of Genetically Engineered Crops.* Union of Concerned Scientists. http://www.ucsusa.org /food_and_agriculture/our-failing-food-system /genetic-engineering/failure-to-yield.html#.Ve _V0K2und5 (accessed September 8, 2015).

University at Buffalo. "Strong Association Between Menopausal Symptoms, Bone Health." *ScienceDaily.* www.sciencedaily.com/releases/2015/01 /150122132849.htm (accessed September 8, 2015).

University of California–San Francisco (UCSF). "Sugared Soda Consumption, Cell Aging Associated in New Study." *ScienceDaily.* www.sciencedaily.com /releases/2014/10/141016165951.htm (accessed September 8, 2015).

University of Cambridge. "Hunter-Gatherer Past Shows Our Fragile Bones Result from Inactivity Since Invention of Farming." *ScienceDaily.* www.sciencedaily .com/releases/2014/12/141222165033.htm.

University of Surrey. "Potassium Salts Aid Bone Health, Limit Osteoporosis Risk, New Research Finds." *ScienceDaily.* www.sciencedaily.com/releases/2015/01 /150114115340.htm (accessed September 8, 2015).

Wallach, S. "Effects of Magnesium on Skeletal Metabolism." *Magnesium and Trace Elements* 9, no. 1 (1990): 1–14.

Weaver, C. M., and Karen Plawecki. "Dietary Calcium: Adequacy of a Vegetarian Diet." *American Journal of Clinical Nutrition* 59, no. 5 (suppl.) (1994): 1238S–41S.

Weaver, Connie M., William R. Proulx, and Robert Heaney. "Choices for Achieving Adequate Dietary Calcium with a Vegetarian Diet." *American Journal of Clinical Nutrition* 70 (suppl.) (1999): 543S–48S.

Wellcome Trust Sanger Institute. "Pathway Between Gut, Liver Regulates Bone Mass: Biological Process Behind Role of Vitamin B_{12} in Bone Formation Unravelled." *ScienceDaily.* www.sciencedaily.com /releases/2014/06/140609205304.htm (accessed September 8, 2015).

Wiley. "Sleep Problems May Impact Bone Health." *ScienceDaily.* www.sciencedaily.com/releases/2015 /02/150203104104.htm (accessed September 8, 2015).

Wilkinson, Emma. "Calcium Pills 'Increase' Risk of Heart Attack." BBC News. http://www.bbc.com/news /health-10805062 (accessed September 8, 2015).

Wu, Wei-Jie, Hwa-Young Lee, Geum-Hwa Lee, Han-Jung Chae, and Byung-Yong Ahn. "The Antiosteoporotic Effects of Cheonggukjang Containing Vitamin K-2 (Menaquinone-7) in Ovariectomized Rats." *Journal of Medicinal Food* 17, no. 12 (2014): 1298–305.

Zand, Janet. "Your Doctor's Bone Treatment Raises Your Risk of Heart Attack by 86%." *Womens Health Letter.* http://www.womenshealthletter.com/Health-Alert-Archive/View-Archive/2471/Your-doctors-bone-treatment-raises-your-risk-of-heart-attack-by-86.htm.

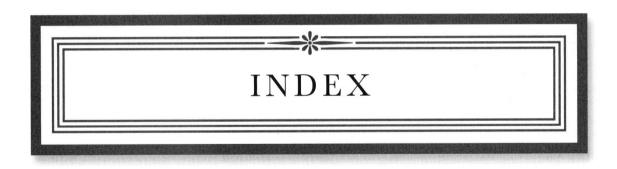

INDEX

Bold page numbers refer to the color insert.

About the Authors

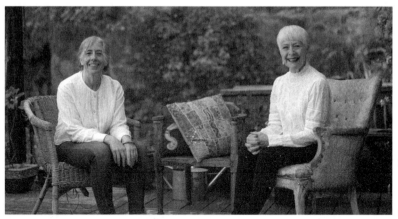

PATRICK FRASER

Dr. Laura Kelly is a licensed Traditional Chinese Medicine practitioner and Doctor of Acupuncture and Oriental Medicine. She completed her medical training and doctorate at Yo San University in Los Angeles. Her private practice focuses on primary care and chronic disease. She is working with a research group to document the biochemical effects of Chinese herbs on fatigue and is leading the investigation on a nonsurgical treatment for paralysis. On her blog, *Case Notes* at laurakellylac .wordpress.com, she writes about her experiences in medical practice. In 2017, she will complete The Institute of Functional Medicine's Certificate Program (IFMCP). She lives and works in Topanga, California.

Helen Bryman Kelly is an award-winning research writer who specializes in medicine and management. She has served as visiting faculty at universities in the United States and the U.K. and is an experienced public speaker. Her client list has included Yale University, IBM, and McGraw-Hill Books. She was the London-based European editor for *theworkingmanager.com* for more than a decade and has been a freelance contributing editor for *Advantage Business Media* since 2008.

About the Foreword Author

Dr. Sidney MacDonald Baker is a graduate and former faculty member of Yale School of Medicine, family practitioner, Gesell Institute of Child Development director, founder of Defeat Autism Now! and Autism360, Linus Pauling Award recipient, and associate editor of *Integrative Medicine: A Clinician's Journal*. He is the author of *Detoxification and Healing*.

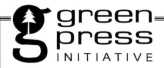

green
press
INITIATIVE

Chelsea Green Publishing is committed to preserving ancient forests and natural resources. We elected to print this title on 30-percent postconsumer recycled paper, processed chlorine-free. As a result, for this printing, we have saved:

14 Trees (40' tall and 6-8" diameter)
6 Million BTUs of Total Energy
1,177 Pounds of Greenhouse Gases
6,381 Gallons of Wastewater
427 Pounds of Solid Waste

Chelsea Green Publishing made this paper choice because we and our printer, Thomson-Shore, Inc., are members of the Green Press Initiative, a nonprofit program dedicated to supporting authors, publishers, and suppliers in their efforts to reduce their use of fiber obtained from endangered forests. For more information, visit: www.greenpressinitiative.org.

Environmental impact estimates were made using the Environmental Defense Paper Calculator. For more information visit: www.papercalculator.org.

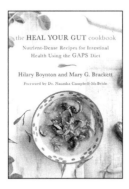
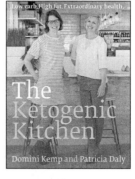
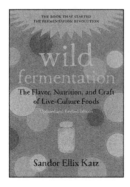
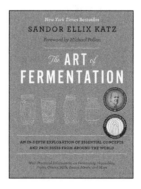
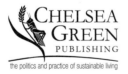

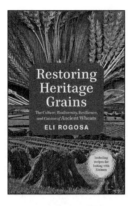
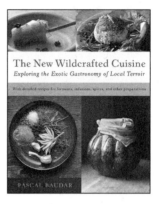
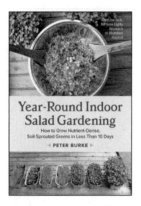
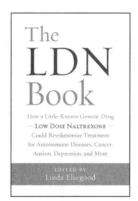
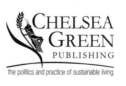